Developmental Disabilities from Childhood to Adulthood

What Works for Psychiatrists in Community and Institutional Settings

Edited by

Roxanne C. Dryden-Edwards, M.D.

and

Lee Combrinck-Graham, M.D.

THE JOHNS HOPKINS UNIVERSITY PRESS

Baltimore

Note: Readers should scrutinize product information sheets for dosage changes or contraindications, particularly for new or infrequently used drugs.

© 2010 The Johns Hopkins University Press
All rights reserved. Published 2010
Printed in the United States of America on acid-free paper
9 8 7 6 5 4 3 2 1

The Johns Hopkins University Press
2715 North Charles Street
Baltimore, Maryland 21218-4363
www.press.jhu.edu

Library of Congress Cataloging-in-Publication Data

Developmental disabilities from childhood to adulthood : what works for psychiatrists in community and institutional settings / edited by Roxanne C. Dryden-Edwards and Lee Combrinck-Graham.

    p. ; cm.
  Includes bibliographical references and index.
  ISBN-13: 978-0-8018-9418-3 (hardcover : alk. paper)
  ISBN-10: 0-8018-9418-2 (hardcover : alk. paper)
  1. Developmental disabilities. 2. Community psychiatry. I. Dryden-Edwards, Roxanne C., 1962– II. Combrinck-Graham, Lee.
  [DNLM: 1. Developmental Disabilities—psychology. 2. Developmental Disabilities—rehabilitation. 3. Community Mental Health Services—methods. 4. Disabled Persons—psychology. 5. Disabled Persons—rehabilitation. 6. Social Adjustment. WM 140 D489 2010]
  RC570.D48 2010
  362.196'8588—dc22   2009024395

A catalog record for this book is available from the British Library.

Special discounts are available for bulk purchases of this book. For more information, please contact Special Sales at 410-516-6936 or specialsales@press.jhu.edu.

The Johns Hopkins University Press uses environmentally friendly book materials, including recycled text paper that is composed of at least 30 percent post-consumer waste, whenever possible. All of our book papers are acid-free, and our jackets and covers are printed on paper with recycled content.

To the true heroes of this book:

people with developmental disabilities and those who love them

Contents

Contributors

Joel D. Bregman, M.D., Director of Clinical Research, Fay J. Lindner Center for Autism, and Associate Investigator, Translational Psychiatry Feinstein Institute for Medical Research, North Shore–LIJ Health System

Robin P. Church, Ed.D., Senior Vice President for Education, Kennedy Krieger Institute; Associate Professor of Education, Johns Hopkins University, Baltimore, Maryland

Lee Combrinck-Graham, M.D., Associate Clinical Professor, Yale Child Study Center, Yale University, New Haven; Medical Director, FSW, Inc., Stamford, Connecticut

John M. de Figueiredo, M.D., Sc.D., Associate Clinical Professor, Department of Psychiatry, Yale University School of Medicine, New Haven, Connecticut

Roxanne C. Dryden-Edwards, M.D., Staff Psychiatrist, Glasser Medical Associates, Gaithersburg, Maryland; Consultant, District of Columbia Department of Youth Rehabilitative Services, Washington, D.C.

Derek Glaaser, Ed.D., Principal, Kennedy Krieger High School Career and Technology Center, Kennedy Krieger Institute, Baltimore, Maryland

Alison A. Golombek, M.D., Attending Psychiatrist, Psychiatry and Behavioral Medicine, Seattle Children's Hospital, Seattle, Washington

Stephanie Hamarman, M.D., Voluntary Faculty, New York Medical College, New York

Craig H. Kennedy, Ph.D., BCBA, Chair, Special Education Department, Professor, Special Education and Pediatrics, Director, Vanderbilt Kennedy Center Behavior Analysis Clinic, Peabody College, Vanderbilt University, Nashville, Tennessee

Bryan King, M.D., Professor and Vice Chair of Psychiatry and Behavioral Sciences, Director of Child and Adolescent Psychiatry, University of Washington and Seattle Children's Hospital, Seattle, Washington

Judith M. Levy, M.S.W., M.A., Acting Director, Maryland Center for Developmental Disabilities; Director, Department of Social Work, Chair, Ethics Committee, Kennedy Krieger Institute, Baltimore, Maryland

Janet A. Martin, M.D., Ph.D., Consultant, Optimum Performance Institute, Woodland Hills; private practice, Los Angeles, California

Gregory J. O'Shanick, M.D., President and Medical Director, Center for Neurorehabilitation Services, Richmond; National Medical Director, Brain Injury Association of America, Inc., McLean, Virginia

Ronald C. Savage, Ed.D., President, North American Brain Injury Society; Senior Consultant, Center for Neurological and NeuroDevelopmental Health, Voorhees, New Jersey; Program Consultant, George Washington University Master's in Traumatic Brain Injury Program, Washington, DC

Ramakrishnan S. Shenoy, M.D., Clinical Professor of Psychiatry, Virginia Commonwealth University Health Services, Richmond; Consultant in Intellectual Disability, Central State Hospital, Petersburg, Virginia

Karen Toth, Ph.D., Assistant Professor, Psychiatry, Seattle Children's Hospital, Seattle, Washington

Maureen van Stone, Esq., M.S., Staff Attorney, Maryland Volunteer Lawyers Service; Director, Project HEAL (Health, Education, Advocacy, and Law), Kennedy Krieger Institute, Baltimore, Maryland

PART I •

The Developmental Disabilities

1

Overview of Developmental Disability

Joel D. Bregman, M.D.

Definition

The concept of *developmental disabilities* (DDs) encompasses a wide range of conditions that involve significant impairments in one or more of the following domains: physical and sensorimotor development, cognitive and psychological processes, verbal and nonverbal communication, social functioning, and adaptive behavior (Rice et al., 2004). The onset of these impairments occurs at some point during the course of physical maturation and neurological development (from gestation through adolescence), although, in the significant majority of cases, the onset is very early in life. The reported prevalence of DDs varies, depending on the definition adopted (including a required degree of severity) and the nature of the population studied. For example, within the general U.S. population, it has been estimated that as many as 17 percent of individuals have some type of DD (Rice et al., 2004) and that 2 percent of all school-age children have a serious DD (Van Naarden Braun, Autry, and Boyle, 2005). Epidemiological monitoring of DDs has been facilitated by such programs as the Centers for Disease Control and Prevention's (CDC) Metropolitan Atlanta Developmental Disabilities Surveillance Program (see Rice et al., 2004).

Although the fundamental aspects of mental retardation (MR) were appreciated by the turn of the twentieth century—namely, childhood onset of significant limitations in cognitive and adaptive functioning—an accurate and meaningful definition remains elusive (Sheerenberger, 1983; Greenspan, 2006). This largely reflects the challenges in deciding when to identify individuals with mild degrees of impairment as manifesting a disabling condition that confers a state of social vulnerability.

Over the years, there have been significant changes in the conception, definition, and characterization of severe cognitive and adaptive impairment. Conceptions have been influenced by neurobiological, sociocultural, and bureaucratic-political factors, with a tendency to adopt a unitary as opposed to a comprehensive and integrated approach. Conceptions have ranged from structure versus function to defect versus difference to transient delay versus permanent impairment to disability versus differential ability.

In recent years, increasing emphasis has been placed on adaptive societal functioning and the supports and services necessary for optimal outcomes. Functional status is judged in relationship to specific sociocultural expectations and requirements for personal independence and responsibility (Luckasson et al., 2002). These efforts are exemplified by the changing definitional emphasis adopted by the American Association for Intellectual and Developmental Disabilities (AAIDD), which until 2007 was known as the American Association for Mental Retardation (AAMR; Schalock et al., 2007). In 1992, the AAMR shifted its focus from viewing mental retardation as a characteristic of the individual to its being a product of nature and the demands of the interactions between the individual and that of the person's sociocultural environment (Smith, 1997). Emphasis was placed on adaptive functioning in areas judged to be critical for successful daily living. In addition, the nature and extent of necessary supportive services were chosen as surrogate indicators of severity, rather than an arbitrary cutoff score on a formal test (Luckasson et al., 2002; Detterman and Gabriel, 2006). The shift from considering tested intelligence to adaptive functioning as the primary indicator of severity was based in part on the expectation that the identified services would compensate for intrinsic limitations to a reasonable extent.

The 2002 edition of *Mental Retardation: Definition, Classification, and Systems of Supports* (Luckasson et al., 2002) continued this emphasis. It defined MR as a condition that "refers to substantial limitations in present functioning. Mental retardation is characterized by significantly subaverage intellectual functioning, existing concurrently with related limitations in two or more of the following applicable adaptive skill areas: communication, self-care, home living, social skills, community use, self-direction, health and safety, functional academics, leisure, and work. Mental retardation manifests before age 18" (Saunders, 2003). In applying this definition, one should consider the following: the community context for peers of similar age and cultural background; assessment procedures that account for cultural and linguistic diversity as well as communication, sensorimotor, and behavioral factors; individual strengths; limitations considered within the context of necessary supportive services; and recognition that, with such services, life functioning is likely to improve (Luckasson et al., 2002).

The *Diagnostic and Statistical Manual of Mental Disorders*, fourth edition, text revision (DSM-IV-TR; American Psychiatric Association, 2000) definition of mental retardation adopts a similar approach but maintains the severity level component present in previous AAMR editions based on IQ (mild, moderate, severe, and profound; Baroff, 2006). In a 2002 interim report, investigators working in collaboration with the AAMR extended the 1992 approach of emphasizing real-life capabilities by proposing that five dimensions be considered in defining MR: intellectual abilities, adaptive behavior, societal participation, interpersonal interactions, and community context.

Despite the comprehensiveness of the AAIDD/AAMR definition and characterization of MR, shortcomings have been described, including inadequate direction for service providers and a lack of clarity for researchers (Detterman and Gabriel, 2006). Approximate IQs and specific adaptive skill domains are included in the criteria (Detterman and Gabriel, 2006). In addition, the severity designations adopted in previous definitions published by the AAMR, as well as the more recent editions of the *Diagnostic and Statistical Manual of Mental Disorders* (such as the DSM-III, DSM-III-R, DSM-IV, and DSM-IV-TR), namely, mild, moderate, severe, and profound, were eliminated in the 1992 and later AAMR descriptions. It has been recommended that future revisions of the definition clarify the conceptualization of a DD, identify the core features of MR, determine the relationship between intelligence and adaptive behavior, and develop criteria for defining MR (Schalock, 2006). Denning, Chamberlain, and Polloway (2000) studied the impact of the changes in the definition and characterization of MR on the public educational system. Departments of Education from all 50 states and from the District of Columbia responded to the investigator's survey. Only 8 percent indicated that they followed the 1992 guidelines. In contrast, more than 85 percent indicated reliance on the 1983 guidelines. Three states reported that they used neither, referring to guidelines developed within their respective localities. Clearly, the shift in conceptualization of mental retardation / intellectual disability (MR/ID) adopted by the AAIDD/AAMR has thus far failed to influence the policies of the country's primary and secondary educational system.

A confusing label that is often used to describe children with developmental problems is *developmental delay.* This term is used in various ways and with varying implications. Although developmental delay is often used as a diagnostic category, it is best conceptualized as a chief complaint or presenting symptom that requires a thoughtful evaluation designed to identify a potential etiology, pathophysiology, functional and societal limitations, and the degree of impairment and disability (Petersen, Kube, and Palmer, 1998).

There also has been an effort to achieve greater international agreement and adopt a more universally applicable system of naming, identifying, and diagnosing DDs. In many countries, the term *intellectual disability* has been adopted in preference to *mental retardation.* Recently, the AAIDD adopted this term, as it more accurately reflects current research findings, provides consistency with international nomenclature, and conveys what many professionals, consumers, and families believe to be a less pejorative connotation than MR (Schalock et al., 2007).

Epidemiology

Determinations of the incidence and prevalence of MR depend on several factors, including definition, diagnostic criteria, sampling procedures, advances in medical science, public awareness of potential biological and environmental risk factors, changes in the level and delivery of health care, and the quality and timeliness of education and training (Simeonsson, Granlund, and Bjorck-Akesson, 2006). With the adoption of intensive early intervention and special educational services during the past several decades, fewer individuals with mild impairment will meet diagnostic criteria, particularly if the presence of functional adaptive skills is emphasized and up-to-date standardized test scores (with large normative and special population sampling procedures) are used. For example, an empirical study identified 0.9 percent of the population as manifesting MR (Baroff, 1991). In a review of epidemiological studies based on total population screening, McLaren and Bryson (1987) reported a prevalence of approximately 1.25 percent. Of those identified as manifesting MR, approximately 90 percent were found to have mild cognitive and adaptive impairments, whereas less than 5 percent had severe-to-profound impairment.

Intellectual disability and autism spectrum disorders are two of the most serious DDs, which in many cases result in significant functional impairment. Reported prevalence rates for MR/ID vary widely on an international basis, in part reflecting differences in definition and diagnosis, sociocultural expectations, and methodological procedures used in epidemiological studies. For example, prevalence rates between 0.5 to 0.7 percent have been reported in the Netherlands (van Schrojenstein Lantman–de Valk et al., 2006; Wullink et al., 2007), 0.6 percent in Ireland (McConkey, Mulvany, and Barron, 2006), 0.8 percent in the United States (Larson et al., 2001), 1 percent in Finland (Heikura et al., 2003), 1 to 2 percent in the People's Republic of China (Sonnander and Claesson, 1997), 3 percent in rural South Africa (Christianson et al., 2002), and approximately 3.5 percent in Leicestershire, United Kingdom (McGrother et al., 2002). Across recent epidemiological studies, the prevalence of autism spectrum disorders has been reported to be between 0.3 and 0.6 percent (probably closer to the higher figure; Fombonne, 2003a, 2003b, 2005; Fombonne et al., 2003, 2006). The prevalence of pervasive developmental disorder (PDD) was determined to be 0.7 percent among 8-year-old children studied in six U.S. states (Centers for Disease Control, 2000).

Etiology and Risk Factors

The search for a likely etiology of intellectual disability in individual cases is a complex endeavor. Wide variations in diagnoses, biological versus environmental factors, and prenatal versus postnatal onset have been reported in the published literature, largely due to key methodological differences. These include the type of population studied; the age and degree of impairment of the individuals; the nature, extent, and technical sophistication of the assessment battery; the focus of the studies (e.g., timing of onset, type of pathology—structural, physiological, functional); and the exclusiveness of the search (e.g., single versus multifactorial etiology; Moog, 2005). Van Karnebeek and colleagues (2005) reported that in their tertiary care center, a specific etiological diagnosis was identifiable in half of the patients evaluated. In a 2005 incidence study of intellectual disability in a 1-year birth cohort in northern

Finland, Heikura and colleagues (2003) reported that in two-thirds of cases a likely biomedical etiology was identified, with prenatal factors being more prominent than postnatal variables.

Despite impressive advances in medical science during the past several decades, a specific etiology for MR can only be identified in only 30 to 50 percent of cases (Curry et al., 1997). Biological factors are often identified in cases of severe intellectual impairment, whereas social and environmental factors often underlie cases of mild impairment. Studies of this type have been based on sampling on the basis of the degree of MR and have assumed that potential risk factors operate consistently across severity. Few epidemiological studies have examined risk factors that may differentiate cases of mild versus severe MR in samples from a population with unknown etiology. In an effort to identify a differential pattern of risk, Croen and colleagues (Croen, Grether, and Hoogstrate, 2002; Croen, Grether, and Selvin, 2001, 2002) investigated risk factors for mild MR (IQ = 50–70) and severe MR (IQ < 50) of unknown etiology among all live births (4.5 million) within an 8-year period in California (1987–94). The population was ascertained from the database of the California Department of Developmental Services. Individuals were excluded if they were diagnosed with cerebral palsy, autism, or medical conditions judged to underlie their intellectual/adaptive impairments (e.g., endocrine/metabolic, chromosomal, infectious, or neurological conditions). Resulting prevalence figures for MR of unknown etiology were 3.6 per 1000 live births, of which 66 percent were of unknown etiology. Of this subgroup, 64 percent had mild, 20 percent has severe, and 6 percent had an unspecified degree of MR. Risk factors for both mild intellectual disability (MID) and severe intellectual disability (SID) included low birth weight (<2500 grams), male gender, multiple births, and mothers >30 years and with less than a high school education. Also within the mentally retarded population of California, risk factors limited to MID included second or later birth order, mother born in California, and mother more likely to be of black heritage, whereas those limited to SID included mother more likely to be of Asian or Hispanic heritage.

The investigators reported that these risk factors were independent of the other variables and were present across the eight birth years of study. The sampling methods may have underestimated the number of those with mild MR (because the sample included children as young as 4 years of age, and a diagnosis of MR is not always able to be made at this young age). However, misclassification of MR severity was judged to be minimal, because the percentages of those with mild and severe MR in these cases of unexplained etiology were similar to those reported in a epidemiological study conducted by the Centers for Disease Control of individuals with a known degree of impairment (Croen, Grether, and Hoogstrate, 2002; Croen, Grether, and Selvin 2001, 2002).

In a review of the epidemiological literature implicating perinatal brain damage as a primary cause of MR and other DDs, Dammann and Leviton (1997b) found that between 8 and 43 percent of cerebral palsy and between 10 and 25 percent of cases of MR are associated with signs of perinatal morbidity that are generally accepted as proxy indicators of brain damage. These variables include abnormalities identified by neuroimaging, neonatal asphyxia, atypical fetal heart rate patterns, and abnormal thyroid functioning.

Clements and colleagues (2006) identified characteristics at birth that predicted the emergence of developmental delays and referral for early intervention services. Of 219,037 births in Massachusetts between 1998 and 2000, 6.8 percent were considered in need of early intervention within the first year of life. Predictors of referral and evaluation included low birth weight (<1500 grams), triplet birth, and the presence of two or more risk factors at birth. These predictors were salient, because 88 percent of infants referred were judged to be appropriate for evaluation and 85 percent of those evaluated were found to be eligible for services.

In a study of diagnoses made later in life, the etiology of ID was investigated among 140 adults consecutively evaluated within inpatient and outpatient services of an Italian neurological institute for MR (Verri et al., 2004). Eighty had MID (IQ = 50–70), and 60 had SID (IQ < 50). A thorough developmental, medical, and family history was obtained and comprehensive physical, neurological, neuroradiological, laboratory, and genetic evaluations were completed. A prenatal etiology was identified among 34 percent of individuals with MID and 28 percent of those with SID. Chromosomal abnormalities and specific syndromes accounted for the highest percentage of this etiological group, present among 19 percent of individuals with MID and 16 percent of those with SID. Congenital anomalies were the next most common etiology, cerebral dysgenesis in 6 percent of people with MID and 3 percent of people with SID and other birth defects in 9 percent of people with MID and 7 percent of people with SID. As might be expected, unidentified metabolic disorders were present in only 1 percent of individuals, all with

SID. A specific etiology could not be identified in 17 percent of the MID group and 10 percent of the SID group. Of associated conditions, 11 percent of the 140 individuals were diagnosed with autism, and 28 percent with other behavioral and psychiatric disorders. It is of note that a new etiological diagnosis was made for 24 percent of the individuals (who were 20 years of age or older). In 11 percent a genetic causation was identified (several of which were inheritable). These findings indicate that etiological diagnoses made later in life can have important implications for treatment and family genetic counseling.

Despite significant advances in the care of preterm and very preterm infants (and a corresponding reduction in mortality figures), rates of premature birth have remained relatively stable, contributing significantly to neurological morbidity (Goldenberg et al., 1996). Immunological mechanisms have been implicated in central nervous system damage in preterm infants (Cowan, Leviton, and Dammann, 2000). For example, immune response factors, including cytokines, have been hypothesized to underlie the development of periventricular leukomalacia (Dammann and Leviton, 1997a; Yoon et al., 1997), which is indicative of cerebral white matter damage and associated with severe cognitive impairments and cerebral palsy. Risk factors for periventricular leukomalacia include extreme prematurity and maternal or placental infection (Zupan et al., 1996).

Among potential risk factors for developmental problems, fetal growth and birth weight have been studied. Follow-up studies of newborns identified as being small for gestational age (SGA) have reported lower intelligence scores compared with appropriate for gestational age (AGA) controls during early childhood (Goldenberg et al., 1996) and during adolescence (Paz et al., 2001). In the latter study, full-term AGA and SGA birth cohorts were evaluated at 17 years of age, controlling for the potentially confounding demographic and clinical variables, including parental education, maternal age, parental smoking, ethnicity, socioeconomic status, birth order, maternal weight gain during pregnancy, maternal height and body mass index, maternal gestational diabetes and hypertension, caesarian section delivery, and newborn asphyxia. Adolescents identified as SGA (<10th percentile for weight) at birth were found to have a small but statistically significant reduction in intelligence test scores compared with AGA controls. However, SGA status was not predictive of low intelligence (defined in this study as IQ < 85) or of decreased academic achievement. These findings contrast with those reported for preterm SGA newborns, who exhibit a greater likelihood of lower cognitive ability and achievement, learning disabilities, and neurological abnormalities (McCarton et al., 1996). The magnitude of the IQ decrement identified in this study was related to the degree of the birth weight disparity. Adolescents identified as being severely SGA (<3rd birth weight percentile) had lower IQ scores than their moderately SGA (3rd–10th birth weight percentile) and AGA peers. This study is significant because of its large sample size and control for a number of confounding variables.

Psychopathology

For several decades, epidemiological studies have reported higher prevalence rates of psychiatric disorders within the ID population than within the general population (for reviews, see Bregman, 1991; Whitaker and Read, 2006). Although the methodological rigor of the studies varies, several adopted sound designs and consistently identified increased prevalence rates within the ID population. For valid comparisons to be made, the methodological procedures should be consistent with those adopted in epidemiological studies of the general population, including similar sampling procedures, as well as definitions and diagnostic criteria of the identified psychiatric disorders (Whitaker and Read, 2006).

The definition of intellectual disability or MR that is adopted significantly affects prevalence rates that are determined in the course of a given study and identifies different, although overlapping subpopulations. Between 1 and 3 percent of the population would meet criteria for MR/ID, depending on whether IQ alone or IQ plus adaptive functioning is considered, as well as on the specific IQ cutoff score selected (e.g., 70, 75, 80). Epidemiological studies examining psychopathology in this population are similarly disparate in their definition of ID, as well as in their interpretation of emotional and behavioral symptoms (for review, see Kerker et al., 2004). Particularly in the past, symptoms considered to be indicative of psychopathology within the general population were attributed to ID or MR rather than to a comorbid neuropsychiatric disorder (diagnostic overshadowing), resulting in an underestimate of psychiatric illness within the MR/ID population. However, an overly descriptive approach to diagnosis could conceivably result in an overestimate, particularly if qualifying variables are not considered, such as medical status, social maturity, cultural context, patient/informant comprehension (especially of questions asked during clinical interviews), communicative ability, or the nature of past experiences with authority figures. Other confounding factors include the social and emotional effects of long-term residential treatment and institutionalization; social rejection and marginalization (especially for those with a mild degree of ID); overdependency fostered by caregivers, teachers, or employers; and limited access to community resources (e.g., social and recreational opportunities, emotional and social support, general guidance).

It is also important to interpret individual symptoms and symptom clusters within the context of the quantitative and qualitative aspects of the individual's cognitive, adaptive, social, cultural, emotional, and personality development (Dosen, 2005). In addition, it is necessary to integrate psychodynamic, developmental phase, and behavioral learning perspectives when determining the significance and meaning of affective and behavioral symptoms, when considering whether they represent a psychiatric disorder, and when planning treatment interventions.

Several methodological issues should be considered when interpreting the findings of research studies, including ascertainment and data-gathering procedures, such as the nature of the population ascertained (e.g., general community versus MR/ID institutions versus outpatient mental health clinics), sampling procedures (e.g., total population, representative sample, administrative sample, random sample), data source (e.g., medical record reviews, hospital or clinic administrative data, parent or caregiver questionnaires, direct interviews or mental status examination—structured, semistructured, or clinical), and the source of psychiatric diagnosis (e.g., past records, current clinical interview, questionnaire algorithms). There also is a lack of professional agreement regarding when to attribute behavioral symptoms or symptom clusters to the effects of developmentally based limitations in frustration tolerance and impulse control and when to attribute such symptoms to a comorbid neuropsychiatric disorder.

Over the years, a number of large-scale psychiatric epidemiology studies have been conducted within the general populations of several countries. Six-month psychiatric prevalence rates for adults in the general populations of Canada and the United States have been reported to be 17 percent and 18 percent, respectively (Myers et al., 1984; Bland, 1988). A report from the office of the U.S. Surgeon General (1999) estimated that about 21 percent of adults in the general population have a mental health condition, for which about 15 percent are being treated. Similar prevalence rates of 18 to 20 percent have been reported for children and young adolescents living in New Zealand, Puerto Rico, and the United States (Anderson et al., 1987; Bird et al., 1988; Costello et al., 1996).

A significant limitation in both research studies and clinical practice involving those with an ID is the dearth of valid and reliable self-report assessment instruments. Direct information regarding the thoughts, feelings, attitudes, and inner experience of patients is most important for accurate diagnosis and effective treatment. The presence of deficits in intellectual areas (e.g., reading comprehension, conceptual understanding) and in communicative ability (both verbal and nonverbal) impedes the development of successful self-report strategies. One type of instrument that is gaining popularity for the population with an ID is the Likert-type scale. In a literature review, Hartley and MacLean (2006) reported that, across studies, a minimum of 50 percent of individuals with borderline-to-mild ID were found to respond appropriately to Likert-type scales. One-third of the reviewed studies of respondents with borderline-to-mild ID reported poor reliability and validity, as opposed to 60 percent of studies involving respondents with moderate to profound ID. Likert-type scales were found to be at least as reliable as yes/no, either/or, and open-ended question formats. The use of pictorial representations of choices increased the response rate by approximately 25 percent among individuals with mild-to-moderate ID. Shorter descriptors and similar choice alternatives across scale items increased response rates. Response bias (choosing the most positive alternative) is less of a problem in Likert-type scales than for yes/no response scales (for which there is a high rate of acquiescence) and similar to either/or scales. Response bias is less of an issue among individuals with a less-severe degree of ID and when assessment questions are presented in a semistructured manner, explaining and paraphrasing items that are poorly understood by the respondents. A significant majority of the studies reviewed reported moderate to high internal consistency, test-retest reliability, and both concurrent and convergent validity. As is the case for response rates, reliability and validity are higher for individuals with a lesser degree of ID who respond appropriately to pretests (to assess for inappropriate and biased response tendencies) for whom items are presented in a semistructured fashion.

The Prevalence of Psychopathology in Adults with Intellectual Disability

Rates of psychopathology have been studied within the adult MR/ID population, drawing from samples ascertained using different methods. Clay and Thomas (2005) investigated the prevalence of psychiatric disorders among 179 adults with MR/ID receiving services from the developmental disabilities department of an Oregon county between 1985 and 2001. Diagnoses were made on the basis of medical record reviews of a stratified random sample of this population. Approximately one-third of the sample was assessed as having an Axis I psychopathology, mood disorders being particularly prominent. Psychiatric disorders were thought to be more prevalent among individuals receiving more intensive developmentally based services (implying that they experienced a greater degree of cognitive and adaptive impairments).

The Prevalence of Psychopathology in Children and Adolescents with Intellectual Disability

Several population-based studies have been conducted within the younger MR/ID population. Emerson (2003) performed a secondary analysis on data collected for a national survey of the mental health status of children and adolescents 5 to 15 years of age living in Great Britain (England, Scotland, and Wales). The original study included a multistage, stratified, random sample that involved interviews with primary caretakers (and youth 11 years of age or older), as well as findings from a teacher questionnaire (collectively referred to as the Development and Well Being Assessment; Goodman et al., 2000). The presence of ID was inferred from information provided by parents and teachers, class placement, and estimates of mental age. The resulting prevalence (2.6% of the total sample) seemed to be equivalent to prevalence estimates of ID in the general population. Thirty-nine percent of children and adolescents with an ID received the diagnosis of a psychiatric disorder based on ICD-10 criteria.

Cormack, Brown, and Hastings (2000) investigated the rate and severity of emotional and behavioral problems in a regional population of children and adolescents 4 to 18 years old attending special schools for youth with moderate-to-severe ID, using data from the parent version of the Developmental Behavior Checklist (DBC; Einfeld and Tonge, 2002). Approximately

50 percent of the children and adolescents for whom data were collected (response rate of 75%) received DBC scores above the checklist's clinical cutoff, suggesting the presence of significant psychiatric disorder.

In a prevalence study of mental health disorders among 8-year-old Finnish children attending special schools for educational subnormality (Linna et al., 1999), one-third were deemed to meet the criteria for a psychiatric disturbance on the Rutter Parent and Teacher Questionnaires (Rutter, 1967).

Wallander, Dekker, and Koot (2006) reported on the stability of psychopathology over a 1-year period. A random sample of 20 percent of children and adolescents, 6 to 18 years of age, attending special schools for students with educable ID (mean IQ = 72) and trainable ID (mean IQ = 56) were evaluated initially, and 58 percent were reassessed one year later. The sample was drawn from 88 percent of all such special schools. Clinical data were derived from the parent version of the Child Behavior Checklist (Achenbach et al., 1991). Although there was assessed to be a statistically significant decrease in psychopathology at 1-year follow-up, neither the severity nor the pattern of psychopathology was judged to have changed in a clinically significant manner. This finding suggests a possible relative stability of emotional and behavioral problems.

Einfeld and Tonge (1996b) reported that 41 percent of 454 4- to 19-year-old children and adolescents with ID who were epidemiologically ascertained met the criteria for a severe emotional and behavioral disorder on the basis of DBC data provided by caregivers (parents in 87% of the cases and residential staff in the remainder; Einfeld and Tonge, 1996b). Studies have demonstrated that the DBC has solid psychometric properties (Tonge et al., 1996; Clarke et al., 2003). The prevalence of psychopathology appeared to remain stable over a 4-year period (approximately 40%; Tonge and Einfeld, 2000). In a 14-year longitudinal follow-up, Einfeld et al. (2006) examined the course of psychopathology as revealed by the DBC. Growth curve analyses for continuous-scale data were performed, which emphasize individual trajectories as opposed to mean values at each data sampling point (there were four sampling points in this longitudinal study). A gradual reduction in the prevalence of serious psychopathology occurred, from 41 percent of the sample at baseline to 31 percent at 14-year follow-up. This contrasts with a 35 percent decline in psychopathology from early childhood to young adulthood reported in a birth cohort study of 221 children in Scotland (Richardson and

Koller, 1996). The severity of emotional and behavioral disturbance was similar regardless of the degree of intellectual impairment. The prevalence of psychopathology declined more in boys than in girls and more in those with mild than those with severe ID. The modest decline may have been related to the lack of treatment interventions for 90 percent of the cohort.

Despite high rates of perceived psychopathology within the childhood ID population, treatment is rarely provided. For those with major psychiatric disorders, treatment has been reported to be provided for 10 percent (Einfeld et al., 2006), 27 percent (Dekker et al., 2002), and 53 percent (only 10% by specialists in both ID and mental health, Tonge and Einfeld, 2000).

Types of Psychopathology

The comparative prevalence of psychopathology between the MR/ID and general populations varies as a function of the specific disorder examined. For example, among adults, the reported prevalence of anxiety disorders and schizophrenia has been reported to be higher in the MR/ID population (Eaton and Menolascino, 1982; Reiss, 1990), whereas substance abuse disorders appear to be more common in the general population (Reiss, 1990). The frequency of anxiety disorder diagnoses was found to be common among persons with ID, affecting 27 percent of those in a clinical community-based population (Stavrakaki and Mintsioulis, 1997). The prevalence of schizophreniform disorders in the ID population has been estimated to be 3 percent (Turner, 1989). The assessment of psychotic symptoms in the ID population is challenging (Hemmings, 2006). For example, true hallucinations must be distinguished from pseudohallucinations, such as self-talk and speaking to "imaginary friends" (Pickard and Paschos, 2005).

Among children, attention deficit hyperactivity disorders (ADHD) and mood disorders have been estimated to be equally prevalent within the MR/ID and general populations (Gillberg et al., 1986). Conduct, anxiety, hyperactivity, and pervasive developmental disorders were found to be significantly more prevalent within the ID population than the general child and adolescent population. In contrast, depressive, eating, and psychotic disorders were diagnosed at equal rates within the ID and general populations (Emerson, 2003).

Masi et al. (1999) compared depressive symptomatology in 60 adolescents and young adults, 12 of whom were unselected consecutively referred adolescents and young adults with mild ID (mean IQ = 61) and 48 who were individuals with average IQ. Assessments were based on the Kiddie-Schedule for

Affective Disorder and Schizophrenia (Geller et al., 1996). Similar symptom profiles were identified in the ID and average IQ subject groups. Those with an ID reported high rates of depressed mood, irritability, low energy, feelings of guilt, and low self-esteem. Comorbid generalized anxiety disorder was assessed as being present in more than 90 percent of those individuals assigned to the dysthymic ID group (versus 70% in the average IQ group). The profiles of the individuals with an ID were more similar to those of prepubertal individuals with average IQ than among the adolescents, suggesting the influence of mental or developmental age. Concordance for reported depressive symptoms between individuals and their parents was significantly higher for the ID than the average IQ group.

Dekker and Koot (2003) studied the 1-year prevalence, degree of comorbidity, and functional impairment of psychopathology within an epidemiological cohort of 7- to 20-year-olds ascertained from a random sample of students attending specialized ID schools within a province of the Netherlands. Mothers were interviewed using selected modules of the Diagnostic Interview Schedule for Children (National Institute of Mental Health, 1997). The investigators found that 22 percent of the sample met the DSM-IV criteria for an anxiety disorder, 4.4 percent for a mood disorder, and 25 percent for a disruptive behavior disorder (whether or not they screened positive for a pervasive developmental disorder). The three most prevalent disorders were thought to be specific phobia (17.5%), ADHD (14.8%), and ODD (13.9%). None of the children was assessed as meeting the symptom criteria for generalized anxiety disorder or post-traumatic stress disorder. Thirty-seven percent met the criteria for more than one neuropsychiatric disorder, and more than half of those with at least one disorder experienced significant functional impairment.

A study investigated the 1-year prevalence of aggressive behavior among 3,065 adults ($\geq$ 19 years of age) with ID/MR (IQ $\leq$ 70) residing in the Leicestershire region of England, which has a population of approximately 700,000; Tyrer et al., 2006). The ascertainment rate was estimated to be 95 percent. Caregivers provided data on adaptive functioning and the frequency and severity of problem behaviors collected by trained interviewers. Approximately 14 percent of the adults with MR/ID were reported to have engaged in aggressive behavior toward others during the previous year. Severe aggression occurring at least once weekly was reported for 12 percent of this population. Of those exhibiting aggression, 18 percent caused serious injury to others. Factors that increased the likelihood of aggressive behavior included male gender, younger adult age, higher degrees of intellectual impairment, institutional residence, low frustration tolerance, and labile affect. The presence of autism and seizure disorders was not associated with aggressive behavior. Individuals with Down syndrome were least likely to engage in aggression.

The Severity of Cognitive and Adaptive Impairments and Psychopathology

The severity of MR/ID also appears to influence reported prevalence rates of psychopathology. For example, within hospital and clinic samples, those with mild-to-moderate cognitive impairment have been reported to have higher rates of psychiatric disorder than those with severe-to-profound impairment (Borthwick-Duffy and Eyman, 1990), particularly for depression, whereas in total population studies, the reverse has been reported (Borthwick-Duffy, 1994). Severity of MR/ID may also influence the assessed prevalence of specific psychiatric disorders. For example, schizophrenia has been reported to occur more often in those with severe than with mild MR/ID (Reiss, 1990) in adults. Among children and adolescents, those with mild-to-moderate ID have been thought to have higher rates of disruptive or antisocial behaviors and anxiety and those with severe ID higher rates of "self-absorbed and autistic" symptomatology (Einfeld and Tonge, 1996b).

Risk Factors and Psychopathology

Investigators have examined demographic, clinical, social, and environmental variables that may influence the development of psychopathology in the population with an ID. Among children and adolescents, significant associations have been reported for various types of biological risk factors (e.g., genetic abnormalities, brain damage, physical symptoms; Moss et al., 1997; Wallander, Dekker, and Koot, 2006); impairment in social, linguistic, and adaptive skills (Iivanainen, Almqvist, and Koskentausta, 2007; Koskentausta, Iivanainen, and Almqvist, 2007); family factors (e.g., single-parent family; Emerson, 2003; Koskentausta, Iivanainen, and Almqvist, 2007); low socioeconomic status (Koskentausta, Iivanainen, and Almqvist, 2007); stern physical discipline or social deprivation (Emerson, 2003); maladaptive family functioning (Emerson, 2003; Wallander, Dekker, and Koot, 2006); mental health of the primary caregiver (Emerson, 2003; Wallander, Dekker, and Koot, 2006; Koskentausta, Iivanainen, and Almqvist, 2007); parental rejection (Moss et al., 1997); and stressful life events (Emerson, 2003).

It also has been reported that children and adolescents with severe physical disabilities may be at significantly lower risk for the development of disruptive behavior and anxiety (Cormack, Brown, and Hastings, 2000). Some investigators have identified a relationship between both age and gender and the prevalence of psychopathology (Cooper, 1997; Emerson, 2003), whereas others have not (Einfeld and Tonge, 1996b; Dekker et al., 2002).

A significant relationship between age and psychopathology has been reported among adults. Cooper (1997) compared the findings of psychiatric examinations (using a semistructured rating scale) on all persons with an ID ≥ 65 years of age and a random sample of persons with an ID 20 to 65 years of age living in the same "defined geographical area." Psychopathology (especially depression and anxiety) was thought to be significantly more prevalent among older adults, affecting approximately 70 percent versus approximately 50 percent among the younger adults. Rates of psychotic and autistic disorders were similar in both age groups.

In a retrospective study spanning 20 years, Tsakanikos and colleagues (2006) compared the psychopathology exhibited by 295 men and 295 women with an ID (85% with mild-to-moderate ID) consecutively referred to a specialty mental health service in southeast London. Personality disorders (primarily antisocial personality disorder) were assessed as being significantly more common among men, whereas dementia and adjustment disorders were deemed more common among women. Rates of depression, anxiety, and schizophrenic disorders were not statistically different between the genders. The finding for depression stands in contrast with other studies, which indicate that women with an ID are thought to be at higher risk for developing depressive disorders than are their male counterparts (Heiman, 2001; Lunsky, 2003).

Psychopathology in Specific Genetic and Clinical Groups:

An increasing number of genetic neurodevelopmental disorders (the result of microdeletions, duplications, or mutations) have been associated with specific patterns of social, affective, cognitive, and behavioral development. The terms *behavioral phenotypes* and *behavioral neurogenetics* have been used to describe this association. Early studies tended to apply standardized psychiatric diagnostic criteria to these associations; however, given the genetic heterogeneity of psychiatric disorders compared with the genetic specificity of neurodevelopmental disorders, it is not surprising that the resulting phenotypes were often not comparable. A more accurate term may be *endophe-*

notype, which refers to inherited state-independent traits that may mirror aspects of a full behavioral phenotype in affected family members (Feinstein and Singh, 2007).

Fragile X syndrome is the most common cause of inherited ID, with a prevalence of 1 in 4,000 in boys and men and 1 in 6,000 to 8,000 in girls and women (Feinstein and Singh, 2007). It results from an abnormally large CGG trinucleotide expansion involving the 5' untranslated region of the *FMR1* gene of the X chromosome (Reiss and Hall, 2007). During the past two decades, studies examining the social and behavioral profile of fragile X syndrome have revealed characteristic features, including gaze aversion, attention deficits, impulsivity, social anxiety, hyperarousal, stereotyped mannerisms, a cluttering speech pattern, and heightened sensory sensitivities. In addition, a higher-than-expected prevalence of ADHD, pervasive developmental disorders, and social phobia have been reported (Bregman et al., 1987, 1988; Reiss and Hall, 2007).

Prader-Willi syndrome (PWS) is a genetic disorder with a prevalence of 1 in 10,000 births, caused by abnormalities within the 15q11-13 region of chromosome 15. The most common abnormality is a deletion of the paternally derived chromosome (~70% of PWS cases). Maternal uniparental disomy (UPD), in which two copies of chromosome 15 are inherited from the mother and none from the father, accounts for approximately 25 percent of cases of PWS, and mutations within the imprinting center (which regulates gene expression) account for the remainder of cases (Venkitaramani and Lombroso, 2007).

PWS has also been associated with social and behavioral problems, including social isolation and withdrawal, food-seeking behaviors, single-mindedness, noncompliance, impulsivity, and temper outbursts, often in response to food restriction (Feinstein and Singh, 2007). In addition, limited flexibility has been described, manifested as overly persistent questioning, intolerance for changes in the daily schedule, and compulsive and ritualistic behaviors like hoarding, hair pulling, skin picking, and placing objects symmetrically or in a certain order (Benarroch et al., 2007). Specific psychiatric disorders may be more common among those with PWS than in the general ID population, particularly ADHD, obsessive compulsive disorder, and bipolar mood disorder (Benarroch et al., 2007).

Prader-Willi syndrome appears to result in a higher-than-expected prevalence of mood disorders. In 2007, Soni and colleagues published a study in which 159 subjects who were recruited from PWS and ID organizations were evaluated using a two-state assessment process and standardized instruments. Seventy-five percent were genetically confirmed to have PWS, 69 percent with the microdeletion, and 28 percent with the UPD subtype (3% had uncommon genetic mechanisms). At $2\frac{1}{2}$ years follow-up, the prevalence of affective disorder remained constant, with a profile consistent with bipolar disorder. In contrast with those manifesting the microdeletion PWS subtype, those with the maternal UPD subtype are reported to have a higher prevalence and more severe course of mood disorders, with a higher number of recurrences and a less-favorable response to antidepressant medication.

Tuberous sclerosis (TS) is another relatively well-characterized genetic disorder that has been associated with various forms of psychopathology (Raznahan et al., 2006). TS is caused by spontaneous mutation or autosomal dominant transmission of two genes that code for proteins that regulate cell division. Resulting hamartomas and neuronal migratory abnormalities underlie the varied clinical manifestations of the disorder, including a 75 percent prevalence of seizure disorders (predominantly infantile spasms) and a 45 to 89 percent prevalence of ID. Associated affective and behavioral symptomatology has been identified for some time, particularly hyperactivity syndromes and autism. The association with autism is particularly strong (Smalley, 1998) and may be linked to temporal lobe pathology (Bolton and Griffiths, 1997).

Raznahan et al. (2006) reported on psychopathology present in a subset of 60 adults with TS, ascertained from a previous population-based study. This subset was found to be representative of the initial sample. Two assessment procedures for psychopathology were used: the Schedule of Affective Disorders and Schizophrenia-Lifetime interview (SADS-L; Endicott and Spitzer, 1978) directly with intellectually capable subjects, and the semistructured informant-based interview; Schedule for Assessment of Psychiatric Problems Associated with Autism and Other Developmental Disorders (SAPPA; Bolten and Rutter, 1994) for less intellectually capable subjects. The latter instrument was developed to assess behavioral change and psychopathology among those developmental disorders. Approximately 70 percent of the study subjects had a seizure disorder, and 40 percent had an ID (IQ < 70). Rates of psychopathology were high. Forty percent met the diagnostic criteria for a mood disorder (three-fourths of whom had major depression), 6.7 percent for alcoholism, and 5 percent for an anxiety disorder. The prevalence of psychopathology was significantly higher for intellectually capable persons with TS than for those with an ID in addition to TS. This disparity may reflect the use of different sources of information and instruments for assessing psychopathology, because the majority of subjects without an ID received the SADS-L interview, whereas the majority of those with an ID were assessed through an informant interviewed with the SAPPA. The presence of a seizure disorder did not affect rates of psychopathology when considering the entire subject sample but did increase the likelihood of psychopathology among those who had TS without an ID.

Autism spectrum disorders are complex neurodevelopmental syndromes that involve qualitative impairments in social reciprocity, semantic and pragmatic communication, and the range and nature of preferred interests and activities, in addition to stereotyped movements, compulsive and ritualistic patterns of behavior, and unusual sensory interests and sensitivities (Bregman, 2005). Although of diverse etiology and pathogenesis, a relatively large percentage of cases are of complex genetic origin. Autism spectrum disorders are often associated with comorbid psychopathology. Brereton et al. (2006) examined patterns of psychopathology exhibited by 367 of 381 consecutive child and adolescent cases of autistic disorder evaluated in centers in five states of Australia during a 2-year period. Comparisons were made with a representative sample of 550 children and adolescents with an ID. The overall degree of psychopathology was significant within the autism group (as reflected by scores on the total behavior problem score of the Developmental Behavior Checklist—Parent, DBC-P; Einfeld and Tonge, 2002). Approximately three-fourths of the autism sample received scores above the clinical cutoff established for the DBC-P. In addition, scores for the autism group were significantly higher than those for the ID normative sample on all but the antisocial behavior subscale of the DBC-P. In particular, children and adolescents with autism scored at or above the 75th percentile on the Self-absorbed, Communication Disturbance, Anxiety, and, Social Relating subscales. In addition, their scores on these subscales were significantly higher than those of the ID comparison group. Clinically significant scores were also present for the Disruptive, Attention Deficit Hyperactivity, and Depression subscales.

Conclusion

Given increased understanding that the term *developmental disabilities* is applied to a wide variety of complex conditions that are the result of a myriad of usually unknown etiologies, the need for collaboration between all health professionals, recipients of services, and their families is clear. The improved life expectancy and independence of individuals with DDs further highlights the need for everyone who works or lives with a person with a DD to work together to enhance the life, well-being, and productivity of the person with the ID. Finally, the difficulties involved with trying to assess whether or not a person with a DD has a psychiatric illness and when to provide treatment highlights how imperative it is for mental health and medical professionals to work together to provide the best care possible (Sovner, 1986; Moss, 1999).

References

Achenbach TM, Howell CT, Quay HC, Conners CK. 1991. National survey of problems and competencies among four- to sixteen-year-olds: Parents' reports for normative and clinical samples. *Monographs of the Society for Research in Child Development* 56(3): v–120.

Anderson JC, Williams S, McGee R, Silva PA. 1987. DSM-III disorders in preadolescent children: Prevalence in a large sample from the general population. *Archives of General Psychiatry* 44(1): 69–76.

Baroff GS. 1991. *Developmental Disabilities: Psychosocial Aspects.* Austin, TX: Pro-Ed.

Baroff GS. 2006. On the 2002 AAMR definition of mental retardation. In HN Switzky and S Greenspan (eds.), *What Is Mental Retardation? Ideas for an Evolving Disability in the 21st Century,* 29–50. Washington, DC: American Association on Mental Retardation.

Benarroch F, Hirsch HJ, Genstil L, Landau YE, Gross-Tsur V. 2007. Prader-Willi syndrome: Medical prevention and behavioral challenges. *Child and Adolescent Psychiatric Clinics of North America* 16(3): 695–708.

Bird HR, Canino G, Rubio-Stipec M, et al. 1988. Estimates of the prevalence of childhood maladjustment in a community survey in Puerto Rico: The use of combined measures. *Archives of General Psychiatry* 45(12): 1120–26. (Erratum appears in *Arch Gen Psychiatry* 51(5): 429.)

Bland RC. 1988. Psychiatric epidemiology. *Canadian Journal of Psychiatry* 33(7): 618–25.

Bolton PF, Griffiths PD. 1997. Association of tuberous sclerosis of temporal lobes with autism and atypical autism [comment]. *Lancet* 349(9049): 392–95.

Bolton PF, Rutter M. 1994. Schedule for Assessment of Psychiatric Problems Associated with Autism and Other Developmental Disorders (SAPPA): Informant Version. Cambridge: Cambridge University and London Institute of Psychiatry.

Borthwick-Duffy SA. 1994. Epidemiology and prevalence of psychopathology in people with mental retardation. *Journal of Consulting and Clinical Psychology* 62(1): 17–27.

Borthwick-Duffy SA, Eyman RK. 1990. Who are the dually diagnosed? *American Journal of Mental Retardation* 94: 586–95.

Bregman JD. 1991. Current developments in the understanding of mental retardation. Part II: Psychopathology. *Journal of the American Academy of Child and Adolescent Psychiatry* 30(6): 861–72.

Bregman JD. 2005. Definitions and characteristics of the spectrum. In D Zager (ed.), *Autism Spectrum Disorders: Identification, Education and Treatment,* 3rd ed., 312–34. Mahwah, NJ: Erlbaum.

Bregman JD, Dykens E, Watson M, Ort SI. 1987. Fragile-X syndrome: Variability of phenotypic expression. *Journal of the American Academy of Child and Adolescent Psychiatry* 26(4): 463–71.

Bregman JD, Leckman JF, Ort SI. 1988. Fragile X syndrome: Genetic predisposition to psychopathology. *Journal of Autism and Developmental Disorders* 18(3): 343–54.

Brereton AV, Tonge BJ, Einfeld SL. 2006. Psychopathology in children and adolescents with autism compared to young people with intellectual disability. *Journal of Autism and Developmental Disorders* 36(7): 863–70.

Centers for Disease Control. 2000. Prevalence of autism spectrum disorders: Autism and developmental disabilities monitoring network, six sites, United States, 2000. *Morbidity and Mortality Weekly Report* 56(1): 1–11.

Christianson AL, Zwane ME, Manga P, et al. 2002. Children with intellectual disability in rural South Africa: Prevalence and associated disability. *Journal of Intellectual Disability Research* 46(2): 179–86.

Clarke A, Tonge B, Einfeld SL, Mackinnon A. 2003. Assessment of change with the Developmental Behavior Checklist. *Journal of Intellectual Disability Research* 47(3): 210–12.

Clay J, Thomas JC. 2005. Prevalence of Axis I psychopathology in an intellectually disabled population: Type of pathology and residential supports. *Journal of Developmental and Physical Disabilities* 17(1): 75–84.

Clements KM, Barfield WD, Kotelchuck M, Lee KG, Wilber N. 2006. Birth characteristics associated with early intervention referral, evaluation for eligibility, and program eligibility in the first year of life. *Maternal and Child Health Journal* 10(5): 433–41.

Cooper SA. 1997. Epidemiology of psychiatric disorders in elderly compared with younger adults with learning disabilities. *British Journal of Psychiatry* 170: 375–80.

Cormack KFM, Brown AC, Hastings RP. 2000. Behavioral and emotional difficulties in students attending schools for intellectual disability. *Journal of Intellectual Disability Research* 44(2): 124–29.

Costello EJ, Angold A, Burns BJ, et al. 1996. The Great Smoky Mountains Study of Youth: Goals, design, methods, and the prevalence of DSM-III-R disorders. *Archives of General Psychiatry* 53(12): 1129–36.

Cowan LD, Leviton A, Dammann O. 2000. New research directions in neuroepidemiology. *Epidemiologic Reviews* 22(1): 18–23.

Croen LA, Grether JK, Hoogstrate J. 2002. The changing prevalence of autism in California. *Journal of Autism and Developmental Disorders* 32: 207–15.

Croen LA, Grether JK, Selvin S. 2001. The epidemiology of mental retardation of unknown cause. *Pediatrics* 107(6): E86.

Croen LA, Grether JK, Selvin S. 2002. Descriptive epidemiology of autism in a California population: Who is at risk? *Journal of Autism and Developmental Disorders* 32: 217–24.

Curry CJ, Stevenson RE, Aughton D, et al. 1997. Evaluation of mental retardation: recommendations of a consensus conference: American College of Medical Genetics. *American Journal of Medical Genetics* 72(4): 468–77.

Dammann O, Leviton A. 1997a. Maternal intrauterine infection, cytokines, and brain damage in the preterm newborn. *Pediatric Research* 42(1): 1–8.

Dammann O, Leviton A. 1997b. The role of perinatal brain damage in developmental disabilities: An epidemiologic perspective. *Mental Retardation and Developmental Disabilities Research Reviews* 3(1): 12–21.

Dekker MC, Koot HM. 2003. DSM-IV disorders in children with borderline to moderate intellectual disability. I: Prevalence and impact. *Journal of the American Academy of Child and Adolescent Psychiatry* 42(8): 915–22.

Dekker MC, Nunn RJ, Einfeld SE, Tonge BJ, Koot HM. 2002. Assessing emotional and behavioral problems in children with intellectual disability: Revisiting the factor structure of the Developmental Behavior Checklist. *Journal of Autism and Developmental Disorders* 32(6): 601–10.

Denning CB, Chamberlain JA, Polloway EA. 2000. An evaluation of state guidelines for mental retardation: Focus of definition and classification practices. *Education and Training in Mental Retardation and Developmental Disabilities* 35(2): 226–32.

Detterman DK, Gabriel L. 2006. Look before you leap: Implications of the 1992 and 2002 Definitions of Mental Retardation. In HN Switzky and S Greenspan (eds.), *What Is Mental Retardation? Ideas for an Evolving Disability in the 21st Century*. Washington, DC: American Association on Mental Retardation.

Dosen A. 2005. Applying the developmental perspective in the psychiatric assessment and diagnosis of persons with intellectual disability. Part I: Assessment. *Journal of Intellectual Disability Research* 49(1): 1–8.

Eaton LF, Menolascino FJ. 1982. Psychiatric disorders in the mentally retarded: Types, problems, and challenges. *American Journal of Psychiatry* 139(10): 1297–1303.

Einfeld SL, Piccinin AM, Mackinnon A, Hofer SM, Taffe J, Gray KM. 2006. Psychopathology in young people with intellectual disability. *Journal of the American Medical Association* 296(16): 1981–89.

Einfeld SL, Tonge BJ. 1995. The Developmental Behavior Checklist: The development and validation of an instrument to assess behavioral and emotional disturbance in children and adolescents with mental retardation. *Journal of Autism and Developmental Disorders* 25(2): 601–10.

Einfeld SL, Tonge BJ. 1996a. Population prevalence of psychopathology in children and adolescents with intellectual disability. Part I: Rationale and methods. *Journal of Intellectual Disability Research* 40(2): 91–98.

Einfeld SL, Tonge BJ. 1996b. Population prevalence of psychopathology in children and adolescents with intellectual disability. Part II: Epidemiological findings. *Journal of Intellectual Disability Research* 40(2): 99–109.

Einfeld SL, Tonge, BJ. 2002. Developmental Behavior Checklist—Parent. Los Angeles: Western Psychological Services.

Emerson E. 2003. Prevalence of psychiatric disorders in children and adolescents with and without intellectual disability. *Journal of Intellectual Disability Research* 47(1): 51–58.

Endicott J, Spitzer RL. 1978. A diagnostic interview: The schedule for affective disorders and schizophrenia. *Archives of General Psychiatry* 35(7): 837–44.

Feinstein C, Singh S. 2007. Social phenotypes in neurogenetic syndromes. *Child and Adolescent Psychiatric Clinics of North America* 16(3): 631–47.

Fombonne E. 2003a. Epidemiological surveys of autism and other pervasive developmental disorders: An update. *Journal of Autism and Developmental Disorders* 33(4): 365–82.

Fombonne E. 2003b. The prevalence of autism (comment). *Journal of the American Medical Association* 289(1): 87–89.

Fombonne E. 2005. Epidemiology of autistic disorder and other pervasive developmental disorders. *Journal of Clinical Psychiatry* 10: 3–8.

Fombonne E, Simmons H, Ford T, Meltzer H, Goodman R. 2003. Prevalence of pervasive developmental disorders in the British nationwide survey of child mental health. *International Review of Psychiatry* 15(1–2): 158–65.

Fombonne E, Zakarian R, Bennett A, Meng L, McLean-Heywood D. 2006. Pervasive developmental disorders in Montreal, Quebec, Canada: Prevalence and links with immunizations. *Pediatrics* 118(1): 139–50.

Geller B, Zimmerman B, Williams M, et al. 1996. Washington University Kiddie Schedule for Affective Disorders and Schizophrenia—Lifetime and Present Episode—DSM IV. St. Louis, MO: Washington University School of Medicine.

Gillberg C, Persson E, Grufman M, Themner U. 1986. Psychiatric disorders in mildly and severely mentally retarded children and adolescents: Epidemiological aspects. *British Journal of Psychiatry* 149: 68–74.

Goldenberg RL, DuBard MB, Cliver SP, et al. 1996. Pregnancy outcome and intelligence at age five years. *American Journal of Obstetrics and Gynecology* 175(6): 1511–15.

Goodman R, Ford T, Richards H, Gatward R, Meltzer H. 2000. The development and well-being assessment: Description and initial validation of an integrated assessment of child and adolescent psychopathology. *Journal of Child Psychology and Psychiatry and Allied Disciplines* 41(5): 645–55.

Greenspan S. 2006. Functional concepts in mental retardation: Finding the natural essence of an artificial category. *Exceptionality* 14(4): 205–24.

Hartley SL, MacLean WE, Jr. 2006. A review of the reliability and validity of Likert-type scales for people with intellectual disability. *Journal of Intellectual Disability Research* 50: 813–27.

Heikura U, Taanila A, Olsen P, Hartikainen AL, von Wendt L, Jarvelin MR. 2003. Temporal changes in incidence and prevalence of intellectual disability between two birth cohorts in Northern Finland. *American Journal on Mental Retardation* 108(1): 19–31.

Heiman T. 2001. Depressive mood in students with mild intellectual disability: Students' reports and teachers' evaluations. *Journal of Intellectual Disability Research* 45(6): 526–34.

Hemmings CP. 2006. Schizophrenia spectrum disorders in people with intellectual disabilities. *Current Opinion in Psychiatry* 19(5): 470–74.

Kerker BD, Owens PL, Zigler E, Horwitz SM. 2004. Mental health disorders among individuals with mental retardation: Challenges to accurate prevalence estimates. *Public Health Reports* 119(4): 409–17.

Koskentausta T, Iivanainen M, Almqvist F. 2007. Risk factors for psychiatric disturbance in children with intellectual disability. *Journal of Intellectual Disability Research* 51(1): 43–53.

Larson SA, Lakin KC, et al. 2001. Prevalence of mental retardation and developmental disabilities: estimates from the 1994/1995 National Health Interview Survey Disability Supplements. *American Journal of Mental Retardation* 106(3): 231–52.

Linna SL, Moilanen I, Ebeling H, et al. 1999. Psychiatric symptoms in children with intellectual disability. *European Child and Adolescent Psychiatry* 8(Suppl 4): 77–82.

Luckasson R, Borthwick-Duffy S, Buntinx WHE, et al. 2002. *Mental Retardation: Definition, Classification, and Systems of Supports,* 10th ed. Washington, DC: American Association on Mental Retardation.

Lunsky Y. 2003. Depressive symptoms in intellectual disability: Does gender play a role? *Journal of Intellectual Disability Research* 47(6): 417–27.

Masi G, Mucci M, Favilla L, Poli P. 1999. Dysthymic disorder in adolescents with intellectual disability. *Journal of Intellectual Disability Research* 43(2): 80–87.

McCarton CM, Wallace IF, Divon M, Vaughan HG, Jr. 1996. Cognitive and neurologic development of the premature, small for gestational age infant through age 6: Comparison by birth weight and gestational age. *Pediatrics* 98(6 Pt 1): 1167–78.

McConkey R, Mulvany F, Barron S. 2006. Adult persons with intellectual disabilities on the island of Ireland. *Journal of Intellectual Disability Research* 50(3): 227–36.

McGrother CW, Bhaumik S, Thorp CF, Watson JM, Taub NA. 2002. Prevalence, morbidity and service need among South Asian and white adults with intellectual disability in Leicestershire, UK. *Journal of Intellectual Disability Research* 46(4): 299–309.

McLaren J, Bryson SE. 1987. Review of recent epidemiological studies of mental retardation: Prevalence, associated disorders, and etiology. *American Journal on Mental Retardation* 92(3): 243–54.

Moog, U. 2005. The outcome of diagnostic studies on the etiology of mental retardation: Considerations on the classification of the causes. *American Journal of Medical Genetics* 137(2): 228–31.

Moss SC. 1999. Assessment: Conceptual issues. In N Bouras (ed.), *of Psychiatric and Behavioural Disorders in Developmental Disabilities and Mental Retardation*, 18–37. Cambridge: Cambridge University Press.

Moss SC, Emerson E, Bouras N, Holland A. 1997. Mental disorders and problematic behaviours in people with intellectual disability: Future directions for research. *Journal of Intellectual Disability Research* 41(6): 440–47.

Myers JK, Weissman MM, Tischler GL. 1984. Six-month prevalence of psychiatric disorders in three communities 1980 to 1982. *Archives of General Psychiatry* 41: 959–67.

National Institute of Mental Health. 1997. Diagnostic Interview Schedule for Children—IV. Bethesda, MD: National Institute of Mental Health.

Paz I, Laor A, Gale R, Harlap S, Stevenson DK, Seidman DS. 2001. Term infants with fetal growth restriction are not at increased risk for low intelligence scores at age 17 years. *Journal of Pediatrics* 138(1): 87–91.

Petersen MC, Kube DA, Palmer FB. 1998. Classification of developmental delays. *Seminars in Pediatric Neurology* 5(1): 2–14.

Pickard M, Paschos D. 2005. Pseudohallucinations in people with intellectual disabilities: Two case reports. *Mental Health Aspects of Developmental Disabilities* 8(3): 91–93.

Raznahan A, Joinson C, O'Callaghan F, Osborne J, Bolton P. 2006. Psychopathology in tuberous sclerosis: An overview and findings in a population-based sample of adults with tuberous sclerosis. *Journal of Intellectual Disability Research* 50(8): 561–69.

Reiss AL, Hall SS. 2007. Fragile X syndrome: Assessment and treatment implications. *Child and Adolescent Psychiatric Clinics of North America* 16: 663–75.

Reiss S. 1990. Prevalence of dual diagnosis in community-based day programs in the Chicago metropolitan area. *American Journal on Mental Retardation* 94: 578–85.

Rice C, Schendel D, Cunniff C, Doernberg N. 2004. Public health monitoring of developmental disabilities with a focus on the autism spectrum disorders. *American Journal of Medical Genetics* 125(1 Pt. C): 22–27.

Richardson SA, Koller H. 1996. *Twenty-two Years: Causes and Consequences of Mental Retardation*. Cambridge, MA: Harvard University Press.

Rutter M. 1967. A Children's Behavior Questionnaire for Completion by Teachers: Preliminary Findings. *Journal of Child Psychology and Psychiatry* 8, 1–11.

Saunders MD. 2003. Mental retardation: Definition, classification, and systems of supports. *Psychological Record* 53(2): 327–29.

Schalock RL. 2006. Scientific and judgmental issues involved in defining mental retardation. In HN Switzky and S Greenspan (eds.), *What Is Mental Retardation? Ideas for an Evolving Disability in the 21st Century.* Washington, DC: American Association on Mental Retardation.

Schalock RL, Luckasson RA, Shogren KA, et al. 2007. The renaming of mental retardation: Understanding the change to the term intellectual disability. *Intellectual and Developmental Disabilities* 45(2): 116–24.

Sheerenberger RC. 1983. *A History of Mental Retardation.* Baltimore: Brookes Publishing Co.

Simeonsson RJ, Granlund M, Bjorck-Akesson E. 2006. The Concept and Classification of Mental Retardation. In HN Switzky and S Greenspan (eds.), *What Is Mental Retardation? Ideas for an Evolving Disability in the 21st Century.* Washington, DC: American Association on Mental Retardation.

Smalley SL. 1998. Autism and tuberous sclerosis. *Journal of Autism and Developmental Disorders* 28(5): 407–14.

Smith J. 1997. Mental retardation as an educational construct: Time for a new shared view? *Education and Training in Mental Retardation and Developmental Disabilities* 32: 167–73.

Soni S, Whittington J, Holland AJ, et al. 2007. The course and outcome of psychiatric illness in people with Prader-Willi syndrome: Implications for management and treatment. *Journal of Intellectual Disability Research* 51(1): 32–42.

Sonnander K, Claesson M. 1997. Classification, prevalence, prevention and rehabilitation of intellectual disability: An overview of research in the People's Republic of China. *Journal of Intellectual Disability Research* 41(2): 180–92.

Sovner R. 1986. Limiting factors in the use of DSM-III with mentally ill / mentally retarded persons. *Psychopharmacology Bulletin* 22:1055–59.

Stavrakaki C, Mintsioulis G. 1997. Implications of a clinical study of anxiety disorders in persons with mental retardation. *Psychiatric Annals* 27(3): 182–89.

Tonge BJ, Einfeld S. 2000. The trajectory of psychiatric disorders in young people with intellectual disabilities. *Australian and New Zealand Journal of Psychiatry* 34(1): 80–84.

Tonge BJ, Einfeld SL, Krupinski J, Mackenzie A. 1996. The use of factor analysis for ascertaining patterns of psychopathology in children with intellectual disabilities. *Journal of Intellectual Disability Research* 40(3): 198–207.

Tsakanikos E, Bouras N, Sturmey P, Holt G. 2006. Psychiatric co-morbidity and gender differences in intellectual disability. *Journal of Intellectual Disability Research* 50(8): 582–87.

Turner TH. 1989. Schizophrenia and mental handicap: An historical review, with implications for further research. *Psychological Medicine* 19: 301–14.

Tyrer F, McGrother C, Thorp C, et al. 2006. Physical aggression towards others in adults with learning disabilities: Prevalence and associated factors. *Journal of Intellectual Disability Research* 50(4): 295–304.

U.S. Surgeon General. *Mental Health: A Report of the Surgeon General.* 1999. Bethesda, MD: National Institute of Mental Health.

van Karnebeek CD, Scheper FY, Abeling NG, et al. 2005. Etiology of mental retardation in children referred to a tertiary care center: A prospective study. *American Journal of Mental Retardation* 110(4): 253–67.

Van Naarden Braun K, Autry A, Boyle C. 2005. A population-based study of the recurrence of developmental disabilities—Metropolitan Atlanta Developmental Disabilities Surveillance Program, 1991–94. *Paediatric and Perinatal Epidemiology* 19(1): 69–79.

van Schrojenstein Lantman–de Valk HM, Wullink M, van den Akker M, et al. 2006. The prevalence of intellectual disability in Limburg, the Netherlands. *Journal of Intellectual Disability Research* 50(1): 61–68.

Venkitaramani DV, Lombroso PJ. 2007. Molecular basis of genetic neuropsychiatric disorders. *Child and Adolescent Psychiatric Clinics of North America* 16(3): 541–56.

Verri A, Maraschio P, Uggetti C, et al. 2004. Late diagnosis in severe and mild intellectual disability in adulthood. *Journal of Intellectual Disability Research* 48(7): 679–86.

Wallander JL, Dekker MC, Koot HM. 2006. Risk factors for psychopathology in children with intellectual disability: A prospective longitudinal population-based study. *Journal of Intellectual Disability Research* 50(4): 259–68.

Whitaker S, Read S. 2006. The prevalence of psychiatric disorders among people with intellectual disabilities: An analysis of the literature. *Journal of Applied Research in Intellectual Disabilities* 19(4): 330–45.

Wullink M, van Schrojenstein Lantman–de Valk HM, Dinant GJ, Metsemakers JF. 2007. Prevalence of people with intellectual disability in the Netherlands. *Journal of Intellectual Disability Research* 51(Pt 7): 511–19.

Yoon BH, Jun JK, Romero R, et al. 1997. Amniotic fluid inflammatory cytokines (interleukin-6, interleukin-1beta, and tumor necrosis factor-alpha), neonatal brain white matter lesions, and cerebral palsy. *American Journal of Obstetrics and Gynecology* 177(1): 19–26.

Zupan V, Gonzalez P, Lacaze-Masmonteil T, et al. 1996. Periventricular leukomalacia: Risk factors revisited. *Developmental Medicine and Child Neurology* 38(12): 1061–67.

2

A Life Cycle Approach to Developmental Disabilities

Lee Combrinck-Graham, M.D.

There is a well-known African saying that it takes a village to raise a child. In Western countries, especially in the United States, where families and individuals are increasingly separated and isolated, it still takes a village to raise a child, especially to raise a child who has developmental disabilities.

A common view of individuals with developmental disabilities (DDs) is that they are somehow stuck, and one cannot expect development in the sense that it occurs in "regular" individuals. Yet development does occur, and individuals with DDs encounter the same psychosocial developmental tasks that "regular" individuals negotiate. At the level of the brain and cognitive output, there is increasing understanding of patterns of development in individuals with intellectual disabilities (Harris, 2005). At the macro, psychosocial level, what is different between individuals with DDs and those without may be the rate of development and the developmentally disabled individual's mental, emotional, and even physical capacities for addressing the concerns posed in different developmental eras.

In a global view, the optimal outcome of child development is becoming an adult who is a contributing member of a community and of adult development is, as a contributing member of a community, leading a fulfilling life with a sense of personal satisfaction and respect for self and others and finally negotiating declining years with dignity. Furthermore, a mentally healthy family is one in which all of the systems are organized for the mutual benefit of its members.

By this definition, it is clear that no one, no matter how sound of mind or body, could develop successfully without interactions with others. Individuals with DDs are more dependent on others to accomplish these life objectives. It takes a village . . .

Another important facet of a developmental approach is that the concept of the life cycle of individuals with DDs actualizes normalization, a model that has been seminal in moving individuals with DDs from institutionalization to community membership.

This chapter will present the life cycle in the context of relationships with individuals who are integral to the person's life, emphasizing that the "normal" development of individuals with DDs is in relationships with others who may begin as caregivers and educators and will become friends, advocates, and admirers.

Stages of Individual Development

Erik Erikson's eight stages of man (1950) is still one of the most descriptive and comprehensive frameworks for understanding individual developmental issues in a psychosocial framework. The stages of development in childhood and adolescence are more elaborated, the theory being that here the changes in growth and maturation are the most dramatic. Also, Erikson was a relatively young man when he developed this framework and had no personal experience of the development in older adulthood. Nevertheless, he posited three adult stages that continue to be valuable models for understanding psychosocial development.

In addition to the psychosocial (driven by individual psychology and physiological development in context) approach, Erikson's model names specific tensions needing to be resolved at each developmental juncture.

Erikson's eight stages and their decision points are

1. Trust versus mistrust
2. Autonomy versus doubt (or shame)
3. Initiative versus guilt
4. Industry (competence) versus inferiority
5. Identity versus identity diffusion (role confusion)

6. Intimacy versus isolation
7. Generativity versus stagnation
8. Integrity versus despair

Recognizing that individuals with DDs go through these stages and that they and their families and caregivers grapple with the tensions of these stages is essential in assessing and promoting their mental health and overall adjustment.

A Family Life Cycle Model

Another framework for examining the development of individuals with DDs is the family life cycle. There have been several approaches to describing evolution of families. The most popular has been to name stages of family development beginning with family formation through marriage, the birth of children, the children's adolescence, children leaving home, and the couple without children.

Combrinck-Graham (1985) proposed a family life cycle in a continuous spiral in which the relationship between one generation's developmental experiences and the others' is reflected in the interactional field. She proposed that in three generations a "regular" family will go through three periods when the family relationship environment is largely "centripetal," that is, close, involved, and nonpathologically enmeshed, and three periods when the environment is primarily "centrifugal," with individuals directed out of the family, involved with interests and relationships in the society outside the family. Between these periods, the family relationships expand from centripetal to centrifugal and then come together from centrifugal to centripetal (see Figure 2.1).

For example, at the birth of a child, the centripetal family draws in all three generations to respond to the care of the relatively helpless infant. A high degree of responsiveness, without need for verbalization, because, after all, babies can't talk, is characteristic of the family interactions while there are infants. Moving out of this intensely intimate environment, the family of school-age children already has greater differentiation between generations, and all three generations are more focused on societal interactions—the children through school and peer experiences, the parents in their occupations and increasing access to socializing with their own peers, the grand-

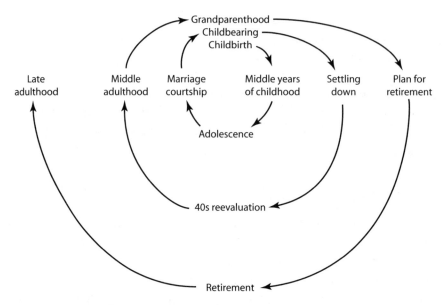

Figure 2.1. Family life spiral. *Source*: Combrinck-Graham, 1985

parents in mentoring and other "philanthropic" roles, often at a leadership level. The centrifugal period is in the overlap of adolescence, midlife reevaluation of the parents, and possible retirement of grandparents. It is important to note that while these developmental forces draw family members away from one another, it is not necessary for the families to come apart for the individuals to accomplish their developmental tasks. Moving back to the centripetal environment may be stimulated by the courtship and marriage, or joining of the youngest generation, a wedding being the rejoining of family members as well as the possible joining of two families. It may also be stimulated by illness and decline in the older generation and the "parent" generation's need to care for them. A new centripetal period begins when new babies arrive, although there may be other events that bring families together in this intimate way.

Combrinck-Graham proposed that centripetal periods were ideal environments for practicing intimacy, and centrifugal periods were ideal for practicing individuation, and in the life span of a normal individual there would be three centripetal (intimacy) and three centrifugal (individuation) periods, each one providing an opportunity to improve over the last.

As individuals with DDs may have different timing in their stages, so family life cycles will be different. However, examining the evolution of individuals and their families can help to focus the mental health professional on what can be available from families and what other resources may be needed to foster optimal development of individuals and their family members.

To reiterate the theme of this chapter, exceptional people require exceptional families and adjustments to developmental timing and expectations of outcome, but the developmental concerns are the same.

Stages of Development in Families with a Member Who Has a Developmental Disability

Developmental disabilities produce differences in developmental rate and trajectory than those that occur in regular individuals and families, and clearly disabilities also have differences among themselves. What follows is a description of how coping with the disability affects the working of developmental tasks in a general way. A developmental approach assumes that everyone involved is growing and changing. This movement has to be recognized to properly assess progress and possible emotional disturbance.

Infancy

Erikson describes the first developmental period as that in which basic trust should be established. Contemporary interest in attachment elaborates what may be understood as basic trust, that is, the infant's expectation that his or her physical and emotional needs will be met in a consistent fashion. This first period could be summarized as a period of forming attachment.

In the family life cycle model, the centripetal, highly involved, and responsive environment fosters attachment and involves both caregivers and the infant. In the family model, the family tends to be so focused inward that its external boundaries (between family and nonfamily) are strong. But with families who have a child with a DD, this is not the case. Of necessity, the family is dependent on health care professionals, developmental experts, and early intervention therapists to assist with diagnosis, treatment of medical problems, and assistance in caring for and facilitating their child's development. The inclusion of these necessary "others" along with the family's own caution and doubt about how to care for their child can threaten the establishment of secure attachment.

Klaus and Kennell (1976), in their early description of maternal-infant bonding, described the tentative approach to a sick or vulnerable infant (in their examples, fragile premature infants in incubators) by touching the child delicately with fingertips, if touching them at all. The delicate touch reflects the parents' concerns that their child will break. Klaus and Kennell report that putting the whole hands in the infant becomes emblematic of the parents' being able to "hold" their infant. Whole hand stroking and soothing is followed by whole body embrace, rocking, and then crooning as the caregivers take charge of the emotional relationship with their vulnerable child.

Parents of medically fragile and vulnerable infants need to learn how to care for them competently and to depend on professionals to support them. Parents of irritable and nonresponsive infants have a different kind of challenge, because there is little or no reciprocal response from the infant to fuel caring and adaptation of caring styles from caregivers. Caregivers need to be rewarded for their efforts at least by feeling effective and in optimal conditions by responses from the infant such as eye contact, smiling, cooing, or cuddling. Without cues from the infant that they are doing the right thing, caregivers need confirmation and encouragement from others, such as professionals and other family members.

Beyond the psychosocial focus of development at this stage are the developments in experience and ability that Piaget (Ginsberg and Opper, 1979) referred to as the sensorimotor stage. This simply means that the infant's acquisition of competence is through the application of primary ego functions of the five senses along with exercising increasingly autonomous motor functions. In this important stage, stimulation is just as critical for babies with DDs, providing experiences for all the senses and exercises to develop motor competence. Ideally parents will provide most of this stimulation, but, again, many parents of infants who have a DD may need input, instruction, ideas about modified equipment, and so on, from professionals.

Engaging all adult caregivers in the process of holding and stimulating their baby takes most effective advantage of the centripetal family environment and may preempt the conflict arising from complex feelings of failure, loss, and guilt that may tear apart families at this most vulnerable stage.

"Toddler" and Preschool Periods

As the child and the family are moving out of the centripetal environment of infancy, both benefit from a wider circle of involvement that includes family friends, professionals, teachers, and other children. These contacts provide additional support for family members and additional opportunities for the child with a DD to experience and interact with others, increasing the child's sense of participation and membership in larger social circles.

These periods collapse the Erikson stages of "autonomy" and "initiative." The failures of development in these periods are doubt, shame, and guilt. Mobility is a crucial factor in "autonomy." A child's ability to move and to move away from caregivers is a major accomplishment. Other kinds of physical control also enhance autonomy, but autonomy also refers to some ability to think independently and to make judgments and decisions. While no preschool child could be expected to make good decisions about where to go, how to cross the street, to stay away from dangers such as hot stoves, or how to deal with another child taking a toy or bothering them, the level of supervision necessary for children with DDs is usually greater than that required for "regular" toddlers and preschoolers. Furthermore, the response and internalization of rules may be limited so that the caregivers have to continue supervision and restating rules for a long time. But, recognition and encouragement of the child who has a DD's increasing autonomy and developing personal initiative is critical to both the child and the family's development.

Joan Goodman, in her study of preschool education for children with intellectual disabilities, *When Slow Is Fast Enough* (1992), contrasts the educational approach that makes children appear to be successful and productive in standard terms, by producing for them (e.g. the card or candy box already constructed on which the child adds glitter), with an approach that encourages a child's initiative and rewards curiosity and exploration. Though her book was a controversial challenge to pedagogical principles, there is no doubt that the approach she recommends supports the increasing sense of personal identity and competence in children with these disabilities, supporting their development at their own rate.

Some parents are reluctant to involve their children in social activities, playgroups, preschools, or to leave them in the care of babysitters or daycare. Some parents report that "no one" will look after my child and consequently feel stuck. If the circle of adults committed to the child is not expanded then all family members may suffer from the negative outcome of this period, shame and guilt.

Professionals must recognize the initiative, accomplishments, and attractions of the child and help parents who are having trouble doing so to see these qualities in their children. Professionals must also assist parents to identify a wider community in which they and their children can be involved. At least this may involve children in therapeutic and educational activities for several hours at a time, sometimes with, but increasingly without, their parent so that both children and parents experience some separation and have some "personal" time. Professionals may also encourage parents to involve their children in other community activities ranging from family get-togethers to religious services, to general circulation in the community, including shopping, haircuts, community parades, visits to Santa Claus, movies and children's theater, and other children's activities such as swimming, dance, gymnastics, and martial arts.

Professionals may have to advocate for providing opportunities in such activities for preschoolers who have DDs. However, they will usually find that parents, given the incentive, encouragement, and connection with like-minded parents, will become formidable advocates themselves.

School Age

Though the previous developmental period requires expanding involvement in the community to facilitate the development of autonomy and initiative, the school-age period is usually considered the significant opportunity for children's development outside of their families, largely in the context of teachers and peers. This social fact that children attend school from age 5 to their late teens fosters the family's further "opening-up" from the centripetal state and allows both child and other family members more interaction outside the family. Parents have more time to themselves while the child is in school, and they can meet other parents through their child's school connections. Children have a more intense diet of experiences and information from sources outside the family, and they bring these new and different practices home without the mediation of the parents. Children begin to have direct influence on how the family members think and respond.

Erikson defines the issues in this stage as industry versus inferiority. Industry means acquisition of knowledge and skills that may be used to contribute to the society. Peer relationships are essential either to feeling successful and competent or to feeling inferior. Critical to a child's finding his or her competent role in the peer group is participation in a learning community that recognizes that each student makes contributions and all students have responsibilities for learning.

Federal laws guaranteeing a free and public education to all children, including those with a handicap, began in 1973. More recent developments in educational policy attempt to reduce discrimination by including special students in regular education. Inclusive education requires that educators do not exclude or discriminate against children with DDs. On the contrary, educators need to find ways to include children in every aspect of student life. Special students may require additional staffing and support. The enterprise of inclusion requires constant advocacy, primarily by parents, but many times also requires attorneys to underscore the guarantee of an appropriate education. Advocates need to be clear about the social and psychological dangers of exclusion and feeling inferior and the necessity of actively promoting the child's competence as well as finding a role for inclusion in the peer group and feeling like a contributing member of the community.

Adolescence

The signal development of adolescence is that of secondary sexual characteristics and the accompanying feelings, which may range from amazement at body changes to active sexual yearnings. In physical growth and sexual development, children at this stage begin to identify themselves as adults. In addition, their growing physical size may enable youngsters to threaten and physically coerce to get what they want when it is hard, or even impossible, to express themselves well in words.

The developmental objective of identity versus identity or role confusion proposed by Erikson is a direct sequel to the previous stage and is very much dependent on it. A child who has developed a secure sense of his or her role in the community may be able to manage the implicit changes in status by increased size and sexual development through adjustments and developments in his or her community functions. But most youngsters with DDs need a lot of help with this.

For children who do not have a DD, the concomitant cognitive and moral developmental accomplishments of the adolescent period help them personally negotiate the changes they experience in role, function, and status. Propositional thinking helps them project into the future, mount an argument, and negotiate rather than having to use force. Developments in adolescence allow youngsters to mentally put themselves into someone else's place and to weigh pros and cons of situations and actions, in terms of not only personal benefit but also larger societal benefit. Most children with DDs can't do this. They may have empathy but usually cannot take a position that could concretely put themselves in a "losing" position.

Because parents have such important functions as advocates and as the ones who push their children to be the best they can be, it is often easier to have someone else educate these youngsters about sex and rules of behavior. While youngsters with disabilities may not be guided by moral judgments, they can follow rules, especially when their experience is that following rules opens doors for more satisfying social relationships.

The requirements of an adolescent who has a DD for supervision, guidance, and constant reminders of the rules, coupled with his or her inability to get around independently, challenges the family development toward individuation and differentiation in what should become a centrifugal stage. Other family members' responsibilities for staying with the adolescent with a DD may restrict their own individuation and differentiation. This may appear to be particularly poignant for siblings, but, in fact, is most confining to mothers who, in general, have borne the major responsibility for advocating for the child's development throughout the life span thus far and are likely to continue to do in subsequent stages in the life cycle.

The challenges, then, for the families of adolescents with DDs are fostering the individual identity of their children while also fostering the differentiation of the other family members. The most developmentally appropriate way to do this is to involve youngsters in more and more activities outside the family, social activities with peers, physical activities, such as sports, and educational activities to prepare them for work. In each of these areas of engagement, the adolescents find themselves in social contexts and define themselves, for example, as someone who is a good dancer, who makes people laugh, who other people like to talk to and be with, who is good at a particular sport, who likes to have fun, who is a good worker, who dresses well, and so on. In this process of identifying and defining themselves, it is usually helpful for youths to have some ability to describe their disability or disabilities.

Early and Middle Adulthood

Though adolescence ends for many at around 18 years old—after they graduate from high school and leave home for college or, having completed school, begin to work independently—education is extended for youngsters with disabilities until the age of 21. This extends the period of adolescence and provides more time to establish several critical functions of young adulthood: a job, a place to live, preferably away from home, and a social context with peers.

Intimacy versus isolation and generativity versus stagnation are the developmental concerns of early and middle adulthood and are no less important concerns for young adults with disabilities. How is intimacy defined in their relationships? And how do they manage their sexual desires and their dreams of having their own families while rarely being able to fulfill them? How do they accept a separate, nonintimate social position without isolation? Largely their individual solutions are built on the accomplishments of the previous developmental stages that include their sense of personal value and accomplishment as well as their understanding of their disability and how it makes their life different.

Generativity may be thought of as bearing children but actually refers to productivity in its broadest sense. Fostering the continuing successful development of adults with DDs means engaging them in activities where they are producing, truly contributing, and seeing the importance of their work. Having a job in which productivity can be measured in hours worked or numbers of items processed or other outcomes can help the individual to value his or her work. Opportunities for performing or exhibiting their creative work foster generativity. Finally, finding ways to help others is a powerful confirmation of personal value. Individuals with DDs can participate in fundraising walkathons or help out with people who are younger, older, or who are more disabled than they are.

The premises of independence, social engagement, and productivity can be realized, but in the current state of our society, only with continuous and staunch advocacy. Arrangements for safe, properly assisted, and convivial living are not easy to come by. In Connecticut, for example, a relatively small state, there are 1,500 to 1,800 adults with mental retardation on the waiting list for places to live outside of their family homes. Social activities are episodic and often seasonal. Individuals with disabilities often can't come and go independently, so social events need to be planned and coordinated. The work they do is often not valued; if it is, its value is not communicated to the worker. But as more people believe in the value of these experiences for individuals with disabilities, and as more persons with disabilities experience respect and dignity inherent in providing supported living and valued work, it becomes easier to locate these individuals into meaningful positions in their communities.

Families stay connected but should not have to continue to run the lives of their adult children. The family moves gradually back toward a more centripetal period from the centrifugal period, when the children move out. This may not be driven by the individual with a disability but will involve him or her, especially when a grandparent needs full-time care and companionship or when a sibling or close relative gets married and then has children. As aunt or uncle, as concerned family member, the now-emancipated adult with a disability contributes to the family, participates in the family emotional field, and benefits from the opportunities provided in the centripetal family to practice the contextual intimacy of that environment.

Older Adulthood

Older adulthood occurs when the individual has less strength, stamina, or ability to continue at the same level of work and participation. Like almost every other developmental stage, when this occurs is different for different individuals with disabilities. For instance there is some evidence that some individuals with Down syndrome age faster and may develop a number of features of senescence at a fairly young age.

Erikson's definition of the concerns of the older adult period is integrity versus despair. Are these core concerns for older adults with disabilities? Of course they are. As individuals get older, have less energy, are less able to think and remember, have some physical problems that are more painful and interfere more and more with their functioning, they need to have some way of handling these losses. Their despair may not be recognizable as such as they withdraw, become more forgetful and dependent, or become more irritable, stubborn, and temperamental. Yet surely their sense of loss with its accompanying fear is no less significant to them than it is to those of us without disabilities.

For many adults with disability, their later life is also affected by the death of their parents who, for most of their lives have been their primary advocates. If the course of their development has been guided "in a village" these losses are far less devastating as there are renewing networks and communities of peers, friends, and professionals who continue to care for and enjoy relating to the individuals with disabilities.

As with all older adults, memories and the opportunities to review them contribute to the integration that allows them to continue to reflect that this was a good and fulfilling life. Again, it is the social network around them that provides pictures and stories for reminiscence, and continues to engage them in activities that reinforce competence and provide pleasure.

Conclusion

Persons with disabilities undergo development in stages that are similar to those that people without disabilities undergo. Recognizing this and facilitating the family's and the individual's negotiation of these stages in a larger context of professionals, peers, and colleagues, can make the life span of an individual with DDs productive and satisfying. This is true even of men, women and children who have limited ability to communicate or function independently. The same principles of wrapping a supportive network around, identifying and facilitating the negotiation of developmental tasks, and according dignity and respect, undoubtedly enhance the quality of their lives.

REFERENCES

Combrinck-Graham LA. 1985. Developmental model for family systems. *Family Process* 24: 139–50.

Erikson EH. 1950. *Childhood and Society.* New York: Norton.

Ginsberg H, Opper S. 1979. *Piaget's Theory of Intellectual Development*, 2nd ed. Englewood Cliffs, NJ: Prentice Hall.

Goodman JF. 1992. *When Slow Is Fast Enough.* New York: Guilford.

Harris JC. 2005. *Intellectual Disability: Understanding Its Development, Causes, Classification, Evaluation, and Treatment.* New York: Oxford University Press.

Klaus M, Kennell J. 1976. *Maternal Infant Bonding: The Impact of Early Separation or Loss on Family Development.* St. Louis: Mosby.

3

Geropsychiatric Aspects of Mental Retardation and Intellectual Disabilities

John M. de Figueiredo, M.D., Sc.D.

This chapter reviews the issues related to the diagnosis and treatment of mental disorders in adults, in particular older adults, with intellectual disabilities. The *Diagnostic and Statistical Manual of Mental Disorders,* fourth edition text revision (DSM-IV-TR; American Psychiatric Association, 2000) defines mental retardation by three criteria: an IQ of about 70 or below; limitations in current adaptive functioning; and onset before 18 years of age. Recently, the expression *intellectual disability* (ID) has been proposed as an alternative to *mental retardation* (MR). An equivalent expression used in the United Kingdom is *learning disability*. This chapter uses the three expressions synonymously and refers to them by the acronym MR/ID. First the increasing demand for health care by an aging population with MR/ID is described. This is followed by a discussion of issues pertinent to psychiatric diagnosis and treatment interventions, with particular emphasis on dementia.

The Scope of the Problem

With rapid closing of institutions for people with mental disorders or mental retardation in the United States, a large majority of adults and older adults with MR/ID live in community groups or at home, often cared for by elderly parents who are themselves struggling with health problems and other disabilities. As a result, these individuals are brought to the family physicians for general health care or to the hospital emergency room when their behavior becomes unmanageable or their health suddenly declines. This increased demand for services is compounded by the scarcity of psychiatrists and other mental health professionals with expertise in the special issues involved in the diagnosis and treatment planning for this population, particularly in rural areas. The MR/ID adult and older adult population remains underserved (Whitaker, 2004). It has been recognized that in the United States, psychiatry residency programs and clinical and counseling psychology graduate programs should offer more intensive training on MR/ID (Syzmanski et al., 1991).

Community placement is not devoid of problems. The transfer from an institution to an unfamiliar setting such as a group home or a foster family can itself be stressful. Advances in the implementation of services that promote full integration and participation in the community are just beginning to be applied to the MR/ID population and in many instances have been hampered by lack of funding. Persons living in the community may have some disadvantages regarding their health care when compared with those living in institutions. Examples of barriers to appropriate health care are dehumanization by social stigma, lack of close supervision for issues related to their health, lack of awareness of issues specifically related to this population among physicians, changes in primary care physician for insurance reasons and the resulting lack of coordination of care, lack of appropriate screening procedures, and lack of health surveillance in general (Harper and Wadsworth, 1992; Carlsen et al., 1994; Kerr, Fraser, and Felce, 1996; Cook and Lennox, 2000; Lennox, Diggens, and Ugoni, 2000; Morgan, Ahmed, and Kerr, 2000). The absence of a community-based integrated system of health care stands out as a serious obstacle to the delivery of adequate physical and mental health services to this population.

Aging and Comorbidity

In the past several decades, the number of older adults with MR/ID has been increasing. This is largely because of advances in medical science and partly because of a more general increase in life span. The average life expectancy for people with all forms of MR/ID increased from about 20 years in the 1930s to about 60 years in 1980. The number of Americans over the age of 60 with MR/ID is estimated at more than 500,000, and this number is expected to double by 2030. At present, persons age 65 or older constitute 12 percent of the MR/ID population; by 2040, they are expected to be 25 percent (Puri et al., 1995; Strauss and Eyman, 1996; Silverman et al., 1998; Shavella et al., 1999; Yang, Rasmussent, and Friedman, 2002). As in the general aging population, increased longevity in individuals with MR/ID is associated with higher morbidity, particularly chronic illnesses, such as cardiovascular disease, cancer, and diabetes (Ryan and Sunada, 1997). Approximately 50 percent of adults with MR/ID have a physical disability, cannot care for themselves, or have trouble ambulating. About 25 percent have no useful speech, and about 10 percent lack basic comprehension skills and are totally dependent on others (Cooper, 1998). Common health problems in people with MR/ID are thyroid disease, obesity, ocular anomalies, hearing loss, poor oral health, bone and joint disease, and mental disorders. These health and behavioral problems increase with age (Jansen et al., 2004).

Several studies have reported that the rates of mental disorders, psychological problems, or problematic behaviors in adults and older adults with MR/ID are higher than those without MR/ID, and that the rates for people with severe and profound MR/ID are higher than in people with mild and moderate MR/ID. However, the studies that support this conclusion have methodological limitations, so the results should be interpreted with caution. A review concluded that there is no good evidence that the prevalence of mental disorders in adults with mild MR/ID is greater than in the population as a whole, though this appears to be the case for those with severe MR/ID (Whitaker and Read, 2006).

A study conducted in New York State examined 1,371 subjects with MR/ID of age 40 years or older living in small group homes and community-based residences for associations of aging with ill health and found psychiatric and behavioral disorders decreased with age. In this study, information was obtained by having nursing staff or service coordinators familiar with the individual complete a questionnaire and use medical records to verify all form entries. The authors recognize that some of the low rates may be due to underrecognition and underreporting of diseases and risk factors (Janicki et al., 2002). It is also possible that older adults with severe mental disorders were excluded from community placement. It may also be a reflection of the value of stability in living situation and its impact on maintenance of behavioral stability and relative comfort.

A comparison of older and younger adults with MR/ID found higher frequency of psychiatric symptoms and psychiatric morbidity among those over age 65 (68.7%, compared with 47.9% among those who were younger). The difference in psychiatric morbidity between the two groups was largely due to higher risk of dementia and its associated psychiatric symptoms in the older group (Cooper, 1997d).

A large-scale epidemiologic study conducted in Scotland found point prevalence rates for psychiatric disorder of 15.7 to 40.9 percent for age 16 or older, depending on the diagnostic method used. In this study, however, "problem behavior" is treated as a subcategory of mental disorder. The study found "problem behavior" to be the most common category of disorder identified (Cooper et al., 2007).

Aging and increasing life expectancy of persons with MR/ID in the United States can be associated with increased cost to the health care system. One component of this increased cost is that individuals with the most common form of MR/ID, Down syndrome (DS), have a greater likelihood of eventually being diagnosed with Alzheimer disease (AD; Janicki et al., 2002) as they age. Caring for individuals with AD require a great deal of financial and human resources. The extent of this increased cost of care is unknown. In the Netherlands, 9 percent of all disease-specific health care expenses are attributed to MR/ID, with two peaks of expenditures, the first between ages 25 and 35, and the second, attributable to dementia, between ages 75 and 85 (Polder et al., 2002).

Diagnostic Challenges

The diagnosis of mental disorders in adults and older adults with MR/ID follows the same principles of history and examination used in the general population. The first and the foremost task in the formulation of a psychiatric diagnosis is a clear, precise, and exhaustive description of the clinical presentation. By "clinical presentation," we mean symptoms, signs, or behaviors that are of psychiatric interest because they are brought to the attention of the psychiatrist for an expert opinion about whether they are a manifestation of a mental disorder. For both verbal and nonverbal patients, the intensity, frequency, duration, and context of the presentation must be described and whether the presentation is a change or departure from the premorbid state. Verbal skills may be poor. Not only mental disorders and other health problems but also normal, homeostatic reactions to changes in daily routines may present as changes in behavior. If the patient is verbal, the clinician should ask questions in a way that matches the level of severity of MR/ID. It may be difficult to distinguish the "normal" from the "abnormal," especially in nonverbal individuals. One way to overcome this problem is by applying successive approximations. This method involves an interpretation of the individual's presentation from various perspectives and reporters. Specifically, the clinician should observe the patient and obtain information from multiple sources (e.g., persons familiar with the patient, such as the caregivers and other health care professionals). The clinician should review the patient's medical record (Moss, 1999). In formulating a diagnosis of a mental disorder in adults and older adults with MR/MD, one must consider the patient and the clinical presentation from several different viewpoints. McHugh and Slavney suggest four viewpoints to guide the diagnostic process: the perspectives of dimensions, behaviors, life stories, and diseases (McHugh and Slavney, 1998; McHugh, 2005; McHugh and Clark, 2006).

One important step in the diagnostic formulation is the reconstruction of the essential characteristics of the person before the development of the clinical presentation. Using dimensions highlights an important distinction, first proposed by Karl Jaspers, between the pathoplastic factors (Jaspers, 1997). Pathoplastic factors are the modifications in the clinical presentation caused by personality and intelligence. The nature of the personality development of individuals with MR/ID is the subject of a debate. Some researchers believe that the development of personality is slower than those without MR/ID, and, therefore, adults with MR/ID are comparable to children without MR/ID. Others believe that personality development takes a different course in individuals with MR/ID (Sturmey, 1995). Irrespective of the nature of the process, it is well established that personality variables play an important role in the manifestations of mental disorders in this population. Besides intellectual capacity measured by IQ, two other types of intelligence are now recognized, emotional and social. The recognition of this perspective leads to the gradation of the developmental delay into levels of severity known as profound, severe, moderate, and mild. These gradations are based on both intellectual capacity as measured by IQ and level of adaptive behavior (American Psychiatric Association, 2000).

Only those clinical presentations that cannot be fully explained by the developmental disability (DD) alone should qualify for consideration of a psychiatric diagnosis. Sovner and colleagues (Sovner, 1986; Sovner and Hurley, 1986, 1987; Sovner and Pary, 1993) noted that many problematic behaviors of persons with MR-ID may be nonspecific effects of the intellectual impairment, such as impaired communication skills. The clinician may have to rely on information from caregivers, family members, and treatment records. He described four pathoplastic factors that may significantly affect the evaluation process: baseline exaggeration, intellectual distortion, psychosocial masking, and cognitive disintegration. *Baseline exaggeration* is the exacerbation of cognitive deficits and aberrant behaviors that predates a clinical presentation and takes place in times of increased stress or following the onset of a mental disorder, making it difficult to identify the onset of clinical presentation. The exaggeration may signal the onset of an episode of a mental disorder, yet the exaggeration itself becomes the focus of clinical attention. Accurate information on baseline functioning at the current place of residence must be available to reduce this bias. *Intellectual distortion* (reduced abstraction or "concrete thinking") refers to a difficulty at describing inner experience in meaningful abstract terms. This difficulty may further compound the reduced ability to communicate clearly leading to difficulty in recognizing the symptoms. *Psychosocial masking* arises from impoverished psychosocial development contributing to lack of depth in descriptions of problematic life experiences. *Cognitive disintegration* refers to increased likelihood of a decrement in cognitive performance and problematic behavior in individuals with limited cognitive capacity, leading to "catastrophic reactions" to relatively minor stressors.

A different perspective is that of behaviors, with the focus not on the cause of the clinical presentation but on its result in terms of loss of function and its impact on the adaptation of the person to the environment. The word *behavior* refers to observable verbal, vocal, or motor activity, not to internal states. From this perspective, certain aspects or forms of psychopathology are negative behaviors perpetuated by reinforcement and contingencies in the environment, following rules of classical or operant conditioning or social learning.

Adaptive behavior includes four major domains: communication, socialization, motor skills, and daily living skills, also known as activities of daily living (ADLs; Sparrow, Balla, and Cicchetti, 1984). Two classes of behavior are of particular concern because they indicate a decline or loss in baseline level of function. One is a decline or loss in ADLs. There are different types of ADLs. *Instrumental activities of daily living* are the ability to work, shop, handle money, clean house, and so forth. Of greater concern is the decline or loss in the *basic activities of daily living*, which refers to personal care, toileting, dressing, and eating. The diagnostic and prognostic value of the decline in ADLs associated with aging is just beginning to be understood. The decline or loss of ADLs should take into consideration the baseline performance because the prevalence of neurological impairments, sensory difficulties or anomalies, particularly with vision and hearing, difficulties with mobility, and poor dentition increases with age (Raitasuo, Taiminen, and Salokangas, 1998; Evenhuis et al., 2001). The other class of behaviors that is of concern is a decline or loss of the capacity for self-regulation. The resulting problematic behaviors, such as aggression or self-injury, may be inappropriate, objectionable, or dangerous and may cause significant distress to the person, to the caregivers, to the family, and to others in the community. To qualify as problematic, the pattern of the behavior should be out of proportion to the level of severity of MR/ID and to the intensity of the stressor. Further, the behavior should be of such frequency, severity, or chronicity that it has an adverse impact on the individual or others concerned and requires special interventions or support. It is important to determine if the problematic behavior is an integral part of the behavioral phenotype and required for the etiological diagnosis of that syndrome (e.g., overeating in Prader-Willi syndrome or self-injurious behavior in Lesch-Nyhan syndrome) or simply associated with the syndrome (Cooper, Melville, and Einfeld, 2003).

Another perspective is that of life stories, an appreciation of the universe of meanings that the illnesses carry with them. Here we focus our attention on the disruption in the assumptions and expectations of the person and the resulting disappointments or surprises. Is the clinical presentation associated with any change in routine, such as cancellation of an activity or treatment program, staff changes, or shifts in the place of residence? Bereavement, for example, has been shown to have a negative impact on both behavioral and psychiatric functioning (Dodd, Dowling, and Hollins, 2005). Recent exposure to stressful life events has been shown to be correlated with higher ratings of aggressive or destructive behavior and of affective or neurotic disorder (Owen et al., 2004).

The fourth perspective, the understanding of the disease, takes us to the disturbance in brain function that has led to the clinical presentation. For example, comorbid MR/ID and epilepsy or in disorders with a demonstrated genetic basis, such as DS and fragile X syndrome, is best understood from this perspective. The practice of applying DSM criteria to this population was based on the untested assumption that patients with and without MR/ID express mental disorder the same way. Whether standard diagnostic criteria are appropriate for the diagnosis of mental disorders in this population has been the subject of debate. Some researchers advocate the application of standard criteria based on consensus among experts, such as the one employed in the DSM, with or without modifications, irrespective of the severity of MR/ID (American Psychiatric Association, 2000; Clarke and Gomez, 1999; Matson et al., 1999; Tsiouris, 2001). Others are of the opinion that standard criteria become less useful as the severity increases and the ability to speak decreases (Holden and Gitlesen, 2004a). The standard criteria are more reliable for people with mild-to-moderate MR/ID (Clarke and Gomez, 1999; Matson et al., 1999; Tsiouris, 2001). The inclusion of behavioral criteria and informant ratings in addition to, or instead of criteria based on expert consensus, aims at making the diagnosis more reliable across the entire MR/ID spectrum (O'Brien, 2003). Unfortunately, informant reports are also subject to bias, being influenced by the needs, beliefs, and levels of tolerance of the informants leading to the challenge of avoiding missing cases because of the patients' inability to report on their internal states (false negatives), and, at the same time, avoiding excessive inclusion due to greater reliance on behavioral manifestations (false positives; Burt, 1999).

Other researchers proposed substitute criteria for mental disorders in the MR/ID population. The identification and use of behavioral equivalents was an important effort to arrive at reliable diagnoses. As originally defined, behavior equivalents were viewed as atypical presentations of mental disorders in the MR/ID population (Sovner and Hurley, 1982, 1983). For example, screaming, self-injurious behavior, and aggression were interpreted as manifestations of depression (Marston, Perry, and Roy, 1997); cyclical self-injurious behavior, unresponsive to behavioral interventions, was viewed as a sign of rapidly cycling bipolar disorder (Osborne et al., 1992); and repetitive, stereotyped, and ritualistic self-injurious behavior was considered as part of obsessive-compulsive disorder (Emerson, Moss, and Kiernan, 1999). Behavioral equivalents, as Charlot noted, may be considered as observable, operational equivalents of psychiatric symptoms in people with MR/ID, but they may also be viewed as alternatives to such symptoms. He noted that problematic behaviors occur in virtually all diagnostic groups studied, and, therefore, they cannot be viewed as syndrome-specific atypical symptoms of mental disorders. The occurrence of problematic behaviors in times of stress, according to Charlot, may be related to central nervous system deficits in people with limited behavioral repertoires (Charlot, 2005). At times it may be difficult, even impossible, to distinguish between a problematic behavior and a manifestation of a mental disorder, and this difficulty may increase with the severity of MR/ID (Moss et al., 1997). The nature of the relationship between specific problematic behaviors and specific psychiatric symptoms or mental disorders remains unclear and is subject to study and debate. Problematic behaviors may occur in the absence of a mental disorder, mental disorders may occur in the absence of problematic behaviors, and problematic behaviors and mental disorders may coexist (Holden and Gitlesen, 2003; Urv, Zigman, and Silverman, 2003; O'Brien, 2003; Charlot, 2005; Allen and Davies, 2007).

The diagnostic challenges and dilemmas outlined above are likely to be more frequent in older patients who may present with complex somatopsychiatric comorbidity (McCarron et al., 2005). The goal is to arrive at a correct diagnosis and a treatment plan by assessing the contribution of each perspective to the clinical presentation. This balanced view should protect the diagnostician against certain well-established biases that may lead to an incorrect formulation. One such bias is *diagnostic overshadowing*, a reduction in the significance of an associated mental disorder in the presence of MR/ID (Reiss, Levitan, and Szysko, 1982). Another is *functional overshadowing*, a lack of recognition of a mental disorder in the presence of normal ADLs for a given level of MR/ID (Raitasuo, Taiminen, and Salokangas, 1998). Yet another bias may be called *comorbid eclipse*, the lack of recognition of somatic comorbidity as the cause of the alteration of baseline behavior and mental status. Avoidance of this bias is particularly important in older adults because the prevalence of somatic comorbidity increases with age. Menopause occurs earlier in women with MR/ID and even earlier in those with DS. It should be kept in mind that behavioral changes in women with MR/ID in later life may be a sign of menopause.

The publication of three manuals—*The Diagnostic Manual—Intellectual Disability* (DM-ID), its accompanying clinical guide, and *The Diagnostic Criteria for Psychiatric Disorders for Use with Adults with Learning Disabilities/Mental Retardation*—is a major advance likely to enhance the reliability and validity of the psychiatric diagnostic process in the evaluation of persons with

MD/IR. At the same time, it opens the way for more rigorous epidemiological studies and clinical trials (Fletcher et al., 2007a, 2007b; Royal College of Psychiatrists, 2001).

Dementia

Consensus has been emerging on the recognition of dementia in individuals with MR/ID. A prerequisite for the diagnosis of dementia is the demonstration of intellectual decline. There should be no evidence from the history, physical examination, or special investigation for any other possible cause of the decline, or a systemic disorder, or alcohol or drug abuse (Seltzer, Schupf, and Wu, 2001). In individuals with MR/ID, cognitive abilities, such as long-term memory, decline with normal aging. Early diagnosis of dementia becomes difficult because of the person's preexisting cognitive limitations inherent to varying underlying severity of the ID (Aylward et al., 1997). Several screening tools are now available for dementia in older adults with MR/ID. Direct evaluation must be supplemented by caregiver interview because caregivers can report on cognitive decline independently of premorbid intelligence (Deb and Braganza, 1999; Bush and Beail, 2004). Measurements of decline have to be sensitive, specific, reliable, and valid, a goal that may be difficult to achieve. They should be used longitudinally over a period of several years to document a decline that is progressive and greater than typical or normative for the age group and the severity of MR/ID (Aylward et al., 1997). Sensory impairment or institutionalization may complicate the testing.

The only known risk factors for the development of Alzheimer disease (AD) in individuals with MR/ID are age and DS (Zigman, Schupf, et al., 1996; Zigman et al., 1997; Schultz et al., 2004, Zigman and Lott, 2007). Alzheimer neuropathy may occur in individuals with MR/ID who do not have DS (Popovich et al., 1990). Age is the strongest risk factor for developing dementia (Seltzer, Schupf, and Wu, 2001). Men with DS develop dementia earlier than women do (Schupf et al., 1998). The etiological contributions of other risk factors to AD found in the general population (attributable risks) such as family history, low educational level, head trauma, cardiovascular disease, stroke, diabetes, apolipoprotein E-epsilon4 (APOE-ε4), and major depression are currently being investigated. The level of MR/ID is unrelated to the risk of dementia or age at onset of dementia.

The overall prevalence of dementia in DS is estimated at 13.3 percent, with a wide range of 6 percent to 75 percent depending on the population studied and the methodology employed. About 40 percent of persons with DS aged 50 and over and 75 percent aged 60 and over have symptoms of dementia. Despite differences in methodology, there is remarkable agreement that the risk of dementia increases after the age of 50. The mean age of onset of dementia in DS is from 50 to 55, with a wide range of 38 to 70. The prevalence of dementia in DS increases with age as follows: 0 to 4 percent for ages under 30, 2 to 33 percent for ages 30 to 39, 8 to 55 percent for ages 40 to 49, 20 to 55 percent for ages 50 to 59, and 29 to 75 percent for ages 60 to 69. The average age of death for persons with DS and AD is 50. The incidence of dementia in DS is estimated at 4 percent. Approximately 50 to 60 percent of individuals with neuropathological changes characteristic of AD may develop dementia of the Alzheimer type by the time they are 60 to 70 years old (Prasher and Krishman, 1993; Zigman, Silverman, et al., 1996; Zigman et al., 2004; Visser et al., 1997; Holland et al., 1998, 2000).

In addition to increasing age, APOE-ε4 has been shown to be a significant risk factor for dementia in people with DS, whereas APOE-ε2 is a protective factor. Estrogen deficiency and increased level of Λ beta 1-42 peptide are associated with increased risk of dementia. Atypical karyotypes that decrease the does of amyloid precursor protein (for example, translocations) are associated with lower risk and lower mortality (Schupf, 2002).

Warning signs of the onset of dementia in DS are the occurrence of seizures, especially in a person who was previously free of seizures, and subtle and progressive changes in behavior and personality, such as indifference, prolonged inactivity or apathy, loss of skills related to ADLs with increased dependence, increase in stereotypy, disorientation, deficits in visual retention, loss of speech, poor pragmatic language function, hyperactive reflexes, and abnormal neurological signs (Cosgrave, Tyrrell, and McCarron, 2000). One of the earliest preclinical signs of dementia is the onset of dyspraxia, a partial loss of the ability to perform purposeful motor acts, though not necessarily lack of knowledge, thus portraying erosion between competence and performance (Dalton and Fedor, 1998).

Early clinical manifestations of dementia are changes in behavior and personality. In addition, signs of frontal lobe dysfunction occur relatively early when compared with the non-MR/ID population (Nelson et al., 2001; Burt et al., 2005; Ball et al., 2006).These include affective and volitional symptoms, such as lack of energy, irritability, slow speech and communication, lack of the sense of danger and sleep disturbance, as well as behavioral symptoms, such as agitation, incontinence, excessive lack of cooperation, social withdrawal, loss of preexisting skills, mealtime or feeding problems, wandering, and aggression (Cooper and Prasher, 1998; Deb, Hare, and Prior, 2007). Disturbances of cognition include forgetfulness, especially decline of immediate memory with relatively intact long-term memory, confusion, and deterioration in learning and orientation, and these symptoms are often associated with increased dependence (Oliver, Crayton, and Holland, 1998). Hallucinations and delusions, particularly delusions of theft or persecution, may also occur, but they appear to be less frequent than in people without DS, and the reasons for this are unclear (Cooper, 1997c). Among patients with MR/ID and dementia, those with DS are more likely to have low mood, restlessness, disturbed sleep, and hallucinations but are less likely to be aggressive (Cooper and Prasher, 1998).

Dementia of the Alzheimer type is suspected when the onset is gradual and the cognitive decline is continuous and other causes of cognitive impairment have been excluded, such as delirium, vascular dementia, dementia of Lewy bodies, hypothyroidism, sensory loss, major depressive disorder and other psychiatric disorders, bereavement, sleep apnea, chronic hepatitis, folic acid abnormalities in patients on anticonvulsants, or cognitive impairment occurring as a side effect of prescribed or nonprescribed medications, particularly anticholinergics (Cosgrave et al., 1999).

Periodic administration of test batteries allows an evaluation of baseline functioning and progression of dementia as well as response to treatment. Several scales and assessment methods are available for this purpose (Deb and Braganza, 1999; Bush and Beail, 2004). Psychological testing with Wechsler Intelligence Scale for Children—Fourth Edition (Wecshler, 2003) reveals that the decline in patients with DS begins with a preclinical stage characterized by memory loss and deficits in the block design and coding subtests; then comes an early stage, involving deficits in object assembly, picture completion, arithmetic and comprehension subtests. This is followed by deficiencies in the information processing, vocabulary, and digit span subtests. At all levels of MR/ID, adaptive behavior of individuals with DS declines more rapidly with age when compared with those without DS (Devenny, 2000).

The laboratory tests for dementia of DS are the same tests that are recommended for those who have dementia without DS. They include CBC and differential, hepatic function tests, renal function tests, thyroid function tests (likely to show hypothyroidism in DS), fasting blood glucose, serum electrolytes, vitamin B12, folate, ESR and C-reactive protein, tests for syphilis and HIV, plasma levels of drugs such as digoxin and anticonvulsants, midstream urine test, EKG, chest x-ray, EEG, vision and hearing tests, CT scan, and MRI. There are abnormalities in EEG, evoked potentials, CT, MRI, SPECT, and PET scans (Pelz et al., 1986; Pearlson et al., 1990; Schapiro et al, 1992; Prasher et al., 1994, 2003; Raz et al., 1995, 1998). These abnormalities are similar to those seen in people without DS but the general conclusion is that the accuracy of the diagnosis is limited and the brain imaging findings should be used in conjunction with clinical assessment. CT scan shows cerebral atrophy in people with DS and dementia. Temporal lobe–oriented CT scan shows reduction in volume in the medial temporal lobe. MRI is useful in identifying vascular lesions and may show neuronal loss in the hippocampus and the amygdala. (Pelz et al., 1986; Weis et al., 1991; Raz et al., 1995, 1998; Pearlson et al., 1998; Prasher et al., 2003).

CASE EXAMPLE

Jerry is a 55-year-old man who was evaluated for a change in behavior and mental status. His record showed that he was born following an uneventful pregnancy and full-term labor to a mother who was 36 years old at the time. He was the youngest of five children. At the age of 10 he was admitted to a large institution for people with DDs in a rural area in the United States. His IQ at the time of admission and subsequent psychometric evaluations 20 and 30 years later placed him in the moderate level of retardation. Chromosomal studies conducted at the age of 40 confirmed the presence of classic trisomy 21. He had the usual childhood illnesses before the age of 10, including mumps (age 4), measles (age 5), German measles (age 7), and chicken pox (age 8). Visual impairment, including cataracts, and hearing loss were noted at the age of 50. However, he continued to participate in daily activities, including shopping, going to church, and doing minor chores in the institution under supervision. He was regularly visited by his family and enjoyed the visits. At the age of 51 he was found to have hepatitis B. Thyroid function tests revealed hypothyroidism, which was treated.

Staff members were concerned about a subtle and gradual decline in function. The decline appeared to have started a couple of years earlier with what was diagnosed as a possible seizure. A 24-hour ambulatory EEG revealed generalized dysrhythmia without definite epileptic activity. Jerry then became incontinent, had frequent bouts of crying for no obvious reason, became afraid of stairs and of taking a shower or coming close to water, and began to dress and undress at inappropriate places and to lose his eating skills. By then, memory loss was evident, because he could not recall names of acquaintances or common objects, words, sentences, names of places, or time of the day. He eventually refused to cooperate even with familiar staff members and did not appear to recognize his family members or enjoy their company. He began wandering aimlessly, requiring constant supervision, until his gait became impaired. Eventually he spent most of his time in bed or sitting in his rocking chair and dozing. At various times there was evidence of behavior suggestive of hallucinations or delusions. A CT scan of the brain revealed cerebral and cerebellar atrophy with partially empty sella turcica. Laboratory investigations failed to reveal a reversible cause of dementia. ▶

Other Mental Disorders

There have been a limited number of epidemiological studies of mental disorders other than dementia in the adult and older adult MR/ID population. Because of differences in methodology, however, the results cannot be easily compared or generalized. These studies were reviewed by Whitaker and Read (2006). Keeping in mind that the studies varied greatly in sampling methods, procedures for arriving at a diagnosis, case definition and identification, and other details, certain conclusions may still be derived that are clinically useful.

There is some evidence that the prevalence of mental disorders is greater for the MR/ID population than for the general population but only for those with severe MR/ID. There is no good evidence that this difference exists for people with mild MR/ID. The prevalence rates of depression and other mood disorders appear to be quite high in the adult MR/ID population. Older people, just as in people without MR/ID, may be more vulnerable to depression than are younger people (Collacott, 1992; Cooper, 1997a, 1997b, 1997c), and depression may be experienced at some stage by one in every 10 people (Meins, 1993).The prevalence rate of depression is estimated at approximately twice that in the general population (Meins, 1993; Cooper, 1997a).

Other studies are focused on the differences in clinical presentations of mental disorders in the population with MR/ID and the feasibility of applying standard diagnostic criteria for depression and other mood disorders (McBrien, 2003). A review of 25 studies conducted 20 years ago established that a diagnosis of mood disorder could be made by applying DSM-III criteria for people with mild or moderate MR/ID. These diagnostic criteria were less effective for those with severe and profound MR/ID on whom the diagnosis could be suspected on the basis of a positive family history and changes in vegetative functioning (Sovner and Hurley, 1982). A retrospective chart review of adults with MR/ID found that bipolar disorder could be identified by applying DSM-IV criteria and that symptoms both related and unrelated to mood were significantly more frequent in bipolar patients than in those with other mood disorders (Cain et al., 2003). It has been noted that severe behavior problems may be a state-dependent phenomenon in rapidly cycling bipolar disorder, with self-injurious behavior being associated only with depressive features and aggression being associated only with manic features (Lowry and Sovner, 1992).

A study examined the presentation and risk factors for depression in 151 adults with a mild-to-moderate ID and found that 39.2 percent of participants had symptoms of depression. Sadness, self-criticism, loss of energy, crying, and tiredness appeared to be the most frequent indicators of depression or risk for depression. Automatic negative thoughts, quality and frequency of social support, self-esteem, and disruptive life events significantly predicted depression scores in people with a mild-to-moderate ID, accounting for 58.1 percent of the variance, thus raising the important question of whether demoralization may be frequent in this population occurring at the subthreshold level of the standard diagnostic criteria (McGillivray and McCabe, 2007).

Although stereotyped as happy, patients with DS are more likely to become depressed than are individuals with other etiologies of MR/ID. This is important to keep in mind because the known progression to dementia may lead to depression's being overlooked, a serious problem because depression is treatable. Depressed individuals with DS function less well in terms of adaptive behavior in subsequent follow-up than do matched controls without a psychiatric history even after the depression is no longer present, suggesting again that demoralization persists after the depression is treated (Collacott and Cooper, 1992). When depression starts later in life, the level of performance in terms of adaptive functioning is higher. Commenting on this finding, Cooper and Collacott (1992) note that depression, even when resolved, may damage a person's confidence and produce a sense of failure, particularly when the first episode takes place earlier in life. This interpretation is in line with our current views about demoralization and calls for additional research on the role of psychotherapy in the treatment of persons with MR/ID (de Figueiredo and Frank, 1982; de Figueiredo, 1993, 2007).

Noncritical family relationships, strong social support, and fewer negative stressful life events are associated with fewer symptoms of bipolar disorder over time. These findings suggest that enhancement of social and adaptive skills should be a critical component of treatment planning in addition to pharmacological interventions (Matson et al., 2006). This is probably also the case with all other mental disorders.

Therapeutic Strategies

The lack of precision in the operational definitions for case identification has made it difficult to design clinical trials of medications for the treatment of mental disorders in the MR/ID population. Psychotropic medications are extensively used for the treatment of both mental disorders and problematic behaviors despite the fact that many studies have significant methodological limitations that preclude definitive conclusions about the efficacy of psychotropic medications for older adults with MR/ID (Cohen-Mansfield, 2001; Matson et al., 2003). The major clinical trials that have led to the approval of available medications explicitly excluded people with MR/ID. With the exception of a few trials for people with dementia of DS, clinical trials specifically targeted at older adults with MR/ID have not been conducted.

A fundamental principle in the treatment of the dually diagnosed is that the treatment has to be multidisciplinary and multimodal, including not only medications but also behavioral interventions, counseling, and environmental changes. This is particularly important in the geriatric population because older patients come with multiple comorbid illnesses and multiple medications. Essential steps before any new prescriptions are written include a review of all medications being taken by the patient and a check for any recent changes. The environment of the patient should be evaluated for level of comfort, structure, temperature, lighting, and excessive stimulation or sensory distortions. Appropriate changes should be made to create a safe, simple, comfortable, predictable, soothing, and pleasant environment. If sleep is a problem, beverages containing caffeine should be reduced and an underlying cause such as pain, sleep apnea, or restless leg syndrome should be ruled out. If hallucinations and delusions are noted, confrontation, conflict, and arguments with the patient should be avoided, and the patient should be provided with reassurance, support, and redirection. Eating and bathing habits and incontinence should be monitored. There is an extensive body of knowledge on nonpharmacological interventions for problematic behaviors in dementia in persons without MR/ID, and such interventions should always be included to meet the needs of persons with MR/ID as a complement or alternative to medication management (Nezu and Nezu, 1994; Cohen-Mansfield, 2001; Rabins, Lyketsos, and Steele, 2006).

Within this framework, it is important to note that psychopharmacological treatment does have an important role in the management of psychopathology in the MR/ID population (Fava, 1997; Reiss and Aman, 1998; Fraser, 1999; Antochi, Stavrakaki, and Emery, 2003; Stanton and Coetzee, 2004). But without a strong support from evidence-based research, recommendations for psychopharmacological treatment are largely based on clinical experience and available knowledge from use in people without MR/ID but with other types of cognitive impairment. Antidepressants are used for the treatment of major depressive disorder, other depressive and anxiety disorders, body dysmorphic syndrome, obsessive-compulsive disorder, and eating disorders. In addition, antidepressants are useful in the treatment of problematic behaviors (Campbell and Duffy, 1995; Troisi et al., 1995; Hellings et al., 1996; Davanzo et al., 1998). Among the antidepressants, paroxetine and sertraline have been reported to be useful in the treatment of problematic behaviors, such as aggression, self-injurious behavior, stereotypy, and distraction, but fluoxetine has been found to aggravate aggression (Lewis et al., 1995, 1996). Clomipramine has also been shown to be effective in the treatment of self-injurious behavior and stereotypy, but concerns have been raised about serious side effects (Lewis et al., 1995, 1996; Brasic et al., 1997). An open trial of citalopram showed that treatment for 1 year at the effective dose prevented recurrence of depression (Verhoeven et al., 2001). An open trial of mirtazapine demonstrated modest response in the treatment of several problematic behaviors, such as insomnia, irritability, aggression, anxiety, hyperactivity, and self-injurious behavior in patients with autistic and other pervasive developmental disorders. The age range of the patients in this trial was 3.8 to 23.5 years, and no study was been done on older adults with MR/ID (Posey et al., 2001). As far as could be determined, no clinical trials have been conducted with escitalopram, venlafaxine, and bupropion in the MR/ID population. Bupropion should be avoided in individuals with MR/ID because of its well-known seizure-inducing potential. Antidepressants should be used with caution, especially in rapid cycling or mixed bipolar disorder or in the depressive phase of bipolar disorder, because they can trigger a switch to hypomania or mania.

CASE EXAMPLE

Emma is a 45-year-old woman who was evaluated for a change in behavior and mental status. Her record showed that she was born following an uneventful pregnancy and full-term labor to a mother who was 27 years of age at the time. She was the third of four children. At the age of 14, she was admitted to a large institution for people with DDs in a rural area in the United States. Her IQ at the time of admission and subsequent psychometric evaluations 20 and 30 years later placed her in the moderate level of retardation. Chromosomal studies conducted at the age of 40 failed to reveal any abnormalities. She had the usual childhood illnesses before the age of 10, including mumps (age 5), measles (age 6), whooping cough (age 7), and chickenpox (age 7). Until 6 months ago, she participated in daily activities, including shopping, going to church, and doing minor chores in the institution under supervision. She was regularly visited by his family and enjoyed the visits.

For the past 6 months, staff members noted that Emma's behavior gradually changed. She became more irritable, grumpy, and argumentative. She did not appear to take pleasure in some of the activities that she had previously enjoyed. She became more withdrawn, preferring to stay in her room and going to day program reluctantly. She had initial insomnia, her appetite was decreased, and she was less able to focus her attention. Slowly she required more assistance with her ADLs. These symptoms and behaviors were a clear departure from baseline, and their course was episodic. The psychiatrist consultant noted that there was no evidence of hallucinations or delusional thinking or any behavior suggestive of hopelessness or helplessness. In fact, Emma was more likely to respond positively to familiar staff. Only rarely she appeared to be somewhat impulsive and had not displayed any act of overt aggression or self-injurious behavior. A thorough medical evaluation failed to reveal any physical or physiological basis for her symptoms or behaviors. A review of the medications being given to the patient led to the conclusion that the clinical presentation could not be interpreted as iatrogenic. The psychiatrist concluded that Emma probably had a depressive disorder, most likely a major depressive disorder. Treatment with citalopram 5 mg daily, later increased to 10 mg daily, alleviated her symptoms significantly after 2 to 3 weeks. This was combined with supportive interventions and reassurance from the staff who attempted to make her immediate surroundings as pleasant and comfortable as possible. ▶

Regarding anxiolytics, buspirone has been shown to be beneficial not only for the treatment of anxiety, particularly generalized anxiety disorder, but also for agitation, aggression, and self-injurious behavior (Ratey, Sovner, and Parks, 1991; Ricketts et al., 1994). Benzodiazepines can reduce irritability and agitation, but they should be avoided due to increased risk for abuse, tolerance, dependence, and paradoxical reactions or behavioral disinhibition. Short-acting benzodiazepines, such as lorazepam or oxazepam, are preferable to the longer-acting ones. When used alone, they should not be used for more than 3 weeks.

Mood stabilizers may be used in the management of acute mania, prophylaxis of bipolar I disorder, cyclothymic disorder, cycloid psychosis, and problematic behaviors. Lithium is useful in the treatment of bipolar I disorder and cyclothymic disorder and is the treatment of choice for cycloid psychosis, which occurs frequently in Prader-Willi syndrome (Verhoeven, Curfs, and Tuinier, 1998). Lithium has also shown to be helpful in the management of aggression, disruptive behavior, and self-injurious behavior (Tyrer et al., 1984; Craft et al., 1987; Pary, 1991). A double-blind placebo-controlled trial of adults revealed that good response was associated with less than one aggressive episode per week before starting treatment, overactivity, stereotypic behavior, being female, and having epilepsy (Tyrer et al., 1984). Lithium works well in bipolar patients with irritability and anger outbursts. Lithium requires close monitoring because people with MR/ID are more prone to developing toxic side effects to it. The length of time lithium lasts in the body increases exponentially as people age; therefore, the dose should be reduced accordingly. Antiepileptic medications would be the treatment of choice when outbursts of rage are associated with abnormal EEG findings. Valproate should be used for rapid cycling and mixed states, disorders that are more common among people with MR/ID than among those without MR/ID

(Sovner, 1989; Ruedrich et al., 1999). As far as we could determine, no studies have been done to evaluate the efficacy of other antiepileptic medications in the adult MR/ID population for psychiatric problems. Though useful, antiepileptic medications may produce behavioral side effects that may be impossible to detect in nonverbal patients without an appropriate behavioral assessment (Kalachnik et al., 1995). Long-term use of high doses of antiepileptic medications, particularly topiramate, may produce memory loss. It is not known if amnesia as a side effect of antiepileptic medications is more likely to occur in people with MR/ID than in those without MR/ID.

Antipsychotic medications (neuroleptics) have been shown to be helpful to some people with MR/ID at reducing self-injurious behaviors, stereotypies, aggression, agitation, and disruptive behavior (Brylewski and Duggan, 2000). Atypical neuroleptics, particularly risperidone and olanzapine, have been shown to be efficacious in the treatment of problematic behaviors and have been used in the treatment of psychotic disorders in people with MR/ID (Vanden Borre et al., 1993; Cohen and Underwood, 1994; Pary, 1994; Khan, 1997; Cohen et al., 1998; Buzan et al., 1998; Antonacci and de Groot, 2000; McDonoough, Hillery, and Kennedy, 2000; Zarcone et al., 2001; Sabaawi, Singh, and de Leon, 2006). Some atypicals are also used for the treatment of bipolar disorder. Olanzapine should be used with caution because it can cause excessive sedation, weight gain, and metabolic syndrome. Clozapine has been shown to be safe, efficacious, and well tolerated for treatment resistant mood and psychotic disorders as well as severe problematic behaviors (Cohen and Underwood, 1994; Pary, 1994; Buzan et al., 1998; Antonacci and de Groot, 2000; Sabaawi, Singh, and de Leon, 2006). If not properly monitored, however, clozapine may produce fatal side effects and therefore a protocol for monitoring should be rigorously followed (Sabaawi, Singh, and de Leon, 2006). Patients who cannot cooperate with blood drawings should not be prescribed clozapine or any medication that requires blood studies. Atypicals have a better side-effect profile than the typicals and appear to be less likely to cause serious undesirable effects, such as tardive dyskinesia, akathisia, or neuroleptic malignant syndrome. However, atypicals can create side effects such as weight gain and metabolic syndrome. Information about other atypicals is unavailable. At this time it is unclear if the concerns expressed about the use of neuroleptic medications in dementia not associated with DS apply to the population with MR/ID. They resulted in a black box warning that neuroleptic medications are not indicated for older persons with behavior disorder associated with dementia and that they have been associated with increased mortality, particularly of cardiovascular events and infections. Antipsychotic medications appear to be effective in the treatment of psychotic aggression, with only a modest effect in controlling pathological aggression in dementia (Antochi, Stavrakaki, and Emery, 2003).

Medications for sleep should be used carefully and with constant monitoring. As far as could be determined, there have been no clinical trials on the use of stimulants in older adults with ADHD and MR/ID. Stimulants may be used, but they can aggravate tics, obsessions, compulsions, epilepsy, anxiety, or symptoms of psychosis. In the absence of evidence to support their use in older adults, they should be avoided. The use of naltrexone and other opioid antagonists for the treatment of self-injurious behavior remains controversial. Beta-blockers are used to manage pathologic aggression, but they can cause hypotension and bradycardia, and their safety and efficacy in older adults with MR/ID have not been adequately assessed. The usefulness of clonidine is also insufficiently documented (Buzan et al., 1995; Willemsen-Swinkels et al., 1995; Casner, Weinheimer, and Gaultieri, 1996; Ruedrich, 1996).

Acetylcholinesterase inhibitors have been shown to be effective in the treatment of cognitive symptoms in dementia of the Alzheimer type and other dementias with cholinergic deficiency (Prasher, 2004). Patients with DS have fewer neurons in the nucleus basalis of Meynert than does the general population, and neuronal loss in that structure is believed to be responsible for the cholinergic deficits found in AD (Casanova et al., 1985). It makes sense, therefore, to attempt to treat the cognitive deficits of DS with acetylcholinesterase inhibitors. Donepezil, rivastigmine, and galantamine have demonstrated efficacy in 3- to 12-month randomized double-blind placebo-controlled trials assessing cognitive, functional, behavioral, and global outcomes in patients with mild to moderately severe AD unrelated to DS. In addition, donepezil has been shown to be efficacious on cognitive and functional measures but not on behavior in severe AD unrelated to DS. Among the acetylcholinesterase inhibitors, donepezil and rivastigmine are the only medications evaluated for use with DS (Prasher, 2004). A number of contraindications and drug interactions should be kept in mind before acetylcholinesterase inhibitors are prescribed (Prasher, 2004).

In general, donepezil appears to be well tolerated by adults with DS and to produce positive effects, such as improvements in cognitive functioning, expressive language, neuropsychiatric symptoms, adaptive behavior, and quality of life (Kishnani et al., 1999, 2001; Lott et al., 2002; Prasher et al., 2002; Johnson et al., 2003; Heller et al., 2003). However, not all patients respond to donepezil, and in some studies the placebo group also showed some improvement. In some cases, donepezil had to be discontinued because of severe side effects, such as agitation, aggression, urinary incontinence, forgetfulness, abdominal pain, vomiting, and diarrhea (Hemingway-Eltomey and Lerner, 1999; Johnson et al., 2003; Cipriani, Bianchetti, and Trabucchi, 2003). Also, some patients tolerated lower but not higher doses of donepezil. Patients with DS appear to be more sensitive to donepezil and apt to develop adverse effects related primarily to peripheral cholinergic overstimulation. Accordingly, a slow titration is recommended (e.g., 5 mg of donepezil daily for 6 weeks before the dose is increased). Administration of a peripherally acting cholinergic antagonist should also be considered.

A retrospective treatment analysis revealed that adults with DS and AD treated with rivastigmine had less of a decline in global and adaptive function over 24 weeks compared with an untreated group; the difference, however, failed to reach statistical significance (Prasher, Fung, and Adams, 2005). Rivastigmine was shown to be safe and efficacious in an open-label study with improvements in overall adaptive function, attention, memory, and language domains. It should be noted that this study included only adolescents (Heller et al., 2006). Similar studies on adults and older adults with DS or other types of dementias in people with MR/ID have not been conducted. The N-methyl-D-aspartate receptor antagonist memantine was shown to be effective in 6-month, randomized, double-blind, placebo-controlled trials, but it has not been evaluated for patients with DS.

A number of other medications or treatment strategies have been used or found to be useful in the symptomatic treatment of AD not associated with DS. These include antioxidants, such as vitamin E (alpha-tocopherol) and selegiline, statins, estrogen replacement, NSAIDs and other COX-2 inhibitors, and antidepressants, particularly SSRIs. A large multicenter trial on vitamin E is currently being undertaken. In a study of adults with DS, among those who had higher total cholesterol levels, those who used statins had less than half the risk of developing dementia of the Alzheimer type than those who did not (Zigman et al., 2007). There is, therefore, compelling reason for further investigating the protective effect of statins for people who have DS.

Noncognitive symptoms are quite prominent in dementia associated with DS. Because individuals with DS are more vulnerable to depression than patients with other types of MR/ID, the noncognitive symptoms could be due to depression, dementia, or both. A study of six adults with DS treated with SSRIs revealed improvements in depressive, apathetic, and compulsive behaviors as assessed by caregivers and on objective measures, such as workplace productivity, and, in some patients, the treatment was associated with concomitant improvement in daily function (Zigman et al., 2007).

Conclusion

The diagnosis and treatment of mental disorders in older adults with intellectual disabilities is of increasing importance, given their increased life expectancy. With this improving life expectancy, more persons with intellectual disabilities are at increasing risk of developing dementia. Assessment and diagnosis for this population must involve interview techniques that are appropriate for their developmental level, multiple sources of information, and observation of the individual when possible. As is generally true for older adults, people with intellectual disabilities in this age group often have multiple comorbid illnesses and medications to consider as part of assessment and treatment. Multidisciplinary, multimodal treatment is fundamental in treating geriatric persons with intellectual disabilities and can make a substantial positive impact on their lives.

References

Allen D, Davies D. 2007. Challenging behavior and psychiatric disorder in intellectual disability. *Current Opinion in Psychiatry* 20(5): 450–55.

American Psychiatric Association. 2000. *Diagnostic and Statistical Manual of Mental Disorders*, 4th ed., text rev. Washington, DC: American Psychiatric Association.

Antochi R, Stavrakaki C, Emery PC. 2003. Psychopharmacological treatments in persons with dual diagnosis of psychiatric disorders and developmental disabilities. *Postgraduate Medical Journal* 79: 139–46.

Antonacci DJ, de Groot CM. 2000. Clozapine treatment in a population of adults with mental retardation. *Journal of Clinical Psychiatry* 61: 22–25.

Aylward EH, Burt DB, Thorpe LU, Lai F, Dalton A. 1997. Diagnosis of dementia in individuals with intellectual disability. *Journal of Intellectual Disability Research* 41(2): 152–64.

Ball SL, Holland AJ, Hon J, et al. 2006. Personality and behavior changes mark the early stages of Alzheimer's disease in adults with Down's syndrome: Findings from a prospective population-based study. *International Journal of Geriatric Psychiatry* 21(7).

Barcikowska M, Silverman W, Zigman W, et al. 1989. Alzheimer-type neuropathology and clinical symptoms of dementia in mentally retarded people without Down syndrome. *American Journal on Mental Retardation* 93(5): 551–57.

Berg JM, Karlinsky H, Holland AJ (eds.). 1993. *Alzheimer Disease, Down Syndrome, and Their Relationship.* Oxford: Oxford University Press.

Blackwood DHR, St Clair DM, Muir WJ, Oliver CJ, Dickens P. 1988. The development of Alzheimer's disease in Down's syndrome assessed by auditory event-related potentials. *Journal of Mental Deficiency Research* 32: 439–53.

Brasic JR, Barnett JY, Sheitman BB, Tsaltas MO. 1997. Adverse effects of clomipramine (letter). *Journal of American Academy of Child and Adolescent Psychiatry* 36: 1165–66.

Brylewski J, Duggan L. 2000. Antipsychotic medication for challenging behavior in people with learning disability. *Cochrane Database of Systematic Reviews* 1(3): 1–26.

Burt DB. 1999. Dementia and depression. In M Janicki, AJ Dalton (eds.), *Dementia, Aging, and Intellectual Disabilities: A Handbook,* 198–216. Philadelphia: Brunner/ Mazel.

Burt DB, Primeaux-Hart S, Loveland KA, et al. 2005. Tests and medical conditions associated with dementia diagnosis. *Journal of Policy and Practice in Intellectual Disabilities* 2(1): 47–56.

Bush A, Beail N. 2004. Risk factors for dementia in people with Down syndrome: Issues in assessment and diagnosis. *American Journal on Mental Retardation* 109(2): 83–97.

Buzan RD, Dubovsky SL, Firestone D, DalPozzo E. 1998. Use of clozapine in 10 mentally retarded adults. *Journal of Neuropsychiatry and Clinical Neuroscience* 10: 93–95.

Buzan RD, Dubovsky SL, Treadway JT, Thomas M. 1995. Opiate antagonists for recurrent self-injurious behavior in three mentally retarded adults. *Psychiatric Services* 46: 511–12.

Cain NN, Davidson PW, Burhan AM, et al. 2003. Identifying bipolar disorders in individuals with intellectual disability. *Journal of Intellectual Disability Research* 47(1): 31–38.

Campbell JJ, III, Duffy JD. 1995. Sertraline treatment of aggression in a developmentally disabled patient (letter). *Journal of Clinical Psychiatry* 56: 123–24.

Carlsen WR, Galliuzzi KE, Forman LF, Cavalieri TA. 1994. Comprehensive geriatric assessment: Applications for community residing, elderly people with mental retardation/developmental disabilities. *Mental Retardation* 32: 334–40.

Casanova M, Walker L, Whitehouse P, Price D. 1985. Abnormalities of the nucleus basalis of Meynert in Down's syndrome. *Annals of Neurology* 18:310–13.

Casner JA, Weinheimer B, Gaultieri CT. 1996. Naltrexone and self-injurious behavior: A retrospective population study. *Journal of Clinical Psychopharmacology* 16: 389–94.

Charlot L. 2005. Use of behavioral equivalents for symptoms of mood disorder. In P Sturmey (ed.), *Mood Disorders in People with Mental Retardation*, 17–45. Kingston, NY: NADD Press.

Cipriani G, Bianchetti A, Trabucchi M. 2003. Donepezil use in the treatment of dementia associated with Down syndrome. *Archives of Neurology* 60(2): 292.

Clarke DJ, Gomez GA. 1999. Utility of DCR-10 criteria in the diagnosis of depression associated with intellectual disability. *Journal of Intellectual Disability Research* 43: 413–20.

Cohen SA, Ihrig K, Lott RS, Kerrick JM. 1998. Risperidone for aggression and self-injurious behavior in adults with mental retardation. *Journal of Autism and Developmental Disorders* 28: 229–33.

Cohen SA, Underwood MT. 1994. The use of clozapine in a mentally retarded and aggressive population. *Journal of Clinical Psychiatry* 55: 440–44.

Cohen WI, Nadel L, Madrick ME (eds.). 2003. *Down Syndrome: Visions for the 21st Century* Hoboken, NJ: Wiley InterScience.

Cohen-Mansfield J. 2001. Nonpharmacologic interventions for inappropriate behaviors in dementia: A review, summary, and critique. *American Journal of Geriatric Psychiatry* 9(4): 361–81.

Cole G, Neal JW, Fraser WI, Cowie VA. 1994. Autopsy findings in patients with mental handicap. *Journal of Intellectual Disability Research* 38: 9–26.

Collacott RA. 1992. Effect of age and residential placement in adaptive behavior in adults with Down's syndrome. *British Journal of Psychiatry* 161: 675–79.

Collacott RA, Cooper SA. 1992. Adaptive behavior after depressive illness in Down's syndrome. *Journal of Nervous and Mental Disease* 180: 468–70.

Cook A, Lennox N. 2000. General practice registrars' care of persons with intellectual disabilities. *Journal of Intellectual and Developmental Disability* 25: 69–77.

Cooper SA. 1997a. Epidemiology of psychiatric disorders in elderly compared with younger adults with learning disabilities. *British Journal of Psychiatry* 170: 373–80.

Cooper SA. 1997b. High prevalence of dementia among people with learning disabilities not attributable to Down's syndrome. *Psychological Medicine* 27: 609–16.

Cooper SA. 1997c. Psychiatric symptoms of dementia among elderly people with learning disabilities. *International Journal of Geriatric Psychiatry* 12(6): 662–66.

Cooper SA. 1997d. Psychiatry of elderly compared to younger adults with intellectual disabilities. *Journal of Applied Research in Intellectual Disabilities* 10: 303–11.

Cooper SA. 1998. Clinical study of the effect of age on the physical health of adults with mental retardation. *American Journal of Mental Retardation* 106: 582–89.

Cooper SA, Collacott RA. 1993. Prognosis of depression in Down's syndrome. *Journal of Nervous and Mental Disease* 181: 204–5.

Cooper SA, Melville CA, Einfeld SL. 2003. Psychiatric diagnosis, intellectual disabilities and diagnostic criteria for psychiatric disorders for use with adults with learning disabilities/mental retardation (DC-LD). *Journal of Intellectual Disability Research* 47: 3–15.

Cooper SA, Prasher VP. 1998. Maladaptive behaviors and symptoms of dementia in adults with Down's syndrome compared with adults with intellectual disability of other etiologies. *Journal of Intellectual Disability Research* 42(4): 293–300.

Cooper SA, Smiley E, Morrison J, Williamson A, Allan L. 2007. Mental ill-health in adults with intellectual disabilities: prevalence and associated factors. *British Journal of Psychiatry* 190: 27–35.

Cosgrave MP, Tyrrell J, McCarron M. 2000. A five year follow-up study of dementia in persons with Down's syndrome: Early symptoms and patterns of deterioration. *Irish Journal of Psychological Medicine* 17: 5–11.

Cosgrave MP, Tyrrell J, McCarron M, Gill M, Lawlor BA. 1999. Age at onset of dementia and age of menopause in women with Down's syndrome. *Journal of Intellectual Disability Research* 43(6): 461–65.

Craft M, Ismail IA, Krishnamurti D, et al. Lithium in the treatment of aggression in mentally handicapped patients: Double blind trial. *British Journal of Psychiatry* 150: 685–89.

Dalton AJ, Fedor BL. 1998. Onset of dyspraxia in aging persons with Down syndrome. *Journal of Intellectual Disability Research* 23: 13–24.

Davanzo PA, Belin TR, Widawski MH, King B. 1998. Paroxetine treatment of aggression and self-injury in persons with mental retardation. *American Journal on Mental Retardation* 102: 427–37.

Deb S, Braganza J. 1999. Comparison of rating scales for the diagnosis of dementia in adults with Down's syndrome. *Journal of Intellectual Disability Research* 43(5): 400–407.

Deb S, da Silva PN, Gemmell HG, et al. 1992. Alzheimer's disease in adults with Down's syndrome: The relationship between regional cerebral flow equivalents and dementia. *Acta Psychiatrica Scandinavica* 86: 340–45.

Deb S, Hare M, Prior L. 2007. Symptoms of dementia among adults with Down's syndrome: A qualitative study. *Journal of Intellectual Disability Research* 51(9): 726–39.

De Figueiredo J.M. 1993. Depression and demoralization: Phenomenological differences and research perspectives. *Comprehensive Psychiatry* 34(5): 308–11.

De Figueiredo J.M. 2007. Editorial: Demoralization and psychotherapy: A tribute to Jerome D. Frank, MD, PhD (1909–2005). *Psychotherapy and Psychosomatics* 76 (3): 129–33.

De Figueiredo JM, Frank JD. 1982. Subjective incompetence, the clinical hallmark of demoralization. *Comprehensive Psychiatry* 23(4): 353–63.

Devenny DA, Krinsky-McHale SJ, Sersen G, Silverman WP. 2000. Sequence of cognitive decline in dementia in adults with Down's syndrome. *Journal of Intellectual Disabilities Research* 44(6): 654–65.

Dodd P, Dowling S, Hollins S. 2005. A review of the emotional, psychiatric and be-
    havioral responses to bereavement in people with intellectual disabilities. *Journal
    of Intellectual Disability Research* 49: 537–43.

Dykens EM. 2007. Psychiatric and behavioral disorders in persons with Down
    syndrome. *Mental Retardation and Developmental Disabilities Research Reviews*
    13(3): 272.

Ebensen AJ, Benson BA. 2006. A prospective analysis of life events, problem behav-
    iors and depression in adults with intellectual disability. *Journal of Intellectual
    Disability Research* 50: 248–58.

Emerson E, Kiernan C, Alborz A, et al. 2001. The prevalence of challenging be-
    haviors: A total population study. *Research in Developmental Disabilities* 2291:
    77–93.

Emerson E, Moss S, Kiernan C. 1999. The relationship between challenging behav-
    ior and psychiatric disorders in people with severe developmental disabilities. In
    N Bouras (ed.), *Psychiatric and Behavioral Disorders in Developmental Disabilities
    and Mental Retardation*, 38–48. Cambridge: Cambridge University Press.

Emerson E, Robertson J, Wood J. 2005. Emotional and behavioral needs of children
    and adolescents with intellectual disabilities in an urban conurbation. *Journal of
    Intellectual Disability Research* 49:16–24.

Engler H, Forsberg A, Almkvist O, et al. 2006. Two-year follow-up of amyloid depo-
    sition in patients with Alzheimer's disease. *Brain* 129: 2856–66.

Epstein CJ, Hassold TJ, Lott IT, Nadel L, Patterson D. 1995. *Etiology and Pathogenesis
    of Down Syndrome.* Hoboken, NJ: John Wiley & Sons.

Evenhuis H, Theunissen M, Denkers I, Verschuure H, Kemme H. 2001. Prevalence
    of visual and hearing impairment in a Dutch institutionalized population with
    intellectual disability. *Journal of Intellectual Disability Research* 45: 457–74.

Eyman RK, Call TI, White JF. 1991. Life expectancy of persons with Down's syn-
    drome. *American Journal of Mental Retardation* 95(6): 603–12.

Fava M. 1997. Psychopharmacologic treatment of pathologic aggression. *Psychiatric
    Clinics of North America* 20(2): 427–51.

Fletcher RJ, Loschen E, Stavrakaki C, First M (eds). 2007a. *Diagnostic Manual—
    Intellectual Disability: A Clinical Guide for Diagnosis of Mental Disorders in Persons
    with Intellectual Disability.* Kingston, NY: NADD Press.

Fletcher RJ, Loschen E, Stavrakaki C, First M (eds.). 2007b. *Diagnostic Manual—
    Intellectual Disability: A Textbook of Diagnosis of Mental Disorders in Persons with
    Intellectual Disability.* Kingston, NY: NADD Press.

Fraser B. 1999. Psychopharmacology and people with learning disability. *Advances
    in Psychiatric Treatment* 5: 471–77.

Geldmacher DS, Lerner AJ, Voci JM, et al. 1997. Treatment of functional decline in
    adults with Down syndrome using selective serotonin-reuptake inhibitor drugs.
    Journal of Geriatric Psychiatry and Neurology 10(3): 99–104.

Gostason R. 1985. Psychiatric illness among the mentally retarded: a Swedish popu-
    lation study. *Acta Psychiatrica Scandinavica* 71 (Suppl. 318): 1–117.

Gottesman II, Gould TD. 2003. The endophenotype concept in psychiatry: Etymology and strategic intentions. *American Journal of Psychiatry* 160: 636–45.

Greenberg JS, Seltzer MM, Hong J. 2006. Bidirectional effects of expressed emotion and behavior problems and symptoms in adolescents and adults with autism. *American Journal on Mental Retardation* 111:229–49.

Harper DC, Wadsworth JS. 1992. Improving health care communication for persons with mental retardation. *Public Health Reports* 107: 297–302.

Hayes C, Johnson Z, Thornton L, et al. 1997. Ten-year survival of Down syndrome births. *International Journal of Epidemiology* 26(4): 822–29.

Heller JH, Spiridigliozzi GA, Crissman BG, et al. 2006. Safety and efficacy of rivastigmine in adolescents with Down syndrome: A preliminary 20-week, open-label study. *Journal of Child and Adolescent Psychopharmacology* 16(6): 755–65.

Heller JH, Spiridigliozzi GA, Sullivan JA, et al. 2003. Donepezil for the treatment of language deficits in adults with Down syndrome: A preliminary 24-week open trial. *American Journal of Medical Genetics* 116(2): 111–16.

Hellings JA, Kelley LA, Gabrielli WF, Kilgore E, Shah P. 1996. Sertraline response in adults with mental retardation and autistic disorder. *Journal of Clinical Psychiatry* 57: 333–36.

Hemingway-Eltomey JM, Lerner AJ. 1999. Adverse effects of donepezil in treating Alzheimer's disease associated with Down's syndrome (letter to the editor). *American Journal of Psychiatry* 156:1470.

Holden B, Gitlesen JP. 2003. Prevalence of psychiatric symptoms in adults with mental retardation and challenging behavior. *Research in Developmental Disabilities* 24: 323–32.

Holden B, Gitlesen JP. 2004a. The association between severity of intellectual disability and psychiatric symptomatology. *Journal of Intellectual Disability Research* 48(6): 556–62.

Holden B, Gitlesen P. 2004b. Psychotropic medication in adults with mental retardation: Prevalence, and prescription practices. *Research in Developmental Disabilities* 25: 509–21.

Holland AJ, Hon J, Huppert FA, Stevens F. 2000. Incidence and course of dementia in people with Down's syndrome: Findings of a population-based study. *Journal of Intellectual Disability Research* 44: 138–46.

Holland AJ, Hon J, Huppert FA, Stevens F, Watson P. 1998. Population-based study of prevalence and presentation of dementia in adults with Down's syndrome. *British Journal of Psychiatry* 172: 493–98.

Hurley AD, Folstein M, Lam N. 2003. Patients with and without intellectual disability seeking outpatient psychiatric services: Diagnoses and prescribing pattern. *Journal of Intellectual Disability Research* 47: 39–50.

Janicki MP, Henderson M, Davidson PW, et al. 2002. Health characteristics and health services utilization in older adults with intellectual disability living in community residence. *Journal of Intellectual Disability Research* 46(4): 287–98.

Jansen DEMC, Krol B, Groothoff JW, Post D. 2004. People with intellectual disability and their health problems: A review of comparative studies. *Journal of Intellectual Disability Research* 48(2): 93–102.

Jaspers K. 1997. *General Psychopathology.* Trans. J. Hoenig and Marian W. Hamilton, with an introduction by Paul R. McHugh. Baltimore: Johns Hopkins University Press.

Johnson N, Fahey C, Chicoine B, Chong G, Gitelman D. 2003. Effects of donepezil on cognitive functioning in Down syndrome. *American Journal on Mental Retardation* 108(6): 367–72.

Kalachnik JE, Hanzel TE, Harder SR, Bauemfeind JD, Engstrom EA. 1995. Antiepileptic drug behavioral side-effects in individuals with mental retardation and the use of behavioral measurement techniques. *Mental Retardation* 33: 374–82.

Kang J, Lemaire HG, Unterbeck A, et al. 1987. The precursor of Alzheimer's disease amyloid A4 protein resembles a cell surface receptor. *Nature* 325: 733–36.

Kerr M, Fraser W, Felce D. 1996. Primary health care for persons with a learning disability. *British Journal of Learning Disabilities* 24: 2–9.

Kesslak JP, Nagata SF, Lott I, Nalcioglu O. 1994. Magnetic resonance imaging analysis of age-related changes in the brains of individuals with Down's syndrome. *Neurology* 44: 1039–45.

Khan BU. 1997. Brief report: Risperidone for severely disturbed behavior and tardive dyskinesia in developmentally disabled adults. *Journal of Autism and Developmental Disorders* 27: 479–89.

Kishnani PS, Spiridigliozzi GA, Heller JH, et al. 2001. Donepezil for Down's syndrome. *American Journal of Psychiatry* 158(1): 143.

Kishnani PS, Sullivan JA, Spiridigliozzi GA, Heller JH, Crissman BG. 2004. Donepezil use in Down syndrome. *Archives of Neurology* 61(4): 605–6.

Kishnani PS, Sullivan JA, Walter BK, et al. 1999. Cholinergic therapy for Down's syndrome. *Lancet* 353: 1064–65.

Klunk WE. 2006. Two-year follow-up of amyloid deposition in patients with Alzheimer's disease. *Brain* 129: 2805–7.

Kondoh T, Amamoto N, Doi T, et al. 2005. Dramatic improvement in Down syndrome-associated cognitive impairment with donepezil. *Annals of Pharmacotherapy* 39(3): 563–66.

Kondoh T, Nakashima M, Sasaki H, Moriuchi H. 2005. Pharmacokinetics of donepezil in Down syndrome. *Annals of Pharmacotherapy* 39(3): 572–73.

Koskentausta T, Livanainen M, Almqvist F. 2007. Risk factors for psychiatric disturbance in children with intellectual disability. *Journal of Intellectual Disability Research* 51: 43–53.

Lai F, Kamman E, Rebeck GW, Anderson A, Nixon RA. 1999. APOE genotype and gender effects on Alzheimer disease in 100 adults with Down syndrome. *Neurology* 53: 331–36.

Lai F, Williams RS. 1989. A prospective study of Alzheimer disease in Down syndrome. *Archives of Neurology* 46:849–53.

Langdon PE, Swift A, Budd R. 2006. Social climate within secure inpatient services for people with intellectual disabilities. *Journal of Intellectual Disability Research* 50:828–36.

Lennox NG, Diggens UJ, Ugoni A. 2000. Health care for persons with an intellectual disability: General practitioner's attitudes and provision of care. *Journal of Intellectual and Developmental Disability* 25: 127–33.

Lewis MH, Bodfish JW, Powell SB, Golden RN. 1995. Clomipramine treatment for stereotype and related repetitive movement disorders associated with mental retardation. *American Journal on Mental Retardation* 100: 299–312.

Lewis MH, Bodfish JW, Powell SB, Parker DE, Golden RN. 1996. Clomipramine treatment for self-injurious behavior of individuals with mental retardation: A double blind comparison with placebo. *American Journal on Mental Retardation* 100: 654–55.

Lott I, Head E. 2001. Alzheimer disease and Down syndrome: Factors in pathogenesis. *Neurobiology of Aging* 26(3): 383–89.

Lott IT, Osann K, Doran E, Nelson L. 2002. Down syndrome and Alzheimer disease, Response to donepezil. *Archives of Neurology* 59: 1133–36.

Lowry MA. 1998. Assessment and treatment of mood disorders in persons with developmental disabilities. *Journal of Developmental and Physical Disabilities* 10(4): 387–406.

Lowry MA, Sovner R. 1992. Severe behavior problems associated with rapidly cycling bipolar disorder in two adults with profound mental retardation. *Journal of Intellectual Disability Research* 36(3): 269–81.

Lubec G. 2003. *Advances in Down Syndrome Research*. New York: Springer.

Mann DMA. 1988a. Alzheimer's disease and Down's syndrome. *Histopathology* 13: 125–37.

Mann DMA. 1988b. The pathological association between Down syndrome and Alzheimer disease. *Mechanisms of Ageing and Development* 43: 99–136.

Marston GM, Perry DW, Roy A. 1997. Manifestations of depression in people with intellectual disability. *Journal of Intellectual Disability Research* 41: 476–80.

Matson JL, Bielecki J, Mayville SB, Matson ML. 2003. Psychopharmacology research for individuals with mental retardation: Methodological issues and suggestions. *Research in Developmental Disabilities* 24: 149–57.

Matson JL, Rush KS, Hamilton M, et al. 1999. Characteristics of depression as assessed by the Diagnostic Assessment for the Severely Handicapped—II (DASH-II). *Research in Developmental Disabilities* 20: 305–13.

Matson JL, Terlonge C, Gonzalez ML, Rivet T. 2006. An evaluation of social and adaptive skills in adults with bipolar disorder and severe/profound intellectual disability. *Research in Developmental Disabilities* 27: 681–87.

McBrien JA. 2003. Assessment and diagnosis of depression in people with intellectual disability. *Journal of Intellectual Disability Research* 47(1): 1–13.

McCarron M, Gill M, McCallion P, Begley C. 2005. Health co-morbidities in ageing persons with Down syndrome and Alzheimer's dementia. *Journal of Intellectual Disability Research* 49(7): 560–66.

McDonoough M, Hillery J, Kennedy N. 2000. Olanzapine for chronic, stereotypic self-injurious behavior: A pilot study in seven adults with intellectual disabilities. *Journal of Intellectual Disability Research* 44(6): 677–84.

McGillivray JA, McCabe MP. 2007. Early detection of depression and associated risk factors in adults with mild/moderate intellectual disability. *Research in Developmental Disabilities* 59–70.

McHugh PR. 2005. Striving for coherence: Psychiatry's efforts over classification. *JAMA* 293 (20): 2526–28.

McHugh PR, Clark MR. 2006. Diagnostic and classificatory dilemmas. In M Blumenfield, JJ Strain (eds.), *Psychosomatic Medicine*, 39–45. Philadelphia: Lippincott, Williams & Wilkins.

McHugh PR, Slavney PR. 1998. *The Perspectives of Psychiatry*, 2nd ed. Baltimore: Johns Hopkins University Press.

Meins W. 1993. Prevalence and risk factors for depressive disorders in adults with intellectual disability. *Australia and New Zealand Journal on Developmental Disabilities* 18: 147–56.

Morgan CL, Ahmed Z, Kerr MP. 2000. Health care provision for persons with a learning disability. *British Journal of Psychiatry* 176: 37–41.

Moss SC. 1999. Assessment: Conceptual issues. In N Bouras (ed.), *Psychiatric and Behavioral Disorders in Developmental Disabilities and Mental Retardation*, 18–39. Cambridge: Cambridge University Press.

Moss SC, Emerson E, Bouras N, Holland A. 1997. Mental disorders and problematic behaviors in people with intellectual disability: Future directions for research. *Journal of Intellectual Disability Research* 41(6): 440–47.

Nelson LD, Orme D, Osann K, Lott IT. 2001. Neurological changes and emotional functioning in adults with Down syndrome. *Journal of Intellectual Disability Research* 450(5): 450–56.

Nezu CM, Nezu AM. 1994. Outpatient psychotherapy for adults with mental retardation and concomitant psychopathology: research and clinical imperatives. *Journal of Consulting and Clinical Psychology* 62: 34–42.

O'Brien G. 2003. The classification of problem behavior in Diagnostic Criteria for Psychiatric Disorders for Use with Adults with Learning Disabilities / Mental Retardation (DC-LD). *Journal of Intellectual Disability Research* 47: 32–37.

Oliver C, Crayton L, Holland A. 1998. A four year prospective study of age-related cognitive change in adults with Down's syndrome. *Psychological Medicine* 28: 1365–77.

Osborne JG, Baggs AW, Darvish R, et al. 1992. Cyclical self-injurious behavior, contingent watermist treatment, and the possibility of a rapid-cycling bipolar disorder. *Journal of Behavior Therapy and Experimental Psychiatry* 23: 325–34.

Owen DM, Hastings RP, Noone SJ, et al. 2004. Life events as correlates of problem behavior and mental health in a residential population of adults with developments disabilities. *Research in Developmental Disabilities* 25:309–20.

Pary RJ. 1991. Towards defining adequate lithium trials for individuals with mental retardation and mental illness. *American Journal on Mental Retardation* 95: 681–91.

Pary RJ. 1994. Clozapine in three individuals with mild mental retardation and treatment-refractory psychiatric disorders. *Mental Retardation* 32: 323–27.

Pearlson GD, Breiter SN, Aylward EH, et al. 1998. MRI brain changes in subjects with Down syndrome with and without dementia. *Developmental Medicine and Child Neurology* 49: 326–34.

Pearlson GD, Warren AC, Starkstein SE, et al. 1990. Brain atrophy in 18 patients with Down syndrome: A CT study. *American Journal of Neuroradiology* 11: 811–16.

Pelz DM, Karlik SJ, Fox AJ, Vinuela F. 1986. Magnetic resonance imaging in Down's syndrome. *Canadian Journal of Neurological Sciences* 13: 566–69.

Polder JJ, Meerding WJ, Bonneux L, van der Maas PJ. 2002. Healthcare costs of intellectual disability in the Netherlands: A cost-of-illness perspective. *Journal of Intellectual Disability Research* 46(2): 168–78.

Popovich ER, Wisniewski HM, Barcikowska M, et al. 1990. Alzheimer neuropathology in non-Down's syndrome mentally retarded adults. *Acta Neuropathologica* 80: 362–67.

Posey DJ, Guenin KD, Kohn AE, Swiezy NB, McDougle CJ. 2001. A naturalistic open-label study of mirtazapine in autistic and other pervasive developmental disabilities. *Journal of Child and Adolescent Psychopharmacology* 11: 267–77.

Prasher VP. 2004. Review of donepezil, rivastigmine, galantamine and memantine for the treatment of dementia in Alzheimer's disease in adults with Down syndrome: Implications for the intellectual disability population. *International Journal of Geriatric Psychiatry* 19(6): 509–15.

Prasher VP, Cumella S, Natarajan K, et al. 2003. Magnetic resonance imaging, Down's syndrome and Alzheimer's disease: Research and clinical implications. *Journal of Intellectual Disability Research* 47 (2): 90–100.

Prasher VP, Fung N, Adams C. 2005. Rivastigmine in the treatment of dementia in Alzheimer's disease in adults with Down syndrome. *International Journal of Geriatric Psychiatry* 20(5): 496–97.

Prasher VP, Huxley A, Haque MS, and the Down Syndrome Ageing Study group. 2002. A 24-week, double-blind, placebo-controlled trial of donepezil in patients with Down syndrome and Alzheimer's disease: Pilot study. *International Journal of Geriatric Psychiatry* 17(3): 270–78.

Prasher VP, Krishnan VHR. 1993. Age of onset and duration of dementia in people with Down syndrome: Integration of 98 reported cases in the literature. *International Journal of Geriatric Psychiatry* 8: 915–22.

Prasher VP, Krishnan VHR, Clarke DJ, Corbett JA, Blake A. 1994. Visual evoked potential in the diagnosis of dementia in people with Down syndrome. *International Journal of Geriatric Psychiatry* 9: 473–78.

Puri BK, Lekh SK, Langa A, Zaman R, Singh I. 1995. Mortality in a hospitalized mentally handicapped population: A 10-year survey. *Journal of Intellectual Disability Research* 39: 442–46.

Rabe A, Wisniewski KE, Schupf N, Wisniewski HM. 1990. Relationship of Down's syndrome to Alzheimer's disease. In SI Deutsch, A Weizman, R Weizman (eds.), *Application of Basic Neuroscience to Child Psychiatry*, 325–40. New York: Plenum Press.

Rabins PV, Lyketsos CG, Steele CD. 2006. *Practical Dementia Care*, 2nd ed. Oxford: Oxford University Press.

Raitasuo S, Taiminen T, Salokangas RKR. 1998. Functioning in activities of daily living of psychiatric inpatients with mental retardation. *Psychiatric Services* 49: 1084–85.

Ratey J, Sovner R, Parks A. 1991. Rogentine: Buspirone treatment of aggression and anxiety in mentally retarded patients: A multiple-baseline, placebo lead-in study. *Journal of Clinical Psychiatry* 52: 159–62.

Raz N, Gunning-Dixon FM, Head D, Dupius JH, Acker JD. 1998. Neuroanatomical correlates of cognitive aging: Evidence from structural magnetic resonance imaging. *Neuropsychiatry* 92: 95–114.

Raz N, Torres IJ, Briggs SD, et al. 1995. Selective neuroanatomic abnormalities in Down's syndrome and their cognitive correlates: Evidence from MRI morphometry. *Neurology* 45: 356–66.

Reiss S, Aman MG (eds.). 1998. *Psychotropic Medications and Developmental Disabilities: The International Consensus Handbook*. Columbus: Ohio State University Nisonger Center.

Reiss S, Levitan DW, Szysko J. 1982. Emotional disturbance and mental retardation: Diagnostic overshadowing. *American Journal of Mental Deficiency* 86: 567–74.

Ricketts RW, Goza AB, Ellis CR, et al. 1994. Clinical effects of buspirone on intractable self-injury in adults with mental retardation. *Journal of the American Academy of Child and Adolescent Psychiatry* 33: 270–76.

Rose D, Rose J. 2005. Staff in services for people with intellectual disabilities: the impact of stress on attributions of challenging behavior. Journal of Intellectual Disability Research 49: 827–38.

Roth GM, Sun B, Greensite FS, Lott IT, Dietrich RB. 1996. Premature aging in persons with Down syndrome: MR findings. *American Journal of Neuroradiology* 17: 1283–89.

Royal College of Psychiatrists. 2001. *Diagnostic Criteria for Psychiatric Disorders for Use with Adults with Learning Disabilities/Mental Retardation*. London: Gaskell Press.

Ruedrich SL. 1996. Beta adrenergic blocking medications for treatment of rage outbursts in mentally retarded persons. *Seminars in Clinical Neuropsychiatry* 1(2): 115–21

Ruedrich SL, Swales TP, Swales TP, et al. 1999. Effect of divalproex sodium on aggression and self-injurious behavior in adults with intellectual disabilities: A retrospective review. *Journal of Intellectual Disability Research* 43(2): 105–11.

Ryan R, Sunada K. 1997. Medical evaluation of persons with mental retardation referred for psychiatric assessment. *General Hospital Psychiatry* 19(4): 272–80.

Sabaawi M, Singh NN, de Leon J. 2006. Guidelines for the use of clozapine in individuals with developmental disabilities. *Research in Developmental Disabilities* 27: 309–36.

Schapiro MB, Haxby JV, Grady CL. 1992. The nature of mental retardation and dementia in Down syndrome: a study with PET, CT and neuropsychology. *Neurobiology of Aging* 13: 723–34.

Schultz J, Aman M, Kelbley T, et al. 2004. Evaluation of screening tools for dementia in older adults with mental retardation. *American Journal on Mental Retardation* 109 (2): 98–110.

Schupf N. 2002. Genetic and host factors for dementia in Down's syndrome. *British Journal of Psychiatry* 180: 405–10.

Schupf N, Kapell D, Nightingale B, et al. 1998. Earlier onset of Alzheimer's disease in men with Down syndrome. *Neurology* 50: 991–95.

Seltzer GB, Schupf N, Wu HS. 2001. A prospective study of menopause in women with Down syndrome. *Journal of Intellectual Disability Research* 45: 1–7.

Shavella R, Strauss D, Baumeister A, Aderson TW. 1999. Mortality in persons with developmental disabilities after transfer into community care: A 1996 update. *American Journal of Mental Retardation* 104(2): 143–47.

Silverman W, Zigman W, Kim H, Krinsky-McHale S, Wisniewski H. 1998. Aging and dementia among adults with mental retardation and Down syndrome. *Topics in Geriatric Rehabilitation* 13: 29–64.

Sovner R. 1986. Limiting factors in the use of DSM-III criteria with mentally ill / mentally retarded persons. *Psychopharmacology Bulletin* 22: 1055–59.

Sovner R. 1989. The use of valproate in the treatment of mentally retarded persons with typical and atypical bipolar disorders. *Journal of Clinical Psychiatry* 50(Suppl.): 40–43.

Sovner R, Hurley AD. 1982. Diagnosing depression in the mentally retarded. *Psychiatric Aspects of Mental Retardation* 1: 1–4.

Sovner R, Hurley AD. 1983. Do the mentally retarded suffer from affective illness? *Archives of General Psychiatry* 40: 61–67.

Sovner R, Hurley AD. 1986. Four factors affecting the diagnosis of psychiatric disorders in mentally retarded persons. *Psychiatric Aspects of Mental Retardation Reviews* 5(9): 45–49.

Sovner R, Hurley AD. 1987. Objective behavioral monitoring of psychotropic drug therapy. *Psychiatric Aspects of Mental Retardation Reviews* 6(10): 47–51.

Sovner R, Pary RJ. 1993. Affective disorders in developmentally disabled persons. In JL Matson, RP Barrett (eds.), *Psychopathology in the Mentally Retarded*, 87–147. New York: Grune & Stratton.

Sparrow SS, Balla DA, Cicchetti DV. 1984. Vineland Adaptive Behavior Scales. Circle Pines, MN: American Guidance Service.

Stanton LR, Coetzee RH. 2004. Down's syndrome and dementia. *Advances in Psychiatric Treatment* 10: 50–58.

Strauss D, Eyman RK. 1996. Mortality of people with mental retardation in California with and without Down syndrome, 1986–1991. *American Journal on Mental Retardation* 100: 643–53.

Sturmey P. 2995. DSM-III-R and people with dual diagnosis: Conceptual issues and strategies for future research. *Journal of Intellectual Disability Research* 39: 357–64.

Syzmanski LS, Madow L, Mallory G, et al. 1991. Task Force Report 30: Report of the Task Force on Psychiatric Services to Adult Mentally Retarded and Developmentally Disabled Persons. Washington, DC: American Psychiatric Association.

Troisi A, Vicario E, Nuccetelli F, Ciani N, Pasini A. 1995. Effects of fluoxetine on aggressive behavior of adult inpatients with mental retardation and epilepsy. *Pharmacopsychiatry* 28: 73–76.

Tsiouris JA. 2001. Diagnosis of depression in people with severe/profound intellectual disability. *Journal of Intellectual Disability Research* 45: 115–20.

Tyrer SP, Walsh A, Edwards DE, Berney TP, Stephens DA: 1984. Factors associated with good response to lithium in aggressive mentally handicapped students. *Progress in Neuropsychopharmacology and Biological Psychiatry* 8: 751–55.

Urv TK, Zigman WB, Silverman W. 2003. Maladaptive behaviors related to adaptive decline in aging adults with mental retardation. *American Journal on Mental Retardation* 108(5): 327–39.

Vanden Borre R, Vermote R, Buttiens M, et al. 1993. Risperidone as add-on therapy in behavioral disturbances in mental retardation: A double-blind placebo-controlled cross-over study. *Acta Psychiatrica Scandinavica* 87: 167–71.

Verhoeven WM, Curfs I.M, Tuinier S. 1998. Prader-Willi syndrome and cycloid psychoses. *Journal of Intellectual Disability Research* 42(6): 455–62.

Verhoeven WM, Veendrik-Meekes MJ, Jacobs GA, van den Berg YW, Tuinier S. 2001. Citalopram in mentally retarded patients with depression: A long-term clinical investigation. *European Psychiatry* 16(2): 104–8.

Visser FE, Aldenkamp AP, van Huffelen AC, et al. 1997. Prospective study of prevalence of Alzheimer-type dementia in institutionalized individuals with Down syndrome. *American Journal on Mental Retardation* 101: 400–412.

Wecshler D. 2003. Wecshler Intelligence Scale for Children, 4th ed. San Antonio, TX: Psychological Corporation.

Weis S, Weber G, Neuhold A, Rett A. 1991. Down syndrome: MR quantification of brain structures and comparison with normal control subjects. *American Journal of Neuroradiology* 12: 1207–11.

Whitaker S. 2004. Hidden learning disability. *British Journal of Learning Disability* 32: 139–43.

Whitaker S, Read S. 2006. The prevalence of psychiatric disorders among people with intellectual disabilities: An analysis of the literature. *Journal of Applied Research in Intellectual Disabilities* 19: 330–45.

Willemsen-Swinkels SHN, Buitelaar IK, Nijhof GJ, van England H. 1995. Failure of naltrexone hydrochloride to reduce self-injurious behavior and autistic behavior in mentally retarded adults: Double blind place controlled studies. *Archives of General Psychiatry* 52: 766–73.

Yang Q, Rasmussen SA, Friedman JM. 2002. Mortality associated with Down's syndrome in the USA from 1983 to 1997: A population-based study. *Lancet* 359 (9311): 1019–25.

Zarcone JR, Hellings JA, Crandall K, et al. 2001. Effects of risperidone on aberrant behavior of persons with developmental disabilities. Part I: A double-blind placebo-controlled crossover study using multiple measures. *American Journal of Mental Retardation* 106: 525–38.

Zigman WB, Lott IT. 2007. Alzheimer's disease in Down syndrome: Neurobiology and risk. *Mental Retardation and Developmental Disabilities Research Review* 13(3): 237–46.

Zigman, WB, Schupf N, Devenny DA, et al. 2004. Incidence and prevalence of dementia in elderly adults with mental retardation without Down syndrome. *American Journal on Mental Retardation* 109: 126–41.

Zigman WB, Schupf N, Haveman M, Silverman W. 1997. The epidemiology of Alzheimer disease in intellectual disability: Results and recommendations from an international conference. *Journal of Intellectual Disability Research* 41(1): 76–80.

Zigman WB, Schupf N, Jenkins EC, et al. 2007. Cholesterol level, statin use and Alzheimer's disease in adults with Down syndrome. *Neuroscience Letters* 416(3): 279–84

Zigman WB, Schupf N, Sersen E, Silverman W. 1996. Prevalence of dementia in adults with and without Down syndrome. *American Journal on Mental Retardation* 100: 403–12

Zigman WB, Silverman W, Wisniewski HM. 1996. Aging and Alzheimer disease in Down syndrome: Clinical and pathological changes. *Mental Retardation and Developmental Disabilities Research Reviews* 2: 73–79.

4

Autism Spectrum Disorders

Alison A. Golombek, M.D., Karen Toth, Ph.D., and Bryan King, M.D.

In 1943 Leo Kanner first described an unusual group of children who appeared congenitally to lack the interest or the ability to "relate themselves in the ordinary way to people and situations" (Kanner, 1973). Language was a struggle for them: they misused pronouns, were excessively literal, or at times were mute or limited to mimicry. Change was fraught with difficulties, as they demonstrated an intense desire and need for sameness, whether in their behavior or interests or in the sequence of words in a sentence or events in their day. Moreover, they struggled to see the forest for the trees, "to experience wholes without full attention to the constituent parts" (Kanner, 1973; Happé, 2005). Last, they reacted to physical sensations unusually, being either too little or too much affected, and often had peculiar interests in the physical world (Volkmar and Klin, 2005). While our conception of autism continues to embrace Kanner's original work, our knowledge of typical and atypical development has grown throughout the intervening years.

From the moment children are born, they are equipped to be part of our larger social world. Within minutes of birth, they can mimic basic human expressions (Meltzoff and Moore, 1977). Within weeks, they recognize their mother's voice, imitate her emotional expressions, and take turns exchanging sounds (Fernand, 1992; Tager-Flusbert, Paul, and Lord, 2005). They naturally look to the human face, especially to the eyes, responding with their own gaze, and within months recognize expressions of happiness, sadness, and surprise. Similarly, they instinctively orient themselves to the human voice and respond with their own coos (Lamb et al., 2002). They watch us constantly and gradually learn to imitate the way our faces look, the way we make sounds, and the way our bodies move. Within the first year, they learn to follow our gaze to see what we are seeing and, of equal importance, learn to catch our eyes to show us something of interest to them. Moreover, they look to us to define the meaning of events, for instance, to decide whether to be afraid or delighted when a flaming object approaches them on their first birthday and they are surrounded by many people and loud noise. As they begin to speak, they use this power of catching and sharing our attention to point to things they wish us to name and bring us things they wish to share (Mundy and Burnette, 2005). In the toddler years they begin to imagine, creating worlds populated by fairy princesses, magical animals, and sometimes monsters. At first pretend play is based on the events of their own lives: the princess gets up, brushes her teeth, gets dressed, and sets off to meet her friends. As children approach school age, however, they begin to imagine not only what other people do, but also what they feel, think, and believe. With this capacity a child understands why his friend is sad when his toy breaks, why the princess might be scared going to the dentist for the first time, or why her mother would be surprised and dismayed to find the cookie jar empty when it was full before she left it in the care of hungry kindergartners. With this powerful tool, the child not only comprehends that there are other minds in this world capable of having their own thoughts, beliefs, and feelings but also begins to use his own cognitive and emotional experience to understand and relate to others (Singer, 2002). At this point he has become fluent in the communication and behavior of the social world.

As complex as this process is, most children negotiate it with relative ease and no special training beyond thousands of hours of interacting with adults and peers. For some children, however, the process goes somehow awry. The infant is somewhat different. He may seem almost unnaturally content, a remarkably easy baby. Or he may be particularly difficult, irritated by the slightest sensation, and not soothed by his mother's touch. As he grows, he may seem less interested in human contact, less likely to look into his mother's eyes or to respond to her voice as she calls his name. His parents may be concerned that he is deaf. He may seem less interested in sharing experiences with others and less likely to catch or direct his parents' gaze or point to something new, although he may point to things he wants his parents to get for him or lead them by the hand to do so. Moreover, he may be drawn to unusual toys, perhaps collecting paperclips and lining them up in a row rather than playing with teddy bears or dolls. Language may also be delayed, at times so significantly that it is limited to mimicry of sounds, or it may appear to progress normally for a time. At some point, however, typically between the 6th and 36th month, the child's development slows or even regresses. At this point parents may become uneasy and bring the child in for assessment. For other children, difficulties may be more subtle initially and become apparent only with age. Parents may note that their child has few friends and does not share the interests of his peers. They wonder why he appears so advanced in language and so gifted in memory, yet lacks the common sense, especially in social situations, of a far younger child. They report that he acts out when his routine is disrupted or when novel situations occur. Last, they worry that he may be anxious or depressed. It is at this point that higher-functioning children may present for evaluation.

The goal of this chapter is to assist the psychiatrist in helping these children and their families. It presents our current understanding of autism spectrum disorders to provide a sound foundation for the psychiatrist, anticipate some of the difficulties associated with this condition, and help educate the families of individuals with autism. It also provides a framework in which to assess not only autism but also the specific difficulties associated with this disorder. Last, it provides guidance in the treatment of these difficulties.

Theory and Evidence

Our conception of autism reflects the impairments in social interaction and communication that isolate an individual from others and the cognitive inflexibility that Kanner first observed. However, our understanding of this disorder has advanced significantly through the development of specific cognitive theories supported by neuropsychological and biological evidence. While these findings have helped us understand the features common to autism spectrum disorders and may help us identify common pathways of pathogenesis, they have clarified that these disorders are heterogeneous in nature and, thus, neither a single cause nor a universal cure for autism is likely.

Numerous theories have been advanced to explain the deficits associated with autism spectrum disorder. Two key theories, the theory of mind, or *mentalizing,* and the theory of weak central coherence, have been especially helpful in explaining the social and cognitive deficits that people with autism struggle with, respectively. The theory of mind recognizes that we develop the understanding that each person has individual thoughts, beliefs, and desires and that these beliefs affect behavior. Neuropsychological experiments using tests of false belief or of deception have revealed that children typically develop this capacity at about 5 years of age or, if development is delayed, about the mental age of 5 (Frith, 2003). Thus, while the preschooler believes his mother automatically knows what naughty thing he did at daycare, the elementary school child recognizes that his experience is not shared by her and that his mother will not find out about it unless he or someone else tells her. In contrast, individuals with autism develop this ability much later or not at all (Frith, 2003). This finding is significant, as this capacity to conceive of other minds allows us to imagine what someone might feel in a certain situation, empathize, and predict what he might do. Without this capacity, the person with autism cannot easily appreciate the emotions of others or understand their behaviors. Such a deficit could account for a person's lack of insight into his or her own emotional states and the actions or reactions that may ensue from them.

In addition to numerous neuropsychological studies, functional neuroimaging is revealing the social brain circuits involved in the process of mentalizing. These circuits include areas within the medial prefrontal cortex that are activated when we think about our internal thoughts and feelings or when others call our name or look at us. They also include areas within the posterior superior temporal sulcus that become active when we observe the movements of others, especially the movements of hands, eyes, and mouth. The temporal pole near the amygdala is also involved in identifying the emotional states of others, especially fear and sadness. Some studies suggest that there are abnormalities in the mentalizing areas of the brain of individuals with autism, including decreased gray matter density in the medial prefrontal cortex and increased density in the amygdaloid area (Frith, 2003).

People with autism also often show impairments in other skills necessary to interact with others, including joint attention, which is the capacity to coordinate another's attention with one's own. In typically developing children, it begins between 6 and 18 months with a child following the mother's gaze. Subsequently, the child begins to point and then bring objects to a parent's attention. The goal of these actions is important. For instance, pointing may signify that the child wants the parent to bring an object to him. It may signify that the child wants the parent to name an object, a critical step in early language development. Alternatively, it may represent the child's desire to share and be social. In contrast to typically developing children, children with autism show significant impairments in joint attention. While they may point to an object they wish a parent to obtain or even take the parent by the hand to the object, they rarely initiate joint attention either with their gaze or with gestures simply for the purpose of sharing. The consequences of this impairment are profound and have been associated with decreased language learning and impaired development of social and cognitive systems. Moreover, these limitations may subsequently alter and limit the child's experiences of the world during critical periods of language and social learning. This difficulty, in turn, may compound the child's isolation and amplify autistic impairments (Mundy and Burnette, 2005).

It is unclear what process undermines this critical capacity of joint attention. Areas of the brain that have been implicated include the dorsal medial aspects of the frontal cortex, which may help regulate visual attention, and the anterior cingulate, which is part of the limbic system and involved in emotions. While our understanding of the role of the anterior cingulated cortex in autism is still imprecise, we do know that impairments in these circuits cause symptoms of lability, apathy, inattention, mutism, and variability in pain sensitivity in illnesses and injuries not related to autism (Busch et al., 2000). Additionally, individuals with autism differ in other areas involved in socialization. For instance, research reveals that persons with autism show a lack of attention to social stimuli but not to nonsocial stimuli such as things (Frith, 2003). They appear less interested in human sounds than in nonhuman sounds (Kuhl et al., 2004) and may show decreased activation in the superior temporal sulcus when listening to vocal sounds rather than nonvocal sounds when compared with typically developing children (Gervais, 2004). They are also less likely to respond to their name, a finding that has strong prognostic value in predicting autism in very young children (Osterling and Dawson, 1994; Werner et al., 2000). Last, individuals with autism show abnormalities in processing faces and facial emotions, capacities that have been associated with an area in the fusiform gyrus (Schultz and Robins, 2005).

While a central defect in neural processing that would explain these various deficits remains the focus of future research, the recent discovery of the function of the mirror neuron system may provide a common pathway for many of the social, communication, and motor deficits seen in autism. The mirror neuron system may allow us to identify with others and develop the skills of reciprocal social interaction, including joint attention, language, and emotion recognition, necessary for empathy and mentalization (J. H. G. Williams et al., 2001).

Even though these findings help us understand the social and communication deficits of autism, they do not explain the cognitive differences. Persons with autism appear to form concepts differently. Their cognitive style focuses on a multitude of concrete details and experiences to form general concepts. Multiple studies demonstrate that children with autism often have greater talents in the recognition of details than do typically developing children. For instance, children with autism, who are often gifted with puzzles, outperform typically developing children when the puzzle lacks a picture. Similarly, children with autism are better at identifying hidden features on embedded feature tests and at block designs that require them to identify smaller shapes within a larger one. They may also display remarkable talent in memory (Frith, 2003). Despite these skills, persons with autism often have difficulty understanding broader concepts or using these concepts to generalize from one situation to another without merely memorizing a rule (Frith, 2003). The theory of weak central coherence offers an explanation for these findings. This theory suggests that there is a continuum between the cognitive style generally seen in individuals with autism, which focuses on details or parts, and the cognitive style seen in typically developing individuals, which focuses on integrating information in the context of a broader and more meaningful concept. This theory helps us understand Kanner's original observation that children with autism struggle to see the forest for the trees (Frith and Hill, 2003).

This concept of central coherence may also be related to the deficits in executive functioning and the peculiarities of attention often found in individuals with autism. It has long been observed that children with autism have difficulties with cognitive flexibility. While they may attend at great length to a particular activity or a particular stimulus, people with autism often struggle to shift their focus or adapt to new events or schedules. These deficits are often categorized as impairments of executive function, include the ability to plan, adapt, and inhibit impulses, and are believed to be under frontal lobe control. Clinical experience and numerous psychological tests demonstrate that children with autism have more difficulty with these abilities (Ozonoff, South, and Provencal, 2005), which may dramatically affect their functioning.

Research strongly suggests that autism is not a static disorder determined at birth. Rather, it is a developmental process that may begin with differences in brain architecture and function or develop secondary to impaired neurodevelopmental processes early in childhood. These changes in brain function alter a child's subsequent interactions, which, in turn, may alter the developing brain. For instance, impairments in joint attention and social orienting may lead to impairments in recognizing and reproducing the movements of other human beings, which, in turn, further isolate the child from human language, emotion, and society (Mundy and Burnette, 2005). In this context of decreased social input, a child's developing brain may be further altered and a child's focus perhaps turned inward. As the child passes by the neurodevelopmental windows that allow for the most efficient learning of various skills, such as language, the trajectory away from human interaction increases. In contrast, intense and early intervention targeted at these fundamental deficits may alter the course of a child's development and, thus, the course of his autism (Dawson et al., 2004).

While these theories and findings help us understand the mind, brain, and experience of the individual with autism, more research is required to understand the fundamental causes of autism, particularly as there are concerns that the prevalence of autism has increased over the past 15 to 20 years to a current prevalence of 10 in 10,000 to 16 in 10,000. Including the broader phenotype (for example, cases that do not meet all of the diagnostic criteria but could be viewed as atypical autism or pervasive developmental disorder, not otherwise specified), estimates approach 60 in 10,000. Whether the prevalence of autism is increasing is controversial, as epidemiological studies have been complicated by changes in the definition of autism, inclusion of broader phenotypes from which most of the increase appears to arise, access to diagnosis, and cultural considerations (Fombonne, 2005). Regardless of whether the increase is real or due to better surveillance, autism is more common than previously believed.

The search for the causes of autism is also complicated by the fact that autism is a disorder defined not by etiology but rather by phenomenology. Moreover, while we are able to identify the core features of autism, we lack an understanding of specific endophenotypes that characterize distinct autistic populations. For instance, approximately 20 percent of children with autism develop macrocephaly. Studies suggest that increased brain volume associated with this abnormality is caused by an early acceleration of brain growth, typically not present at birth, that may plateau in the later years (Minshew et al., 2005). Yet not all children with autism fit this pattern. Similarly, children with autism may have different developmental trajectories. For instance, approximately 25 percent of children ultimately diagnosed with this disorder develop normally until sometime in the second year, when a regression in social and language skills occurs. For others, the lack of appropriate development occurs far earlier (Dawson, 2007). Similarly, epilepsy, intellectual disability, the lack of speech, or known associated medical comorbidities may represent alternative pathways to this disorder. Further clarification of possible endophenotypes may explain differences in neuroanatomical studies in autism.

There is a strong genetic component in autism. Twin studies suggest a concordance in monozygotic twins ranging from 37 percent, if autism is narrowly defined, to 90 percent, if a broader phenotype is considered. Additionally, investigations using the broader phenotype reveal a concordance of approximately 10 percent in dizygotic twins (Frith and Hill, 2003). Other studies have found a monozygotic concordance rate as high as 60 percent and a dizygotic concordance rate of 10 percent, representing a heritability rate of more than 90 percent (Yang and Gill, 2007). Moreover, evidence suggests that the broader phenotype may be present in 10 to 20 percent of first-degree relatives (Yang and Gill, 2007). These results indicate that although there is a significant genetic component to autism, it is associated with the interaction of multiple genes rather than a single one. At least five to 20 genes have been suggested, although the number may be far greater (Yang and Gill, 2007). Chromosomes 2, 7, 16, and 17 have been consistently implicated (Frith and Hill, 2003). Other genetic abnormalities associated with autism are those that cause fragile X syndrome, tuberous sclerosis, neurofibromatosis type I, Cowden and other hamartoma syndromes, Smith-Magenis syndrome, and Angelman and Prader-Willi syndromes (Zafeiriou, Ververi, and Vargiami, 2007). Duplications of a small region of chromosome 15 are associated with autism and may increase the risk for sudden death. Because of this and other known physical problems associated with certain genetic etiologies, the imperative to pursue appropriate genetic testing in the autism workup is being articulated. Last, in contrast to autism associated with multiple genetic hits, evidence demonstrates that Rett disorder is caused by a single mutation of the *MECP2* gene that affects approximately 1 in 10,000 girls. This mutation causes a progressive lost of skills, including speech and social skills, after a period of normal development generally lasting until the 6th to the 18th month. Children with this mutation also develop microcephaly, seizures, ataxia, loss of purposeful hand use, and intermittent hyperventilation (Rutter, 2005).

Additional attention has been directed to the role of neurotransmitters and other substances in the etiopathogenesis of autism. These agents of interest include serotonin, dopamine, norepinephrine, acetylcholine, glutamate, gaba-aminobutyric acid, and cortisol, thyroid hormones, sex hormones, opioid peptides (such as endorphins and enkephalins), amino acids, and purine pathway products (including uric acid). With the exception of known metabolic syndromes, no clear relationship has been established (Anderson and Hosino, 2005). Metabolic syndromes associated with autism include phenylketonuria, a treatable amino acid disorder, and Smith-Lemli Opitz syndrome, characterized by impairments in cholesterol metabolism (Zafeiriou, Ververi, and Vargiami, 2007). Mitochondrial abnormalities have also been increasingly recognized and may be present in as many as 7 percent of individuals with autism (King and Bostic, 2006). Maternal illness, specifically first-trimester exposure to rubella, has also been associated with autism (Chess, 1977). However, meta-analysis has revealed no evidence to support a causal role in autism for measles, mumps, and rubella vaccination (Demicheli et al., 2007). Last, autism spectrum disorders have also been associated with fetal anticonvulsant syndromes among other prenatal toxins (Moore et al., 2000). It is important to note that meta-analysis has also revealed no evidence to support a causal role for mercury levels (Hussain et al., 2007). Research is ongoing in these areas as well as in areas of autoimmune dysfunction, allergies, and inflammatory processes.

Evaluation

An individual ultimately diagnosed with an autism spectrum disorder may present with a vast array of symptoms ranging from subtle dysfunction to severe impairment. While a comprehensive evaluation is recommended, the heterogeneity of this disorder and those affected by it requires that both evaluation and treatment be individualized and guided by function. Moreover, each person must be understood as an individual with strengths and vulnerabilities who exists within the context of a family with its own level of adaptive coping skills and within the broader systems of school and society. Neither evaluation nor treatment can proceed without this understanding. The following three case studies illustrate some of the challenges individuals with autism face that must be considered in an evaluation.

CASE EXAMPLES

Charlie is a 10-year-old child diagnosed with autism who now presents to a clinic for concerns of extreme behavior. His parents are worried that he continues to bang his head so frequently and so hard that a helmet is required for safety. Charlie lives with his mother, father, and 7-year-old brother, David, who has also been diagnosed with autism. His mother states that Charlie was not exposed to prenatal drugs or alcohol or to maternal illness. She reports that Charlie's delivery was without complications, but that he was a fussy baby and picking him up or singing to him appeared to make him more upset. She does not remember his making much eye contact with her or with others and recalls that he seemed happiest when alone in his crib watching his mobile. She became concerned around his first birthday when she realized Charlie was not progressing like other children. He appeared less coordinated, fell more often, did not walk until 18 months, and had difficulty using crayons. She reports that he never learned to talk, although he makes sounds, at times repeating the same syllable over and over. These limitations have not changed over the years. Although his mother continues to speak to him, she does not know how much he understands. She admits that she and her husband are often overwhelmed because they don't know what Charlie wants. She states that Charlie will lead her by the hand to something that he wants and will flap his hands when he seems excited, but otherwise does not communicate. She reports that Charlie is calmest when he can play with the wheels on his cars.

Tantrums often occur during which Charlie screams and bangs his hand against his head or his head against a wall. His head-banging is worse when they take him shopping or to visit relatives. He also has tantrums when he has to change what he is doing or when he can't have something he wants. She admits that sometimes Charlie hits others, especially when they try to touch him. She also reports that Charlie screams, arches his neck, or twists his head several times during the day, but it is unclear why this occurs. He also picks his skin sometimes. Charlie continues to function at the level of a much younger child and is not toilet trained.

Charlie was diagnosed with grand mal seizures that started when he was in preschool. He therefore takes antiseizure medication. His mother believes he is no longer experiencing seizures. His head-banging caused frequent and extensive bruising before he started wearing a helmet. His skin picking continues to cause frequent localized skin infections, which are treated with topical antibiotics. She states that there are no other medical concerns but admits that her son has had no dental exams and only limited physical exams because of tantrums. She cannot recall when he had a vision or hearing test. When asked about her family's medical history, she revealed that Charlie's uncle was diagnosed with mental retardation and lives in a group home. Charlie's brother was also diagnosed with autism and mental retardation, although he can speak and function better than Charlie does.

The first diagnosis of autism and developmental delays came when Charlie was 4 years old. Although he received speech therapy early in his life, he no longer is doing so owing to a failure to progress over several years. Charlie is now in a classroom for children with severe behavioral problems but does not seem to be progressing in skills. ▶

Noah is a 13-year-old boy who initially presented to the emergency room because he told his mother that he would rather be dead. He lives with his mother, father, and 11-year-old brother. Noah's mother states that there were no concerns with her pregnancy or with Noah's delivery. He achieved milestones on time, although his language was slightly delayed at first, with few words until the age of 2, but he then progressed rapidly, teaching himself to read by the age of 4. He has always done well academically, and recent testing performed by a school psychologist reveals that he is academically performing above the 90th percentile in all his subjects. However, earlier testing with a psychologist unfamiliar with Noah, who did not allow him breaks, reported significant delays.

Although Noah does well intellectually, he struggles socially and emotionally. His mother states that Noah was always an affectionate child within the family and still hugs his parents in public even at his current age. She reports Noah is outgoing, often seeking people out to tell them about his interests, which have included trains and sports scores. While he is knowledgeable about these subjects, Noah often does not realize that other people are not as interested in them as he is and has difficulty interpreting their behavior. Noah has always been awkward with people, especially with those his own age, and has not been able to keep friends.

His mother is worried that Noah may be depressed. In a separate interview, Noah states that he often is unhappy and feels guilty over many things, including not finishing his homework, but also over little things, such as not knowing how to use a new vacuum cleaner. He reports that he has always been teased and doesn't understand why. While he consistently stated he would never kill himself, he admits he bangs his head against the wall sometimes when he is unhappy. He does not think things will change much for him in the future. He states that recently he has not been sleeping well and often worries about things like school, what would happen if his parents got sick, global warming, and the plight of homeless people.

Noah's mother also reports that her son has always had trouble in school, where, until recently, he was mainstreamed with no additional support. When he was younger, he often had tantrums, especially during transitions. His teachers learned to prepare him for transitions, and he, in turn, became more accustomed to the routine. They also allowed him to skip music class, which was a challenge, and let him play with trains, which he enjoyed. Last, they reported that the school's well-established buddy system helped include Noah in peer activities. However, Noah began to have more difficulties when he advanced to middle school. He had problems moving from one class to another and often lost homework assignments. His grades suffered and he became more emotional, at times crying in class. He was also teased by other children. His increasing distress and difficulty learning prompted his family to move him from the classroom to an Internet-based curriculum. While his mother observes that he is no longer teased, she also reports he is more reluctant to engage in social pursuits or play with peers his own age. He continues to have difficulty organizing homework and doing assignments on time. She admits that she struggles to keep him on task.

Noah's mother did not cite any medical concerns. Her son has always been healthy and enjoys going to the doctor and dentist because he is fascinated by the technical equipment in the examining rooms. She reports that the family has a psychiatric history of some anxiety and depression but no serious mental health issues. She states that Noah's father and uncles are somewhat awkward socially but are all talented engineers or computer scientists. ▶

Eric is a 24-year-old man who was brought to a psychiatric emergency room by the police. They were called by Eric's neighbor, who reported that Eric wanted to have sex with her 13-year-old daughter. In the course of the investigation, the police also became concerned when Eric admitted that he had thoughts of hurting people.

Eric lives with his mother and younger brother. His mother stated that her son had never been sexually inappropriate or violent with anyone. She reported that he did well in special education and in a job-transitioning program. However, after this program ended, Eric was able to get only a part-time job bagging groceries. He stays at home the rest of the time, helping out with family chores, such as gardening, or reading alone. She admitted that she wanted more for her son when he was younger but now thinks that nothing can be done for him.

When interviewed alone, Eric admitted that he thought about sex when he saw his 13-year-old neighbor sunbathing in her backyard. His neighbor saw him outside and asked what he was doing. He told her that he was thinking about sex. Eric confessed that he has been thinking about sex a lot lately, which makes him feel ashamed and guilty. However, he can't stop thinking about sex and has started rubbing himself. He began to cry when discussing this. He denied talking to anyone about his feelings or his behavior. However, when asked explicit questions about whether he would act on his thoughts, he appeared shocked. He stated that he knows that thoughts are different from actions and that he would never hurt anyone or even touch them. His school taught him never to touch people without asking and also taught him about not touching "private places."

Eric also admitted that he told the police he had been thinking about killing people when they asked him. However, he denied that he would ever hurt anyone because he knew hurting people is wrong. He admitted that he had been reading a book about mass murderers and could not stop thinking about the topic, although his thoughts made him upset. He admitted that he often has thoughts that occur over and over in his mind and that he cannot stop no matter how much he wants to. However, he denied acting on his thoughts and repeated that he knew the difference between right and wrong. Last, Eric admitted, that since school ended, he has had no friends.

He reported that he stays at home a lot and reads books. He would like to have friends. ▶

Diagnosis of Autism

The most comprehensive and reliable method of diagnosing autism is evaluation by a multidisciplinary team, which may include physicians, psychologists, speech and language pathologists, and occupational and physical therapists, among others (Ozonoff, Goodlin-Jones, and Solomon, 2005; Filipek et al.,1999). This type of evaluation, often conducted within a research setting or through specialty clinics, typically reflects multiple sources of information, including parents, teachers, and other professionals. It may draw heavily from diagnostic tools such as the Autism Diagnostic Interview—Revised (ADI-R; Lord et al., 1994), a semistructured parent interview, and the Autism Diagnostic Observation Scale (ADOS; Lord et al., 1989; Lord, 1997), a semistructured direct observation measure. While these tools help guide diagnosis, they are not intended to be used by themselves to make a diagnosis. Tools such as the ADI-R and the ADOS can provide the clinician with necessary information to apply criteria from the revised fourth edition of the *Diagnostic and Statistical Manual of Mental Disorders* (DSM-IV-TR; American Psychiatric Association, 2000). However, even without the benefit of such tools, the DSM-IV-TR criteria can help the practitioner identify areas of concern that affect function. It is important to note that the diagnosis of autism may be more difficult to make if a child is younger than 3 years old. The Modified Checklist for Autism in Toddlers (Robins and Dumont-Mathieu, 2006) may be of particular use in these cases to identify those children who should go on to have a more comprehensive evaluation for autism (Coonrod and Stone, 2005). As early diagnosis and treatment are critical for optimal outcomes and may alter the course of autism, referral to a specialty clinic when concerns first arise is always appropriate. Similarly, assessing autism in someone with mental retardation or severe speech and language disorders may be especially challenging and more appropriate for a multidisciplinary team.

The diagnosis in adults may also be challenging. Reference to the fourth module of the ADOS may be especially helpful in providing age-appropriate diagnostic questions. The Social Communication Questionnaire (Eaves et al., 2006) may similarly be of use. This instrument is a parent-report questionnaire derived from the ADI-R and is available in two forms, one of which evaluates a child's lifetime symptoms and the other targets a child's current symptoms. Thus, this tool may be used not only for diagnosis and screening but also to assess progress or change over time (Ozonoff, Goodlin-Jones, and Solomon, 2005). Last, the Diagnostic Interview for Social and Communication Disorders (DISCO; Wing et al., 2002) may be useful in clinical settings and in caring for adult patients. While the DISCO was not designed to diagnose autism, it is a tool to evaluate development and function, provide recommendations for treatment of adults with autism, and help track improvement (Lord and Corsello, 2005).

DSM-IV-TR criteria focus on the three domains that define the presentation of autism: impairments in reciprocal social interaction, impairments in communication, and restricted repetitive and stereotyped patterns of behavior. For a diagnosis of autistic disorder, at least six total symptoms must be present, of which least two symptoms must be present within the domain of social interaction and at least one of which must be present in each of the domains of communication and behavior. The onset of delay or dysfunction in social interaction, language as used in social communication, or symbolic or imaginative play must occur before age 3. DSM-IV-TR also requires that the presentation is not better accounted for by Rett disorder or childhood disintegrative disorder. The latter is exceedingly rare. Qualitative impairments in social interaction may be manifested by impairment in the use of non-verbal gestures such as eye gaze, facial expression, body posture, and other gestures; failure to develop peer relations appropriate to the child's developmental level; a lack of spontaneous seeking to share enjoyment, interests, or achievements (for instance, by pointing out, showing, or bringing objects to another's attention); or a lack of social or emotional reciprocity. Qualitative impairments in communication may present as a lack of language or delays in spoken language acquisition without compensation by other modes of communication; marked impairment in the ability to initiate or sustain conversation in those with language; stereotyped repetitive or idiosyncratic language; or a lack of imaginary play or imitative play appropriate to the child's developmental level. Characteristic abnormalities in behavior are manifested by encompassing preoccupations with restricted patterns of interest that are abnormal in intensity or focus; inflexible adherence to nonfunctional routines or rituals; stereotyped and repetitive motor mannerisms such as hand flapping, finger flicking or twisting, or complex whole body movements; or a persistent preoccupation with parts of objects (American Psychiatric Association, 2000).

Although research has not been able to clearly differentiate Asperger disorder from autism without intellectual disability (Ozonoff and Griffith, 2000), the DSM-IV-TR allows the diagnosis of Asperger disorder when an individual presents with no significant delay in language but has a qualitative impairment in social functioning and restricted and repetitive patterns of behavior, interests, and activities that significantly impair function. Additionally, individuals with this diagnosis must have average or above average cognitive ability and not meet the criteria for another pervasive developmental disorder.

In contrast, Rett disorder and childhood disintegrative disorder require a period of normal development before the loss of skills. Rett disorder is characterized by apparently normal prenatal, perinatal, and postnatal development through the first 5 months of life with a normal head circumference at birth that then decelerates in growth rate between 5 and 48 months and is accompanied by the loss of previously acquired purposeful hand skills between the ages of 5 and 30 months and the subsequent development of abnormal and stereotyped movements. Children with this disorder also present with impairments in gait or trunk movement, psychomotor retardation, and limited receptive and expressive language. Childhood disintegrative disorder requires normal development for a longer period of time, specifically through the age of 2, followed by a loss of previously acquired skills before the age of 10. These include motor skills, bowel and bladder control, receptive and expressive language skills, social skills and adaptive behavior, and play. The child with this disorder must also have impairments in the core autistic domains of social interaction, communication, and restricted repetitive behavior (American Psychiatric Association, 2000). Suspicion of either of these disorders warrants a full medical workup including neurological assessment and genetic evaluation.

While the diagnosis of autism may help explain someone's struggles, the diagnosis is just a starting point. A clear understanding of the individual's strengths and weaknesses, particularly in those domains associated with autism, is necessary. An assessment of these domains is essential in guiding treatment, not only to target deficits specific to autism, but for the difficulties in function, behavior, and mood that are often associated with the disorder. These domains include those of communication and socialization, cognitive ability including intellectual and executive functions, academic and adaptive functions, motor deficits and sensory-based behaviors, and emotional and behavioral functioning. Assessing pertinent medical and psychiatric concerns is also required. Last, it is important to realize that individuals with autism function within the context of their own development, their families, and the larger social world, all of which must be taken into account to provide effective treatments.

Communication and Socialization

Understanding an individual's capacity for communication and socialization is essential not only in the diagnosis and treatment of autism but in the evaluation and treatment of multiple problems associated with it. Not unexpectedly, impairments in communication often underlie anxiety, frustration, tantrums, aggression, and self-injurious behavior. Impairments in socialization also lead to further isolation and increased severity of autistic characteristics.

Like Charlie in the above case study, a person who cannot tell us about his pain, desires, frustrations, or fears may act out or become aggressive. Moreover, an individual isolated from the world may turn inward for stimulation and meaning. For the approximately 30 to 40 percent of individuals with autism who are mute or severely limited in verbal communication, speech and language testing is essential (Paul, 2005). Only through this type of assessment can alternative or augmentative forms of communication be developed. Often drawing on relatively preserved or even enhanced skills of visual perception, these strategies include systems such as the Picture Exchange Communication System (Frost and Bondy, 1994). Paired with a visual schedule, this approach may enable the severely impaired person to communicate his needs to others and understand what is expected of him for the first time in his life.

Individuals with less severe impairments, such as Noah, may still have deficits in receptive language or auditory processing skills that cause them to be overwhelmed and frustrated by more complex verbal statements. They may misunderstand language that is not literal and concrete and fail to notice or adequately interpret nonverbal communication such as gestures. As a result, they may shut down or become frustrated or angry. In these cases, they may be perceived as stubborn or defiant when, in fact, they simply do not understand what is expected of them. Additionally, individuals with intact receptive language may also struggle with complex verbal statements owing to deficits in verbal processing. As with Eric, they may fail to understand the intent of a question or interaction. While Eric appeared to understand the policeman's questions, his concrete and painfully honest responses revealed his misunderstanding of the situation.

Even generally high-functioning children like Noah suffer from rejection and teasing because they do not understand the subtle pragmatics of communication, especially in social situations. For instance, they may not coordinate eye contact and facial expressions with speech and their speech may be abnormal in prosody and terse or pedantic in word choice. They may also demonstrate stereotyped or repetitive language. Moreover, they struggle to understand the reciprocal nature of social interaction. While they may want to make friends, they have difficulties making social overtures that are not limited to their own particular interests and do not grasp the need for—nor do they find reinforcing—reciprocal conversation and sharing. Last, their understanding of emotions and social relationships are often limited and characteristic of children of far younger ages.

In all of these cases, a speech and language evaluation is necessary to assess a child's receptive, expressive, pragmatic, or social language skills. Additional information may be provided by the social and communication domains of the Vineland Adaptive Behavior Scales (Sparrow, Balla, and Cicchetti, 1984), which have supplementary norms developed specifically for individuals with autism (Carter et al., 1998). This type of comprehensive speech and language evaluation can teach us how to best to communicate with an individual and how best to help him communicate with us. In doing so, this type of intervention may significantly reduce the profound frustration and isolation experienced by some children and adults with autism.

Cognitive Function

Of equal importance is an understanding of intellectual, executive, academic, and adaptive functions. In each of these areas, the person with autism has strengths that serve as the foundation of treatment and weaknesses that must be addressed. If adequately targeted in treatment, an individual with autism may make significant progress in each of these domains. As cognitive ability is one of the strongest predictors of prognosis, effort must be made to facilitate progress in this area. Moreover, cognitive testing may reveal a degree of delay or disability that will allow an individual access to additional supports or services. This is especially critical in the adult years. Last, evaluation of cognitive function is necessary as social and communicative deficits are also present in individuals with intellectual disability. The diagnosis of autism requires that social and communicative deficits exceed those that would be expected in an individual with impaired cognitive function (Klin et al., 2005).

Impaired intellectual function is linked with increased limitations and dependence and has long been associated with autism. Historically, the prevalence of intellectual disability or mental retardation has been estimated between 70 and 80 percent in people with the disorder (Fombonne, 1999). However, studies suggest that the current prevalence is much lower. It is possible that our use of a broader diagnostic phenotype has affected these estimates. However, it is also believed that this change reflects progress due to early intervention and special education (Shea and Mesibov, 2005). In fact, while intelligence scores are generally more stable and predictive the older a person is, scores may improve with both development and intervention (Ozonoff, Goodlin-Jones, and Solomon, 2005).

In assessing intellectual function in an individual with autism, it is important to choose the appropriate measure and attempt to assess his best performance in multiple domains including verbal and performance intelligence, working memory, and processing speed. While individuals with autism may demonstrate higher performance scores than verbal scores, this split often depends on the severity of autism and is not present in the majority of those with this diagnosis (Ozonoff, Goodlin-Jones, and Solomon 2005). Measures that have been helpful in assessing intellectual function in children with autism include the Wechsler scales (Wechsler Intelligence Scale for Children—Fourth Edition; Wecshler, 2003; Wechsler Preschool and Primary Scale of Intelligence—Third Edition; Wecshler, 2002) if a child has adequate verbal skills, the Differential Abilities Scale (Elliot, 1990) or the Kaufman-Assessment Battery for Children (Kaufman and Kaufman, 2004) for those with impaired verbal skills, and the Leiter International Performance Scale-Revised (Roid and Miller, 1997) for individuals with low or no language skill from ages 2 years to 20 years, 11 months (Klin et al., 2005).

Executive Function

The assessment of executive functioning is critical, as these skills are important to school or vocational success and affect both treatment response and prognosis (Ozonoff, Goodlin-Jones, and Solomon 2005). Executive functions are the operations that direct and organize behavior and include the skills of planning, organization, attention, cognitive flexibility, and impulse inhibition. They also affect the ability to organize and sequence thoughts and language. Measures that assess executive function include the Wisconsin Card Sorting Test (Heaton et al., 2000), which is available in both an examiner-administered and a computer version. The Behavioral Rating Inventory of Executive Function (Gioia et al., 1993), a parent or teacher questionnaire, may also assist in understanding the impact a child's deficits in executive functions have on his daily life.

Individuals with autism often have impairments in executive function. They may succeed at simple, one-step tasks, but then become overwhelmed by more complex, multistep tasks. It is critical to understand that tasks that appear simple, such as setting the table, getting dressed, cleaning one's room, completing one's homework, or writing a book report, are actually composed of multiple steps that must occur in specific sequences. To aid the person with autism these tasks must be broken down into discrete steps, and teaching strategies that build on the individual's strengths in visual processing and memory should be used to help the individual better organize and manage his or her approach.

As the cause of much anxiety and frustration in the person with autism, limitations in executive functions are often at the root of many maladaptive behaviors. Addressing these deficits may result in better behavioral control and increased ability to learn new skills and concepts for all people with autism. In Charlie's case, deficits in executive function compound his limitations in language. Tantrums or self-injurious behavior may be one of the few coping skills he has learned to deal with the anxiety and frustration of an incomprehensible and unpredictable world. While Noah is higher functioning than Charlie, his limitations in organization, attention, cognitive flexibility, and inhibitory control make him more likely to be overwhelmed by new situations and task demands. He struggles to adapt to the demands of middle school that require a child to organize himself and his work and seamlessly transition from one situation to the next. In this circumstance, he may easily miss or not understand important instructions or information and fall behind in his work.

Attention

People with autism often have problems both with sustained attention and with selectively attending to specific input while ignoring other stimuli and switching attention from one mode of information to another. Thus, focusing on schoolwork while sitting in a noisy room or switching attention from verbal instructions to the written word may be especially challenging. Similarly, the adult who competently learned a task in a calm environment may struggle when asked to perform it on a noisy factory floor or in a grocery store where he is constantly interrupted. Moreover, as Kanner originally noted, individuals with autism tend to overfocus on specific details but miss the larger meaning. These deficits make it harder for an individual with autism to stay on task and make it more likely that he or she will be overwhelmed, particularly in environments with a lot of stimulation or on tasks that require multiple inputs. People with autism may also lack significant cognitive flexibility that enables them to generate more than one problem-solving strategy or generalize information from one arena to another. This deficit is often apparent in the response to transitions or to novel situations. Someone who relies on a well-established routine or a single coping skill will flounder when something new occurs or when something different is required. Those who live with autism may struggle with impulse inhibition and act without necessary reflection. In this situation, an individual may engage in maladaptive behavior not with intent, but simply because it was his first or only response.

Academic Function

Individuals with autism may struggle in specific academic domains but may excel and even demonstrate astonishing abilities in others. They may possess good memory and precocious reading skills but struggle with reading comprehension. Additionally, some individuals with autism demonstrate impairments in psychomotor coordination, visuospatial organization, nonverbal problem solving, and mathematics. These deficits are sometimes characterized as a nonverbal learning disorder and indicate the need for additional educational services (Ozonoff, Goodlin-Jones, and Solomon, 2005). Instruments that have proven useful in assessing both the academic strengths and weakness of children with autism include the Woodcock-Johnson Test of Achievement—Third Edition (Mather and Schrank, 2003).

Adaptive Function

As individuals with autism often show profound deficits in daily functioning, a measure of adaptive skills in the areas of communication, daily living, socialization, and motor skills is strongly recommended. The most commonly used scale to assess adaptive functioning is the Vineland Adaptive Behavior

Scales, which provides normative scales for individuals with autism (Sparrow, Balla, and Cicchetti, 1984; Carter et al., 1998). This measure can be especially helpful in designing individual education programs and treatment goals that identify the steps to greater independence. Adaptive measures also play a pivotal role in obtaining services, especially when an individual's cognitive measures do not fully demonstrate the degree of functional impairment (Klin et al., 2005). Adaptive measures should be used to assess both functional strengths and weaknesses, to develop meaningful treatment goals, including greater independence, and to monitor progress toward those goals.

Sensory and Motor Function

It is estimated that 42 to 88 percent of children with autism have unusual responses to sensations (Baranek, Parham, and Bodfish, 2005). The Sensory Experiences Questionnaire (Baranek et al., 2006) or the Sensory Profile (Dunn, 1999) may be helpful in evaluating sensory differences. Altered sensitivities, for instance, hypersensitivity to sound, may place an individual at much greater risk of being overwhelmed in noisy or overstimulating environments. These sensitivities may also affect a child's ability to regulate emotions and tolerate transitions. For instance, Charlie in the above case study may act out when getting dressed because he cannot tolerate a scratchy tag. Similarly, children with autism may be drawn to potentially maladaptive sensory experiences, such as sniffing inappropriate things or shredding papers. Replacement behaviors, such as smelling perfumes (Bregman, Zager, and Gerdtz, 2005) or shredding napkins, may satisfy the functional need of the maladaptive behavior in a more adaptive manner. All of these examples, however, rely on a careful functional analysis of the behavior and underlying stressors of a person with autism. In general, people with autism may be more distracted and overwhelmed by sensory stimulation. A calm, relatively quiet, and lower stimulation environment may maximize a person's ability to regulate his or her emotions and behavior and allow for optimal functioning at school or at work. When difficulties processing sensory information affect an individual's ability to regulate emotions and manage transitions, targeting these needs in school, work, and home settings is important. The Alert Program (M. S. Williams and Shellenberger, 1996) may be a useful resource in addressing this issue.

Motor impairments may also be common in individuals with autism. Impairments may include problems with motor imitation, including oral and facial movements that affect speech and language skills (Rogers et al., 2003) and with motor praxis, specifically learning new and complex movements (Baranek, Parham, and Bodfish, 2005). Evaluation and treatment by occupational and physical therapists may reduce these deficits, particularly if function is the primary goal, and will also guide modifications in the environment.

Emotional and Behavioral Function

An assessment of an individual's temperament or emotional reactivity and skills of emotional self-regulation is necessary in anticipating difficulties in function and in developing treatment strategies. This evaluation may rely primarily on a history of the person's function with particular emphasis on his tolerance to change, transitions, and frustration. Alternatively, the Behavioral Assessment System for Children—Second Edition (BASC-2; Reynolds and Kamphaus, 2004), which is designed to measure numerous aspects of emotional and behavioral functioning in the community and home settings, may be helpful. This tool assesses both internalizing and externalizing problems. Areas assessed include anxiety, withdrawal, depression, inattention, and hyperactivity as well as other behavioral topics of particular concern to persons with autism including social withdrawal, limited adaptability, poor functional communication, and atypical interpersonal relating skills.

Deficits in emotion regulation often compound deficits in other domains, including social interaction, communication, cognitive ability, and executive function. It is important to realize that these difficulties affect a person's ability to function in the everyday home, work, school, and other social environments. It is also critical to recognize the impact these struggles have on an individual's ability to learn and benefit from instruction and intervention. In particular, difficulties adjusting to change and managing transitions combined with poor organizational skills and attention deficits may cause great stress and extreme frustration for someone with autism. When combined with poor insight into the emotional state of oneself and others, concrete concept formation, and limited mental flexibility, stress and frustration may then lead to maladaptive behaviors.

Behavior is often the presenting concern in those with autism spectrum disorders. Understanding the behavior of people with autism in the context of the strengths and vulnerabilities that uniquely characterize them and in the context of specific situations is necessary. It is critical that caregivers, teachers, or job coaches recognize that behaviors do not exist in a vacuum but identify, communicate, and serve specific needs. In people with autism, particularly with significantly impaired communication skills, stereotypies, tantrums, or self-injurious behavior may be their only way of expressing distress when overwhelmed by the environment, of getting attention, of avoiding unpleasant tasks, or of communicating frustration, fears, pain, and desires. Instruments that may aide in identifying behaviors include the Vineland Adaptive Behavior Skills (Sparrow, Balla, and Cicchetti, 1984; Carter et al., 1998), the BASC-2 (Reynolds and Kamphaus, 2004), and the Aberrant Behavior Checklist (Aman and Singh, 1985), which are often used to monitor treatment responses (Ozonoff, Goodlin-Jones, and Solomon, 2005). Similarly, DISCO (Wing et al., 2002) may be helpful to guide treatment recommendation and monitor progress in adults with autism. The approach that is most useful in assessing behavior is functional analysis. This process first evaluates environmental factors that make a behavior more or less likely to occur, for instance, hunger, fatigue, or overstimulation. Second, it assesses the contingencies that reinforce maladaptive behavior such as attention and escape from unpleasant task as well as the contingencies that reinforce positive behaviors such as attention, praise, and reward. It also develops adaptive alternative behaviors and skills (Powers, 2005). The text, *Functional Assessment and Program Development for Problem Behavior: A Practical Handbook,* is an excellent resource for those wishing to perform a functional analysis of behavior (O'Neill et al., 1997).

For instance, Charlie's head-banging in the context of shopping may occur because he is overwhelmed and overstimulated by the shopping mall; his screaming and neck-arching may occur because he is in pain; and he may pick his skin to soothe himself when he is anxious. Identifying the factors that provoke these behaviors, understanding the communicative intent of them, and helping him develop alternative behaviors are necessary steps in reducing maladaptive behaviors. Similarly, for Noah, tantrums at the end of a day may reflect fatigue compounded by the frustration of being asked to perform a task he cannot. Alternatively, his tantrums in group activities have been reinforced by his escape from them and from the reward of engaging in his favorite hobby. Restructuring his day and providing tasks that build slowly on previous success may reduce tantrums in this context. Providing an alternative when in group activities, while recognizing his difficulties with social circumstances, for instance, by letting him sit at the edge of the group, may decrease both anxiety and his motivation to escape. Similarly, Noah's tantrums in music class may reflect his intolerance of noise. His withdrawal from school may indicate distress over being teased, but his avoidance of other social situations may also indicate growing social anxiety. A functional analysis of all of these behaviors is required to develop a treatment program that will be most effective.

Last, while some children may experience increased cognitive and behavioral deterioration in adolescence, several longitudinal studies suggest that for many adolescents with autism, difficulties improve over time (Shea and Mesibov, 2005). However, problematic behaviors, including tantrums, self-injury, aggression, compulsions, unacceptable sexual behavior, and resistance to change may persist or may become more concerning when carried out by children who are bigger and stronger (Shea and Mesibov, 2005). Early intervention guided by functional analysis supports a more positive outcome by providing a child and his family with more effective tools to cope.

Medical and Psychiatric Evaluation

The recommended medical evaluation for individuals with autism remains unclear but groups like the Autism Treatment Network are actively working to help establish standards. In general, the approach must be individualized. However, all persons with autism should receive definitive hearing evaluations. Other tests that are recommended include lead levels and karyotype and DNA analysis for fragile X syndrome if there is a concern for developmental delay and if these tests have not been previously performed. Additional neonatal screening tests, such as for phenylketonuria, should be considered if caring for an older adult or a child born outside the United States where routine tests may not have been available. Furthermore, a loss of cognitive or adaptive skills warrants consideration of seizures as do seizure symptoms or dramatic changes in behavior (Filipek, 2005). Epilepsy can occur in up to one-third of individuals with autism, has peak onsets before 5 and between 10 and 12 years of age, and may be more difficult to detect as symptoms associated with some kinds of seizures, including detachment and stereotypies, also may occur in autism (Minshew et al., 2005). As a loss of skills is also associated with a myriad of conditions, genetic, biochemical, and neurological studies must be determined by presentation. At this time, routine genetic, biochemical, and imaging studies are controversial when there is an absence of pertinent family history, dysmorphic features or focal neurological findings, clinical symptoms, or a clear loss of previously acquired skills. Similarly, routine screening for celiac antibodies, allergies to gluten, casein, molds or abnormalities in vitamins, trace elements, intestinal permeability, or stool in connection with a diagnosis of autism is not supported by evidence. In summary, the medical evaluation of autism must be individualized and directed by clinical judgment (Filipek, 2005).

In contrast, every person with autism requires routine medical and dental care. While examinations may be difficult, it is essential that no one is deprived of normal care owing to their disability. Moreover, individuals who lack the capacity to communicate their needs and feelings are at much higher risk of experiencing undiagnosed and untreated medical, dental, and psychiatric illnesses. These illnesses may dramatically affect their behavior. For instance, a person with a headache or toothache who cannot communicate may grab or bang his head in an attempt to deal with untreated pain. Additionally, individuals with autism may have increased rates of gastrointestinal and sleep disturbances. A person with undiagnosed and untreated gastroesophageal reflux disorder may hold his stomach, arch his neck, or twist in pain as in the example of Charlie. He may also develop a chronic dry or nighttime cough, hoarseness, or dental erosions. Rates of gastroesophageal reflux disorder may be as high as 25 percent for individuals with autism spectrum disorders. Other gastrointestinal symptoms that are more common in persons with autism include abnormal stool patterns and food selectivity but may also include constipation, vomiting, and abdominal pain (Valicenti-McDermott et al., 2006).

Similarly, people with autism experience sleep disturbances more frequently than those in the general population. Problems with sleep include delayed onset of sleep, decreased sleep duration, higher levels of sleep anxiety, and increased parasomnias. The causes of these problems remain unclear but may be related to abnormalities in developing circadian rhythms owing to the early inability to read social cues or to increased arousal and anxiety (Couturier et al., 2005). Additionally, concerns of sleep apnea must also be considered in the individual with autism who is obese, snores heavily at night, or has episodes when he or she stops breathing. Impaired sleep affects daytime performance. Moreover, someone who does not get adequate rest will have increased difficulty regulating himself and his environment. Use of the BEARS technique, a five-item questionnaire, may provide detailed information about sleep. This questionnaire asks about *B*edtime problems, *E*xcessive daytime sleepiness, *A*wakenings at night, *R*egularity and duration of sleep, and *S*noring (Owens and Dalzell, 2005). Additionally, a sleep diary may help quantify disturbances and monitor changes with treatment. Recommendations for improved sleep rely primarily on increasing sleep hygiene, as there are no FDA-approved medications at this time despite routine use of various agents.

A pediatrician or other primary care physician specially trained in developmental or behavioral disorders may be of significant help in providing and coordinating medical care, usually within the context of a child's medical home. Similarly, dentists with training in caring for the developmentally disabled may also be necessary. A functional analysis of any behavior, particularly those of new onset or involving self-injurious behavior, must consider underlying medical causes and receive appropriate medical evaluation.

Additional Psychiatric Evaluation

Individuals with autism have psychiatric symptoms more often than typically developing peers. While epidemiological studies vary widely, some psychiatric disorders, such as anxiety and depression, are believed to be present in as many as one-third of people with autism spectrum disorders. In contrast, the prevalence of schizophrenia does not appear to differ from that of the general population. However, the prevalence of other disorders such as obsessive-compulsive disorder may be far more difficult to detect owing to similar symptoms present in autism, including stereotyped behavior and insistence on sameness (Howlin, 2005). The diagnosis of psychosis is also fraught with difficulty, as many of the diagnostic features of autism might also be suggestive of psychosis in individuals without autism spectrum disorders. These characteristics include flat affect, poor eye contact, echolalia, impoverished thought content, concrete thought processes, and unusual movements. Individuals with autism who interpret language literally may misinterpret common psychiatric diagnostic questions such as, "Do you hear voices?" and may lack the understanding to meaningfully answer questions such as "Have you ever thought of hurting someone?" as in the case of Eric (Howlin, 2005). In these situations, it is imperative for the professional to consider an individual's thoughts and behaviors within the context of autism to prevent misdiagnosis. Moreover, relying on self-reports by persons with autism may underestimate the presence of symptoms because of inherent difficulties the individual has with identifying emotional states, recognizing symptoms, communicating distress, and understanding abstract concepts. It is important to recognize that psychiatric disorders evolve over the course of the development of an individual. Despite these difficulties, early diagnosis and treatment are warranted owing to the severity of the effect of psychiatric disorders on function and the difficulty of altering maladaptive patterns that are established during an illness (Howlin, 2005). Instruments that may be of assistance in diagnosis include the BASC-2 (Reynolds and Kamphaus, 2004) that rely on self-report, parent report, and teacher report. Self-report measures of inadequacy and atypicality in high-functioning children may be most suggestive of affective disorders (Ozonoff, Goodlin-Jones, and Solomon, 2005). While medication may be helpful, it is rarely adequate without also providing practical behavioral suggestions on how to deal with problems (Howlin, 2005).

Psychiatric disorders in individuals with autism may present with changes in function or with specific symptoms including changes in sleep, appetite, mood, and behavior. Anxiety may be especially common and problematic. Provoked by any number of circumstances including changes in routine, novel situations, too much stimulation, or difficult task demands, anxiety may be further exacerbated by other deficits common in persons with autism including impaired understanding of social situations and emotional states and limited self-regulation skills. Anxiety may present as fearfulness, agitation, irritability, tantrums, self-injurious behavior, aggression, and other maladaptive behaviors (Loveland and Tunali-Kotoski, 2005) or unusual fears, obsessive questioning, insistence on sameness, and stereotypies (Ozonoff, Goodlin-Jones, and Solomon, 2005). In the adolescent, particularly the high-functioning adolescent, anxiety may become even more problematic as an individual recognizes that he is different and struggles to fit into a world that continues to confuse him. The effort to maintain the appearance of being "normal" may be exhausting. Last, some individuals with autism spectrum disorders may experience a constant state of physiological hyperarousal and anxiety that further impairs daily functioning (Arick et al., 2005).

Depression may also be more common in individuals with autism, especially in adolescence (Howlin, 2005) and among higher-functioning individuals (Loveland and Tunali-Kotoski, 2005). Provoked by increasing awareness of being different, repeated lack of success in making friends, and increased academic demands, depression in an adolescent with autism spectrum disorders may present as decreased desire for social interaction and decreased function characterized by disorganization and inattention and increased isolation and insistence on routines. Once again, the effort to appear "normal" may lead to persistent fatigue (Loveland and Tunali-Kotoski, 2005).

As noted above, it is well known that individuals with autism struggle with impairments in executive functioning. While symptoms of attention deficit hyperactivity disorder (ADHD) such as inattention, distractibility, or hyperactivity have been reported in up to a third of persons with autism, DSM-IV-TR currently does not allow a separate diagnosis of ADHD. Although individuals with autism and those with ADHD share some symptoms, persons with autism typically have lower functioning owing to additional problems with social interaction and communication. Moreover, the etiology of these executive function deficits may be somewhat different in this population and may reflect problems with information processing, processing speed, and cognitive flexibility rather than deficits in sustained attention. However, in common with people with ADHD, those with autism and ADHD symptoms often struggle in work or school, require additional supports such as highly structured classrooms and lower stimulation environments, and perform best when tasks are broken down into smaller steps.

Development across the Life span

It is important to consider a child's function in the context of the developmental stage. While the trajectory of development may differ for a child with autism, the goals of development are the same as for typically developing children. These include individual growth, integration into society, and greater independence. Assessing both an individual's current abilities and his or her future needs is necessary for continued progress at each developmental stage. This is especially true in adolescence, when consideration of future options become important. Federal law mandates that a child receive assistance with transition planning and services that may begin as early as the 14th birthday, but no later than the 16th, to prepare the child for future endeavors, including supported or independent living and work or additional education. Both a child's preference and abilities must be taken into consideration (Gerhardt and Holmes, 2005). Most people with autism do not live totally independently as adults but continue to live with their parents or in supported living environments (Howlin, 2005). Thus, planning for the future is often a family function.

Unfortunately, many adults with autism struggle to find work. Others, like Eric, are underemployed. While part of this struggle may be due to impairments in communication and social interaction, up to 75 percent of adults with any disability are unemployed despite the fact that the vast majority wish to work (Gerhardt and Holmes, 2005). Advocacy for increasing independence and work skills should be included in any treatment plan as a child transitions to adulthood. The main agency that provides vocational assistance to individuals with disabilities is the Rehabilitation Service Administration, which is present in each state. Options may include employment in a sheltered facility, supported employment (employment in a competitive environment but with the additional supervision and support of a job coach), and independent work (Dawson and Toth, 2006). Despite these challenges, programs such as Treatment and Education of Autistic and Related Communication Handicapped Children (TEACCH) in North Carolina, Eden WERC's in New Jersey, and Community Services for Autistic Adults and Children in Maryland, have been extremely successful at providing employment opportunities for the majority of individuals with autism. Other programs using the supported employment model have also demonstrated remarkable success at placing adults with autism who also have limited language, low intellectual ability, and challenging behavior (Gerhardt and Holmes, 2005).

While our knowledge about the child with autism has increased dramatically, our understanding of the adult with autism remains minimal. In contrast to the extensive literature on autism in children, a 2001 review of the literature for autism and adults found less than 30 papers. These included investigations of diagnosis, genetics, neurobiology, behavioral and psychological research, and treatment and outcome. The majority of these investigations focused on specific topics or were limited to a small sample size or to only high-functioning individuals (Brereton and Tonge, 2002). However, additional research has been conducted in the intervening years. While some studies have focused on pharmacological interventions, others have evaluated the evolving presentation of autism, prognosis and progress, and the need for ongoing care. A recent review of 405 patients revealed significant progress over time in communication, reciprocal social interaction, and restrictive repetitive behaviors and interests. However, it also revealed that nearly two-thirds of participants lived with their parents while another third lived in a residential home and suggested that, while symptoms may evolve and diminish over time, improvement of symptoms did not eliminate the need for developmentally appropriate care and support (Setlzer et al., 2003). Additionally, research continues to demonstrate that overall outcome still tends to be poor (Billstedt, Gillberg, and Gillberg, 2005), despite models of both care and work that have proved successful. More research into treatment and outcome is necessary.

Families and Community

An evaluation of the individual with autism must extend to an evaluation of the strengths and weaknesses of his or her family and community, as the majority of treatment will occur within these contexts. Families of a person with autism often experience increased stress and depression and do so to a degree that exceeds that of families of children with other developmental disabilities. The Parenting Stress Index (Abidin, 1983) may be a useful tool for assessing these difficulties (Ozonoff, Goodlin-Jones, and Solomon, 2005). Increased family stress may impair care, treatment, and advocacy, as the family often plays the primary role in these areas. Providing early parent education and skills training has been shown to significantly improve parental mental health and adjustment (Tonge et al., 2006). Helping individuals to learn functional routines that are of assistance to the family, such as setting the table, may also help both the people with autism and their caregivers appreciate their unique contribution to family life. Providing a list of resources for an individual's family, teachers, and others involved in his care may be of great assistance. A list of resources is included at the end of this chapter.

Treatment

Treatment Programs

There are multiple approaches to the treatment of autism. Although no particular treatment demonstrates significant success in more than 50 to 70 percent of children (Schreibman and Ingersoll, 2005), early and intense education has been shown to modify the course of autism in many children (Faja and Dawson, 2006). While more research is needed to determine which children will benefit most from a particular course, programs based on the principles of applied behavioral analysis are recommended. This method emphasizes the building of skills through techniques such as prompting, shaping, chaining (breaking down tasks into constituent components and then linking them together), and teaching functional routines. Both discrete trial training and pivotal response training teach new skills by building on previously learned ones using a sequence of a cue, the child's response and a consequence that is generally a positive reinforcer. In discrete trial training, the choice of task is generally left to the instructor and can be effective in teaching specific new skills. Pivotal response training allows the individual to initiate activity so that learning occurs in a more functional and naturalistic setting. Functional routines draw on existing strengths to learn specific patterns of behavior. These routines teach complex behaviors, such as going to the bathroom or knowing what to do in a day, by breaking them down into smaller tasks the individual can master. Once mastered, steps are linked together to provide a behavioral routine that may be used in daily life (Arick et al., 2005).

Many of these techniques have been incorporated in variety of programs or curricula, each with their own particular emphasis or style. These include Strategies for Teaching based on Autism Research (STAR), an instructional curriculum for teachers, the Denver Model, which focuses on development, Learning Experiences—An Alternative Program for Preschoolers and Parents (LEAP), and TEACCH, which is based on structured teaching. Depending on the program, care may be delivered in a specialized center, school, or home. As we cannot yet compare the efficacy of these various programs (Harris, Handleman, and Jennett, 2005), the choice of a particular program must reflect an individual's needs, the resources available in the community, and a family's preference. Regardless of program, however, identifying target skills and monitoring progress is most likely to lead to success.

In addition to more formal treatment programs, recommendations that present practical suggestions to improve a person's life are often highly valued by his family, school, work site, and other social settings. Recommendations are of particular use when combined with a comprehensive evaluation of a child's strengths and weaknesses and an explanation of autism spectrum disorders. The next sections describe specific interventions targeted at the core deficits of communication and socialization, executive function, motor and sensory abnormalities, and emotional regulation and behavioral control. Also, as treatment of underlying psychiatric symptoms may not only treat mood and behavior but also facilitate greater learning and progress, a review of medication strategies is discussed in the chapter on psychopharmacology. A list of resources is provided for both families and providers at the end of this chapter.

Strategies to Improve Communication and Social Interaction

Communication is an issue of concern for all individuals with autism spectrum disorders. Strategies to improve communication with others include gaining attention, preferably using eye contact, before delivering instruction; using simple, short, and concrete verbal phrases; and pairing verbal instruction with written instructions and visual aides in the form of pictures or words. Examples include using calendars to organize a person's daily schedule and providing a written list of specific tasks to be accomplished that the individual may then check off as he performs them. Avoiding idioms, double meanings, and sarcasm is also helpful, although these skills should be taught directly in structured settings to help him understand these frequently elusive concepts. As individuals with autism may struggle to read facial expressions and interpret body language, conveying information in a calm and explicit manner may help him understand. Moreover, because people with autism may process information more slowly than others and may have more difficulty integrating different modalities of information, repeating verbal information, pairing verbal information with visual cues, and allowing the person more time may be essential in helping him comprehend specific expectations. Last, demonstrating tasks before asking the individual to perform them draws on the often preserved or enhanced strengths of visual learning.

Social interactions are also impaired in persons with autism but are amenable to treatment. Individual and group social skills training targeted at developing appropriate social interactions with same-age peers can be useful. These therapies improve social skills by teaching conversational skills, reciprocal social interactions, perspective taking, and emotional expression and regulation. Individual therapy may also help a person cope with a particular situation by providing him strategies that will improve him understanding of social situations and give him specific behaviors to use when he is interacting with others. Strategies that have proved effective for many individuals with autism are social stories, such as Comic Strip Conversations, by Carol Gray, Ph.D. These stories are scripts that aid in the understanding of various social situations including activities of daily living such as toileting, dressing, and sleeping; social skills such as greetings and manners, turn-taking and sharing; smiling and giving hugs; and specific situations including what to do when unexpected noises occur, how to have a play date, and what to do when your family goes out to dinner. Such stories should be individualized for each person and reviewed on a regular basis so that the individual gains an understanding of how to behave in certain situations. Other strategies include role-playing and concrete problem solving, for instance, making a list of who to speak with when teased. It may also be helpful to create a written set of individualized social rules that clearly define which behaviors are appropriate and which are not. For instance, "When I don't want to do something at work, I will ask my supervisor for a break. I will not scream or hit people." Teaching safety phrases such as "I'm sorry I upset you" or "Can you explain that to me again?" or "I don't understand. Why should I do that?" is also important. This technique provides a person a way to gain important social information readily apparent to many but elusive to those who struggle to read social cues and to understand language.

Many individuals with autism have difficulty in unstructured, especially social, situations. Providing structured activities or assigning a particular role to play may alleviate the anxiety caused by the situation and allow a person with autism to more easily fit into the larger world. Developing social stories or social rules may also help him understand what is expected of him in these situations or be used to explain social games and routines. Role-playing may also be useful. These strategies should be individualized to a person's particular needs and reviewed frequently. Finally, using some random means of assigning partners should be considered in social games and routines to prevent a child from always being the one nobody picks.

Using a buddy system can help the person with autism negotiate social difficulties. Buddy systems have been used in various school systems and tend to be most effective when they are well established within the school and within the classroom routine and include a variety of peers to avoid unintentionally setting a child up for further teasing or isolation. The best buddies are responsible, good-natured children who are tolerant and accepting. Buddy programs have also been used to help the child with autism improve his social skills. In these settings, it is helpful to provide the peer and, at times, other classmates, with an understanding of autism and to teach the peer to give easy instructions, demonstrate skills, give praise and supports, and ignore inappropriate behaviors (Handelman, Harris, and Martins, 2005). The buddy system can also be adapted to adults with autism by engagement of a job coach and through the involvement of home caregivers.

Strategies to Improve Executive Function

Strategies that successfully target deficits in executive function may significantly increase an individual's ability to work and learn and significantly decrease maladaptive behaviors. Assigning a one-to-one aide may be necessary to provide adequate support. Other techniques may also help significantly. As persons with autism are often visual and concrete learners, organizational techniques of calendars, day programs, and task lists can be of immense benefit. A computer schedule may be helpful as it provides an over-all template in which modifications can be made. Reviewing this schedule at the beginning of a day will help the person orient himself to his day and often greatly improves transitions as he knows what to expect and when. Using task lists and checking off tasks as they are completed allows a person to feel successful and to monitor his progress to the overall goal, a key strategy especially when the task is not one he enjoys. Having a fun task at the end of a project may also be motivating and rewarding, especially when the person can see the task listed on his calendar after the less preferable work. Additionally, individuals with autism often struggle with deficits in central coherence that affect their ability to comprehend a task in its entirety.

Breaking down large tasks into individual components, ideally arranged visually to clarify in what order to proceed, will also help the person organize himself and his work and decrease his anxiety. Using concrete examples and hands-on activities, demonstrating projects ahead of time, and pairing visual cues to concepts will also draw on the visual strengths of a child with autism and facilitate learning. Moreover, allowing the individual to learn new skills in a familiar environment, reducing his work load, and emphasizing quality rather than quantity of work, maximizes learning and minimizes frustration, anxiety, and maladaptive behaviors. Those with executive function difficulties often struggle in new situations. Using schedules, structured activities, assigning specific roles, or using social stories or social rules help the person prepare for and adapt more easily to new situations. In time, the anxiety associated with the unexpected and the new may also decrease as the individual recognizes he has multiple strategies to use when dealing with new and scary situations.

Strategies for Sensory and Motor Abnormalities

Individuals with autism spectrum disorders are often irritated or overwhelmed by sensations. A functional analysis of behavior combined with an understanding of the person's sensitivities can be effective in reducing distress and maladaptive behavior by directing modifications in the environment. Examples of modifications include providing earmuffs to those with low tolerance to noise when riding a raucous school bus and removing scratchy tags from clothing for someone with tactile sensitivities. Alternatively, for those drawn to inappropriate sensory experiences either as self-stimulation or as a coping skill, teaching replacement behaviors may be especially effective.

It is important that any intervention be guided by a functional analysis and monitored for progress or lack thereof. While many alternative therapies target particular sensory impairments using techniques such as sensory integration, vision therapy, or auditory integration therapy, there is no clear evidence at this time that these approaches will improve functioning, especially in more natural settings (Baranek, Parham, and Bodfish, 2005).

Similarly, motor impairments are common in autism and may frustrate a person and decrease her function. Modifying the environment or using adaptive strategies, such as allowing the person who struggles with handwriting to type or dictate, should be considered.

Strategies to Improve Emotional Regulation

Strategies that foster emotional regulation by modifying the environment and teaching new coping skills may have profound impact on learning and functioning. Environmental alterations include using visual supports, increasing structure through the use of calendars or activity schedules, decreasing workload during periods of increased frustration and fatigue, providing frequent breaks, alternating difficult tasks with easier or more pleasant ones, providing concrete instruction and feedback, and reducing environmental stimulation. Providing intermittent opportunities throughout the day for arousal regulation, including sensory activities, relaxation techniques, and quiet time is often necessary. Coping skills designed to improve emotional regulation may include techniques that also improve communication and social interaction. These strategies include developing safety plans, such as, "When I get upset, I can take a break in the quiet room," using social stories to explain complex social situations and teach adaptive responses to new situations, and teaching self-regulation skills such as distraction, deep-breathing, or taking a break. It is important that the specific techniques chosen are appropriate to the individual's developmental level and, ideally, reflect his own preferences and input. The Alert Program (www.alertprogram.com) provides useful strategies for self-regulation.

Strategies to Improve Behavior

Individuals with autism often struggle with behavior. Behavior is most effectively modified through the use of incentives and reinforcement of positive behaviors. It is critical to understand that positive behaviors are established slowly over time through training, modeling, shaping, prompting, and incentives. In these situations, it is essential that those working with a person with autism understand his strengths and vulnerabilities and adapt their expectations accordingly, especially in challenging circumstances. Expectations should be applied with flexibility, taking into consideration the fact that the person with autism may have different needs and abilities than his peer group. This is equally true for high-functioning individuals with autism who may struggle far more than their parents, caregivers, or others appreciate. Furthermore, behavior within social situations must be assessed carefully as those with autism are likely to misread social cues and misunderstand verbal instruction.

It is helpful to establish a behavioral intervention program to address these needs. A behavioral program should increase support and predictability in the environment to decrease stress and frustration and subsequent acting out. It should provide concrete and immediate reinforcement and clear guidelines for success in small steps for prosocial skills and prosocial behavior. Moreover, reinforcement and rewards should be provided when the individual attempts or approximates a desired skill or behavior as this will further shape his behavior. It is important to choose reinforcers that are motivating to the individual and to provide a variety of reinforcers such as praise, pleasant activities, food, or stickers to make it more likely that he will continue to anticipate something rewarding and not become satiated.

Given the challenges inherent in autism, daily feedback and positive reinforcement should be provided for appropriate social interactions with peers, work supervisors, or teachers and for compliance with rules in each setting. Establishing a home note system between work or school and home may be especially helpful in developing consistency of approach and assessing the efficacy of a program. Additionally, minimizing the affect in one's voice to maintain a neutral tone when giving consequences for actions or redirections, remaining as calm as possible, being as predictable as possible, and demonstrating compassion and patience is essential in shaping behavior in persons with autism.

Functional behavioral assessments are essential in evaluating and treating negative behaviors. These assessments should be conducted regularly in the home and in the workplace or school as needed, but particularly at onset of a school year, job, or program. This approach identifies the antecedents and consequences to behavior, including predisposing, precipitating, and perpetuating factors. Both factors and consequences are then modified to shape behavior, and alternative functional behaviors are taught. Progress is monitored, and the behavioral program adjusted accordingly (Powers, 2005).

Psychopharmacology

While there is no current pharmacological treatment for autism, multiple treatments exist for the psychiatric symptoms that may arise in the context of autism. As the approach to psychopharmacology in autism is similar to that for any individual with a developmental disorder, this information is presented in the chapter dedicated to this topic.

Conclusion

Autism spectrum disorders describe a wide range of deficits that strike at the core of social communication and interaction. While we have learned much about these disorders, it is now clear that there is neither a single cause nor a single cure for autism. Research directed at understanding both specific endophenotypes and possible common pathways is necessary. Regardless of etiology, early multidisciplinary diagnosis and treatment are necessary, as early and intensive treatment will enable the child to progress in multiple domains and may change the trajectory of this lifelong developmental disorder. Moreover, it is essential to remember that an individual with an autism spectrum disorder is a person first and presents with unique strengths and vulnerabilities. Treatment must always occur in the context of individual abilities, desires, and goals. While autism may isolate the individual from the broader world, persons with autism do not exist in isolation. We must do what we can to ensure that they lead enriching and fulfilling lives even as we recognize that the world is a better place, a more enriched place, by virtue of their presence in it.

RESOURCES

There are many books that help families and other caregivers understand the nature of autism. These include *A Parent's Guide to Asperger Syndrome and High-functioning Autism,* by Sally Ozonoff, Geraldine Dawon, and James McPartland; *Children with Autism, A Parent's Guide,* by Michael D. Powers; *The Autistic Spectrum: A Parent's Guide to Understanding and Helping Your Child,* by Lorna Wing, Ami Klin, and

Fred Volkmar; and *Asperger's Syndrome: A Guide for Parents and Professionals,* by Tony Atwood.

Resources for intervention include the Alert Program for emotional self-regulation (www.alertprogram.com), the Gray Center for social stories and comic strip conversations (www.thegraycenter.org), and Use Visual Strategies.com at www.use visualstrategies.com for visual strategies. Resources for teaching social skills include *Social Skills Stories: Functional Picture Stories for Readers and Nonreaders K–12,* by Anne Marie Johnson and Jackie L. Susnik; *Autism and PDD Social Skills Lessons,* by Nena C. Challenner; *SSS: Social Skills Strategies Book A and B,* by Nancy Gajewski and Patty Mayo; and *RAPP: Resource of Activities for Peer Pragmatics,* by Nancy McConnell and Carolyn M. Bladgen. The Autism Society of North Carolina also maintains a bookstore and hundreds of resources on autism and related disorders. They can be reached at 800-442-2762.

There are many organizations that are useful to primary caregivers, teachers, and parents. These include the National Autism Society of America at www.autism-society.org and Autism Speaks at www.autismspeaks.org. These advocacy sites provide education on autism and autism research. The Parent to Parent Program (www.p2pusa.org) offers support for parents of children with disabilities. Other organizations include the Source, a resource on Asperger disorder at http://asperger .org, and Learning Disabilities Online at www.ldonline.org.

For the professional, the *Handbook of Autism and Pervasive Developmental Disorders,* edited by Fred Volkmar, Rhea Paul, Ami Klin, and Donald Cohen, is recommended. Additionally, institutional resources include Division TEACCH at www.teacch .com, the Yale Developmental Disabilities Clinic at www.info.med.yale.edu/chldstdy/ autism, and the Kennedy Krieger Institute at www.IANproject.org.

References

Abidin R. 1983. Parenting Stress Index: Manual, Administration Booklet, and Research Update. Charlottesville, VA: Pediatric Psychology Books.

Aman MG, Singh NN. 1985. Psychometric characteristics of the Aberrant Behavior Checklist. *American Journal of Mental Deficiencies* 89(5): 492–502.

American Psychiatric Association. 2000. *Diagnostic and Statistical Manual of Mental Disorders,* 4th ed., text rev. Washington, DC: American Psychiatric Association.

Anderson GM, Hoshino Y. 2005. Neurochemical studies of autism. In F Volkmar, R Paul, A Klin, D Cohen (eds.), *Handbook of Autism and Pervasive Developmental Disorders,* 3rd ed., 1:453–72. Hoboken, NJ: Wiley.

Arick JR, Krug DA, Fullerton A, Loos L, Falco R. 2005. School-based programs. In F Volkmar, R Paul, A Klin, D Cohen (eds.), *Handbook of Autism and Pervasive Developmental Disorders,* 3rd ed., 2:1003–28. Hoboken, NJ: Wiley.

Baranek GT, David FJ, Poe MD, Stone WL, Watson LR. 2006. Sensory Experiences Questionnaire: Discriminating sensory features in young children with autism, developmental delays, and typical development. *Journal of Child Psychology and Psychiatry* 47(6): 591–601.

Baranek GT, Parham LD, Bodfish JW. 2005. Sensory and motor features in autism: Assessment and intervention. In F Volkmar, R Paul, A Klin, D Cohen (eds.), *Handbook of Autism and Pervasive Developmental Disorders*, 3rd ed., 2:831–57. Hoboken, NJ: Wiley.

Billstedt E, Gillberg IC, Gillberg C. 2005. Autism after adolescence: Population-based 13- to 22-year follow-up study of 120 individuals with autism diagnosed in childhood. *Journal of Autism and Developmental Disorders* 35(3): 351–60.

Bregman JD, Zager D, Gerdtz J. 2005. Behavioral interventions. In F Volkmar, R Paul, A Klin, D Cohen (eds.), *Handbook of Autism and Pervasive Developmental Disorders*, 3rd ed., 2:897–924. Hoboken, NJ: Wiley.

Brereton AV, Tonge BJ. 2002. Autism and related disorders in adults. *Current Opinion in Psychiatry* 15(5): 483–87.

Busch G. Luu P, Posner M. 2000. Cognitive and emotional influences in the anterior cingulated cortex. *Trends in Cognitive Science* 4: 214–22.

Carter M, Volkmar F, Sparrow S, et al. 1998. The Vineland Adaptive Behavior scales: Supplementary norms for individuals with autism. *Journal of Autism and Developmental Disorders* 28: 287–303.

Chess S. 1977. Follow-up report on autism in congenital rubella. *Journal of Autism and Childhood Schizophrenia* 7(1): 69–81.

Coonrod EE, Stone WL. 2005. Screening for autism in young children. In F Volkmar, R Paul, A Klin, D Cohen (eds.), *Handbook of Autism and Pervasive Developmental Disorders*, 3rd ed., 2:707–29. Hoboken, NJ: Wiley.

Couturier J, Speechley K, Steele M, et al. 2005. Parental perception of sleep problems in children of normal intelligence with pervasive developmental disorders: Prevalence, severity, and pattern. *Journal of the American Academy of Child and Adolescent Psychiatry* 44(8): 815–22.

Dawson G. 2007. Despite major challenges, autism research continues to offer hope. *Archives of Pediatrics and Adolescent Medicine* 161: 411–12.

Dawson G, Toth K. 2006. Autism spectrum disorders. In D Cicchetti, D Cohen (eds.), *Developmental Psychopathology*. Vol. 3: *Risk, Disorder, and Adaptation*, 2nd ed., 317–57. Hoboken, NJ: Wiley.

Dawson G, Toth K, Abbott R, et al. 2004. Early social attention impairments in autism: Social orienting, joint attention, and attention to distress. *Developmental Psychology* 40(2): 271–83.

Demicheli V, Jefferson T, Rivetti A, Price D. 2007. Vaccines for measles, mumps, and rubella. Cochrane Database of Systematic Reviews. Available at www.cochrane.org/reviews.

Dunn W. 1999. *Sensory Profile*. San Antonio: Psychological Corporation.

Eaves LC, Wingert HD, Ho HH, Mickelson EC. 2006. Screening for autism spectrum disorders with the social communication questionnaire. *Journal of Developmental and Behavioral Pediatrics* 27(Suppl. 2): S95–103.

Elliot CD. 1990. *Differential Abilities Scales: Introductory and Technical Handbook.* New York: Psychological Corporation.

Faja S, Dawson G. 2006. Early intervention for autism. In J Luby (ed.), *Handbook of Preschool Mental Health: Development, Disorders and Treatment,* 338–416. New York: Guilford Press.

Fernand A. 1992. Human maternal vocalizations to infants as biologically relelvant signals: An evolutionary perspective. In JH Barkon and L Casmides, eds., *Adapted Mind: Evolutionary Psychology and the Generation of Culture,* 391–428. Oxford: Oxford University Press.

Filipek PA. 2005. Medical aspects of autism. In F Volkmar, R Paul, A Klin, D Cohen (eds.), *Handbook of Autism and Pervasive Developmental Disorders,* 3rd ed., 1:534–78. Hoboken, NJ: Wiley.

Filipek PA, Accardo PJ, Baranek EH, Cook G. 1999. Screening and diagnosis of autistic spectrum disorders. *Journal of Autism and Developmental Disorders* 29(6): 439–84.

Fombonne E. 1999. The epidemiology of autism: A review. *Psychological Medicine* 29: 769–86.

Fombonne E. 2005. Epidemiological studies of pervasive developmental disorders. In F Volkmar, R Paul, A Klin, D Cohen (eds.), *Handbook of Autism and Pervasive Developmental Disorders,* 3rd ed., 1:42–69 Hoboken, NJ: Wiley.

Frith U. 2003. *Autism: Explaining the Enigma,* 2nd ed. Malden, MA: Blackwell.

Frith U, Hill E. 2003. Understanding autism: Insights from mind and brain. In U Frith, and E Hill (eds.), *Autism: Mind and Brain,* 1–19. Oxford: Oxford University Press.

Frost LA, Bondy AS. 1994. *The Picture Exchange Communication System Training Manual.* Cherry Hill, NJ: Pyramid Educational Consultants.

Gerhardt PF, Holmes DL. 2005. Employment: Options and issues for adolescents and adults with autism spectrum disorders. In F Volkmar, R Paul, A Klin, D Cohen (eds.), *Handbook of Autism and Pervasive Developmental Disorders,* 3rd ed., 2:1087–1101. Hoboken, NJ: Wiley.

Gervais H, Belin P, Boddaert N. et al. 2004. Abnormal cortical voice processing in autism. *Nature Neuroscience* 7(8): 801–2.

Gioia GA, Isquith PK, Guy SC, Kenworthy L. 1993. *Behavior Rating Inventory of Executive Function (BRIEF).* Lutz, FL: Psychological Assessment Resources.

Handelman JS, Harris SL, Martins MP. 2005. Helping children with autism enter the mainstream. In F Volkmar, R Paul, A Klin, D Cohen (eds.), *Handbook of Autism and Pervasive Developmental Disorders,* 3rd ed., 2:1029–42. Hoboken, NJ: Wiley.

Happé F. 2005. The weak central coherence account of autism. In F Volkmar, R Paul, A Klin, D Cohen (eds.), *Handbook of Autism and Pervasive Developmental Disorders,* 3rd ed., 1:640–49. Hoboken, NJ: Wiley.

Harris SL, Handleman JS, Jennett HK. 2005. Models of educational intervention for students with autism: home, center, and school-based programming In F Volkmar, R Paul, A Klin, D Cohen (eds.), *Handbook of Autism and Pervasive Developmental Disorders,* 3rd ed., 1:1043–54. Hoboken, NJ: Wiley.

Heaton RK, Chelune GJ, Talley JL, Kay GG, Curtiss G. 2000. *Wisconsin Card Sorting Test, Revised and Expanded (WCST)*. Lutz, FL: Psychological Assessment Resources.

Howlin P. 2005. Outcomes in autism spectrum disorders. In F Volkmar, R Paul, A Klin, D Cohen (eds.), *Handbook of Autism and Pervasive Developmental Disorders*, 3rd ed., 1:201–20. Hoboken, NJ: Wiley.

Hussain J, Woolf AD, Sandel M, Shannon M. 2007. Environmental evaluation of a child with developmental disability. *Pediatric Clinics of North America* 55(1): 47–62.

Kanner L. 1973. *Childhood Psychosis: Initial Studies and New Insights*. Hoboken, NJ: Wiley.

Kaufman AS, Kaufman NL. 2004. *Kaufman Assessment Battery for Children: Manual*, 2nd ed. Circle Pines, MN: American Guidance Service.

King BH, Bostic JQ. 2006. An update on pharmacologic treatments for autism spectrum disorders. *Child and Adolescent Psychiatric Clinics of North America* 15(1): 161–75.

Klin A, Saulnier C, Tsatsanis K, Volkmar F. 2005. Clinical evaluation in autism spectrum disorders: Psychological assessment within a transdisciplinary framework. In F Volkmar, R Paul, A Klin, D Cohen (eds.), *Handbook of Autism and Pervasive Developmental Disorders*, 3rd ed., 1:772–98. Hoboken, NJ: Wiley.

Kuhl PK, Coffey-Corina S, Padden D, Dawson G. 2004. Links between social and linguistic processing of speech in preschool children with autism: Behavioral and electrophysiological measures. *Developmental Science* 8(1): F1–12.

Lamb ME, Teti DM, Bornstein MH, Nash A. 2002. Infancy. In M Lewis (ed.), *Child and Adolescent Psychiatry*, 3rd ed., 293–323. Philadelphia: Lippincott Williams & Wilkins.

Lord C, Corsello C. 2005. Diagnostic instruments in autistic spectrum disorders. In F Volkmar, R Paul, A Klin, D Cohen (eds.), *Handbook of Autism and Pervasive Developmental Disorders*, 3rd ed., 2:730–71. Hoboken, NJ: Wiley.

Lord C, Rutter ML, Goode S, et al. 1989. The Autism Diagnostic Observation Schedule: A standardized observation of communicative and social behavior. *Journal of Autism and Developmental Disorders* 19(3): 363–67.

Lord C, Rutter ML, Le Couteur. 1994. The Autism Diagnostic Interview—Revised: A revisedversion of a diagnostic interview for caregivers of individuals with possible pervasive developmental disorders. *Journal of Autism and Developmental Disorders* 24(5): 659–85.

Loveland, KA, Tunali-Kotoski, B. 2005. The school-age child with autism spectrum disorder. In F Volkmar, R Paul, A Klin, D Cohen (eds.), *Handbook of Autism and Pervasive Developmental Disorders*, 3rd ed., 1:247–87. Hoboken, NJ: Wiley.

Mather N, Schrank FA. 2003. *Using the Woodcock-Johnson III Discrepancy Procedures for Diagnosing Learning Disabilities*. San Diego: Academic Press.

Meltzoff AN, Moore MK. 1977. Imitation of facial and manual gestures by human neonates. *Science* 198(4312): 75–78.

Minshew N, Sweeney JA, Bauman ML, Webb SJ. 2005. Neurological aspects of autism. In F Volkmar, R Paul, A Klin, D Cohen (eds.), *Handbook of Autism and Pervasive Developmental Disorders*, 3rd ed., 1:473–514. Hoboken, NJ: Wiley.

Moore SJ, Turnpenney AQ, Glover S, et al. 2000. A clinical study of 57 children with fetal anticonvulsant syndromes. *Journal of Medical Genetics* 37: 489–97.

Mundy P, Burnette C. 2005. Joint attention and neurodevelopmental models of attention. In F Volkmar, R Paul, A Klin, D Cohen (eds.), *Handbook of Autism and Pervasive Developmental Disorders*, 3rd ed., 1:650–81. Hoboken, NJ: Wiley.

O'Neill R, Homer RH, Albin RW, et al. 1997. *Functional Assessment and Program Development for Problem Behavior: A Practical Handbook*. Pacific Grove, CA; Brooks/Cole.

Osterling JA, Dawson G. 1994. Early recognition of children with autism: A study of first birthday home videotapes. *Journal of Autism and Developmental Disorders* 24(3): 247–57.

Owens JA, Dalzell V. 2005. Use of the "BEARS" sleep screening tool in a pediatric residents' continuity clinic: A pilot study. *Sleep Medicine* 6(1): 63–69.

Ozonoff S, Goodlin-Jones BL, Solomon M. 2005. Evidence-based assessment of autism spectrum disorders in children and adolescents. *Journal of Clinical Adolescent Psychology* 34(3): 523–40.

Ozonoff S, Griffith EM. 2000. Neuropsychological function and the external validity of Asperger syndrome. In A Klin, F Volkmar, S Sparrow (eds.), *Asperger Syndrome*, 72–96. New York: Guilford Press.

Ozonoff S, South M, Provencal S. 2005. Executive Functions. In F Volkmar, R Paul, A Klin, D Cohen (eds.), *Handbook of Autism and Pervasive Developmental Disorders*, 3rd ed., 1:606–27. Hoboken, NJ: Wiley.

Paul R. 2005. Assessing communication in autism spectrum disorders. In F Volkmar, R Paul, A Klin, D Cohen (eds.), *Handbook of Autism and Pervasive Developmental Disorders*, 3rd ed., 1:799–816. Hoboken, NJ: Wiley.

Powers MD. 2005. Behavioral assessment of individuals with autism: A functional ecological approach. In F Volkmar, R Paul, A Klin, D Cohen (eds.), *Handbook of Autism and Pervasive Developmental Disorders*, 3rd ed., 2:817–30. Hoboken, NJ: Wiley.

Reynolds CR, Kamphaus RW. 2004. *Behavioral Assessment System for Children*, 2nd ed. San Antonio, TX: Pearson Assessments.

Robins DL, Dumont-Mathieu T. 2006. The Modified Checklist for Autism in Toddlers (M-CHAT): A review of current findings and future directions. *Journal of Developmental and Behavioral Pediatrics* 27(Suppl. 2): S111–19.

Rogers SJ, Hepburn SL, Stackhouse T, Wehner E. 2003. Imitation performance in toddlers with autism and those with other developmental disorders. *Journal of Child Psychology and Psychiatry* 44(5): 763–81.

Roid GM, Miller LJ. 1997. *Leiter International Performance Scale-Revised: Examiner's Manual*. Wood Dale, IL: Stoelting.

Rutter M. 2005. Genetic influences and autism. In F Volkmar, R Paul, A Klin, D Cohen (eds.), *Handbook of Autism and Pervasive Developmental Disorders*, 3rd ed., 1:425–52. Hoboken, NJ: Wiley.

Schreibman L, Ingersoll B. 2005. Behavioral interventions to promote learning in individuals with autism. In F Volkmar, R Paul, A Klin, D Cohen (eds.), *Handbook of Autism and Pervasive Developmental Disorders*, 3rd ed., 2:882–96. Hoboken, NJ: Wiley.

Schultz RT, Robins DL. 2005. Functional neuroimaging studies of autism spectrum disorders. In F Volkmar, R Paul, A Klin, D Cohen (eds.), *Handbook of Autism and Pervasive Developmental Disorders*, 3rd ed., 1:515–33. Hoboken, NJ: Wiley.

Seltzer MM, Krauss MW, Shattuck PT, et al. 2003. The symptoms of autism spectrum disorders in adolescence and adulthood. *Journal of Autism and Developmental Disorders* 33(6): 565–81.

Shea V, Mesibov G. 2005. Adolescents and adults with autism. In F Volkmar, R Paul, A Klin, D Cohen (eds.), *Handbook of Autism and Pervasive Developmental Disorders*, 3rd ed., 1:228–311 Hoboken, NJ: Wiley.

Singer JL. 2002. Cognitive and affective implications of imaginative play in childhood. In M Lewis (ed.), *Child and Adolescent Psychiatry*, 3rd ed., 252–63. Philadelphia: Lippincott Williams & Wilkins.

Sparrow S, Balla D, Cicchetti D. 1984. *Vineland Adaptive Behavior Scales: Interview Edition*. Circle Pines, MN: American Guidance Service.

Tager-Flusbert T, Paul R, Lord C. 2005. Language and communication in autism. In F Volkmar, R Paul, A Klin, D Cohen (eds.), *Handbook of Autism and Pervasive Developmental Disorders*, 3rd ed., 1:335–64. Hoboken, NJ: Wiley.

Tonge B, Brereton A, Kiomall M, et al. 2006. Effects on parental mental health of an education and skills training program for parents of young children with autism: A randomized controlled trial. *Journal of the American Academy of Child and Adolescent Psychiatry* 45(5): 561–69.

Valicenti-McDermott M, McVicar K, Rapin I, et al. 2006. Frequency of gastrointestinal symptoms in children autistic spectrum disorders and association with family history of autoimmune disease. *Journal of Developmental and Behavioral Pediatrics* 27(2): S128–36.

Volkmar FR, Klin A. 2005. Issues in the classification of autism and related conditions. In F Volkmar, R Paul, A Klin, D Cohen (eds.), *Handbook of Autism and Pervasive Developmental Disorders*, 3rd ed., 1:5–41. Hoboken, NJ: Wiley.

Wecshler D. 2002. Wecshler Preschool and Primary Scale of Intelligence, 3rd ed. San Antonio, TX: Psychological Corporation.

Wecshler D. 2003. Wecshler Intelligence Scale for Children: Technical and Interpretative Manual, 4th ed. San Antonio, TX: Psychological Corporation.

Werner E, Dawson G, Osterlin J, Dinno N. 2000. Brief report: Recognition of autism spectrum disorder before one year of age—A retrospective study based on home videotapes. *Journal of Autism and Developmental Disorders* 30(2):157–62.

Williams JHG, Whiten A, Suddendorf T, Perrett DI. 2001. Imitation, mirror neurons, and autism. *Neuroscience and Behavioral Reviews* 25: 287–85.

Williams MS, Shellenberger S. 1996. *How Does Your Engine Run? A Leader's Guide to the Alert Program for Self-Regulation*. Albuquerque, NM: TherapyWorks.

Wing L, Leekam SR, Libby SJ, Gould J, Larcombe M. 2002. The Diagnostic Interview for Social and Communication Disorders: Background, inter-rater reliability and clinical use. *Journal of Child Psychology and Psychiatry and Allied Disciplines* 43(3): 307–25.

Yang MS, Gill M. 2007. A review of gene linkage, association and expression studies in autism and assessment of convergent evidence. *International Journal of Developmental Neuroscience* 25(2): 69–85.

Zafeiriou DI, Ververi A, Vargiami E. 2007. Childhood autism and associated comorbidities. *Brain and Development* 29(5): 257–72.

PART II ◆

Etiology and Assessment

5

Genetic Causes of Mental Retardation

Janet A. Martin, M.D., Ph.D.

Mental retardation (MR) is estimated to affect approximately 2 percent of the population and is understood to have a multifactorial etiology, involving both genetic and environmental factors. Although in the majority of cases the exact cause is never identified, family histories indicate that about 50 percent of moderate-to-profound MR has a genetic etiology (Raynham et al., 1996). It is therefore important for the psychiatrist in the community to have a working knowledge of these disorders, to know how to screen for these conditions, and to be able to diagnose and treat or appropriately refer affected individuals to get the help they need and deserve.

Countless genes are involved in intelligence and cognitive functioning. Because of this polygenic etiology of intelligence, many genetic alterations can have dramatic effects on cognitive function. These include chromosomal abnormalities, such as spontaneous or inherited translocations, deletions, inversions, duplications, and trisomies. Mutations affecting cognitive ability can be sex-linked or autosomal and can be inherited in a dominant or recessive pattern. While most of the exact genes involved in mental deficiency are not known, many syndromes are associated with abnormalities in particular regions of the genome, which are readily identifiable. For example, the most common inherited form of MR is fragile X syndrome, and the most common chromosomal abnormality causing MR is trisomy 21. This chapter presents an overview of these and other common syndromes involving MR in order of prevalence, covering their phenotype and genotype. It then provides guidance

Table 5.1.   Common genetic disorders causing mental retardation

Syndrome	Prevalence	Genetic abnormality	Distinguishing features
Angelman	1:12,500	15q11-13 (maternal)	Happy disposition, ataxia, seizures, impaired verbal skills
Down	1:650–1:1,000	trisomy 21 (21q22)	Characteristic dysmorphism, cardiac and bowel problems
Fragile X	1:4,000 in men 1:12,000 in women	X-linked (FMR1 gene)	Prominent ears and jaw, macroorchidism
Prader-Willi	1:16,000–1:25,000	15q11-13 (paternal)	Initial hypotonia, hyperphagia, hypogonadism
Rett	1:10,000– 1:15,000 in women	X-linked (MECP2 gene)	Loss of functional hand movements
Smith-Magenis	1:25,000	17p11.2	Tented upper lip, nail pulling, insertion of foreign objects into body
VCF	1:5,000	22q11.2	Cleft palate, retrognathia, socially withdrawn
Williams	1:10,000	17q11.23	Elfin features, friendliness, musical prowess

for how the general psychiatrist can adequately assist affected persons in getting high-quality care. Table 5.1 summarizes the more common conditions.

Genetic Conditions

Down Syndrome

Down syndrome (DS; Down, 1887) occurs in more than 1 in 1,000 births. The vast majority of cases of DS are due to nondysjunction of chromosome 21 during formation of the ovum, but occasionally the extra chromosome is of paternal origin. Additionally, about 5 percent of cases are due to a translocation of part of chromosome 21 onto another chromosome, usually 13 or 15. The risk of occurrence increases with maternal age, from 1 in 200 at age 35, to 1 in 100 at age 37, to 1 in 20 at age 45 (Benke, 2005).

Individuals with DS tend to have moderate-to-severe MR and language delay, particularly in expressive language. Typically, those who are affected by this disorder are sociable and good tempered, although some may experience hyperactivity, impulsivity, or aggression. Characteristic dysmorphisms includes short anterior-posterior head diameter, slanted eyes with epicanthal folds, a flattened nasal bridge, enlarged tongue, single palmar crease, and short stature. Medical problems are common in this population, including hearing impairment, visual problems, congenital heart disease, bowel obstruction, celiac disease, thyroid dysfunction, and delayed bone maturation.

Psychiatric conditions of depression, obsessive-compulsive disorder, and conduct disorder occur more frequently in individuals with DS than in the general population. Clinicians should be aware that depression is a significant cause of decreased functioning in this population; thus, it is important to address such conditions. Given that psychotherapy may be a greater challenge in these cases, selective serotonin reuptake inhibitors (SSRIs) become more important in the treatment regimen. These medications also become important for treating pseudodementia (symptoms that appear consistent with dementia but are caused by a psychiatric condition), which is not uncommon in DS (Moldavsky, Len, and Lerman-Sagie, 2001; Tyler and Edman, 2004).

Furthermore, as these individuals age, there is an exponential increase in the prevalence of Alzheimer disease (AD), with approximately 9 percent of persons with DS younger than 50 having dementia, increasing to 32 percent in their late 50s (Coppus et al., 2006). It is thus incumbent on the general psychiatrist to develop a working knowledge of any special considerations that may be involved in treating AD in this population. It is important to get a thorough medical workup of those developing symptoms of dementia, because many conditions (including depression, substance abuse, medication effects, infection, delirium, and systemic illnesses, such as hypothyroidism) must be ruled out before a diagnosis of dementia can be made. Although many people with DS are living longer as a result of improved medical care, most die in their 50s (D. S. Smith, 2001; Benke, 2005).

Fragile X Syndrome

Clinicians have been aware of sex-linked MR for many decades, with the Martin-Bell syndrome initially being described in the 1940s. However, only in the past two decades have specific genes on the X chromosome been identified as responsible for causing MR (Chelly, 1999). The most common of these mutations is a fragile site on the X chromosome, Xq27.3, where the fragile X mental retardation (FMR-1) gene has been delineated (Verkerk, Pieretti, and Sutcliffe, 1991). Fragile X syndrome is now known to be the most common inherited form of MR, affecting 1 in 4,000 men and 1 in 4,000 to 1 in 6,000 women.

Individuals with fragile X syndrome present with mild-to-severe MR, language skills that have peaked about age 4, perseverative speech, hyperactivity, distractibility, and mood lability. They often avoid eye contact, have stereotypic movements when excited or agitated, and may lack interest in social interaction. Their phenotypic features include flat feet, hyperextensible finger joints, double-jointed thumbs, and a high arched palate. They less frequently have single palmar creases, hand calluses, and heart murmurs or clicks. Most men with fragile X syndrome have macroorchidism and a long, thin face with prominent ears and jaw. Also, they often have a hypersensitivity to sensory stimulation, such as tactile, auditory, or visual stimulation. About 15 percent meet the criteria for autism, and about 70 percent of men with the syndrome fulfill the diagnostic criteria for attention deficit hyperactivity disorder (Hagerman, 1997; de Vries et al., 1998; Moldavsky, Len, and Lerman-Sagie, 2001).

Affected women generally do not develop the typical facial features seen in men and have milder degrees of MR. Fifty percent of women with the full mutation have a normal IQ. They often have impaired social behavior, demonstrating reduced eye contact, shyness, social isolation, odd patterns of communication, and occasionally selective mutism (de Vries et al., 1998; Moldavsky, Len, and Lerman-Sagie, 2001).

Medical problems that are more common in this population include strabismus, hernia, scoliosis, mitral valve prolapse, frequent otitis media and sinusitis, and gastroesophageal reflux. Seizures occur in about 20 percent of men and 5 percent of women.

Fragile X syndrome occurs when the *FMR1* gene is disrupted by a trinucleotide expansion. Normally, there are between six and 54 CGG repeats in an untranslated region of the first exon. These CGG repeats can expand with subsequent generations to the permutation form with 43 to 200 repeats or the full mutation with >200 repeats. The likelihood of expansion increases with larger permutations, such that the risk of a woman with a permutation having an affected offspring is less than 20 percent for permutations with less than 70 repeats but greater than 80 percent for permutations with more 80 repeats. When the gene has the full mutation, it usually becomes hypermethylated, preventing its transcription. The exact mechanism by which a lack of *FMR1* protein causes MR is not fully understood, but some individuals with fragile X syndrome have reduced size of the cerebellar vermis and enlargement of the caudate, thalamus, and hippocampus in neuroimaging studies. Furthermore, neuropathological studies have found reductions in the dendritic spines of neurons with consequent reductions in synaptic connections (Hagerman, 1997; de Vries et al., 1998).

Velocardiofacial Syndrome

Velocardiofacial syndrome is an autosomal dominant disorder involving microdeletion of chromosome 22q11.2. Most mutations occur sporadically, affecting approximately 1 in 5000 births (Moldavsky, Len, and Lerman-Sagie, 2001). Fewer than half of affected individuals have mild MR (Swillen et al., 1997).

Persons with velocardiofacial syndrome typically have long faces with narrow palpebral fissures, bulbous tips of tubular noses, cleft palate, recessed jaw (retrognathia), and small open mouths. They are typically short and have slender fingers. Many had feeding problems and speech difficulties as children as a result of the cleft palate and velopharyngeal insufficiency. More typical medical problems include hypocalcemia, immunodeficiency, and cardiac malformations, such as ventricular septal defect or tetralogy of Fallot. Cognitively, verbal IQ is typically higher than performance IQ, and individuals have problems with abstract thinking and distractibility. Many have poor social skills and lack normal facial expressions and prosody of speech. They may also develop psychiatric conditions, especially bipolar spectrum disorders and schizophrenia, which generally respond poorly to medication (Shprintzen et al., 1981; Moldavsky, Len, and Lerman-Sagie, 2001).

Williams Syndrome

Williams syndrome (Williams, Barrett-Boyes, and Lowe, 1961) results from a microdeletion of chromosome 7q11.23 and consequent loss of the LIM-kinase and elastin genes. It generally occurs sporadically in 1 in 10,000 births and can then be transmitted as an autosomal dominant condition (Moldavsky, Len, and Lerman-Sagie, 2001; Fisch, 2005).

Facial features typically associated with this condition are described as "elfin," such as a wide mouth with dental anomalies, a long, flat philtrum, upturned nose with flat nasal bridge, and small chin. Affected individuals may also have stellate irises, mild microcephaly, slender limbs and trunk, and short stature. Medical problems can include stenosis of the aortic, pulmonary, or renal arteries, hypertension, hypercalcemia, and hypotonia. Cognitively, they usually have mild-to-moderate MR or low normal intelligence, with verbal skills higher than performance IQ. Visuomotor integration is particularly poor, although face-processing and musical abilities are usually very good. People with Williams syndrome typically have a history of being overly friendly, talkative, hyperactive, easily distracted as children, and may have shown autistic symptoms when very young. Many also have a hypersensitivity to sound. They typically had poor progress in school and are rarely able to work as adults. Psychiatrically, affected individuals are often anxious, obsessing about the future or somatic concerns, and may experience depressive symptoms (Moldavsky, Len, and Lerman-Sagie, 2001; Fisch, 2005).

Angelman Syndrome

Angelman syndrome (Angelman, 1965), which used to be referred to as the "happy puppet syndrome," is caused by the absence of a maternal copy of the chromosome region 15q11-13, usually as a spontaneous deletion and rarely as a result of uniparental disomy (two paternal copies of the chromosome and absence of the maternal copy). About a fourth of cases result from mutations in a ubiquitin-protein ligase gene and can be familial. This syndrome occurs in about 1 out of 12,500 births and contributes to at least 1.4 percent of cases of moderate-to-severe MR (Moldavsky, Len, and Lerman-Sagie, 2001).

Affected individuals may present with a large, wide mouth revealing the tongue, a happy disposition, and motor and speech delays. One study focusing on cases of deletional mutations found that all of the 27 individuals observed were nonverbal, had severe MR, and had delays in ambulation, with five being nonambulatory into adulthood (A. Smith et al., 1996). Common medical problems associated with Angelman syndrome include epilepsy, ataxia, abnormal sleeping patterns, and hypopigmentation. Behaviorally, these individuals are usually smiling and may have sudden attacks (paroxysmal) of laughter, although hyperactivity and aggressive behaviors have been noted. Many show autistic features, such as repetitive or stereotypic behaviors, and some meet the criteria for autistic disorder (A. Smith et al., 1996; Moldavsky, Len, and Lerman-Sagie, 2001).

Rett Syndrome

Rett syndrome (Rett, 1966) is an X-linked disorder caused by mutations in the methyl-CpG-binding protein 2 (*MECP2*) gene and almost exclusively affects girls and women. Most mutations are sporadic, occurring in 1 out of 10,000 to 15,000 female births (Amir et al., 1999; Moldavsky, Len, and Lerman-Sagie, 2001). Girls with this condition usually have a history of normal development for the first 6 to 18 months of life before experiencing a slowing of head growth and development of autistic features. They lose purposeful hand movements and develop stereotypic movements, such as hand-wringing, clapping, tapping, washing, and mouthing. They also commonly develop gait apraxia, truncal ataxia or apraxia, psychomotor retardation, and severe impairment of expressive and receptive language. Their autistic features tend to subside with age, but they eventually lose motor function and become nonambulatory. Although verbal and motor skills are significantly impaired, visual function is maintained, and they sometimes communicate via "eye-pointing" to objects. In different variations of this syndrome, speech may be preserved or individuals may present with an Angelman-like phenotype (Moldavsky, Len, and Lerman-Sagie, 2001; Laccone et al., 2002). The medical problems associated with this condition include seizures, growth retardation, scoliosis, spasticity, dystonia, periodic apnea or hyperventilation, and peripheral vasomotor conditions (Moldavsky, Len, and Lerman-Sagie, 2001).

Many different mutations in the *MECP2* gene can lead to Rett syndrome in girls and women and may account for the variations in phenotype. It was once thought that these mutations were lethal in boys and men due to the lack of male individuals with this disorder, but several have been identified with these mutations. If they survive to birth, boys with this syndrome present with a lethal encephalopathy or with varying degrees of MR (Laccone et al., 2002; Turner et al., 2003).

Prader-Willi Syndrome

Prader-Willi syndrome (Prader et al., 1956) results predominantly from a deletion of 15q11–13 on the paternal copy of chromosome 15, although about one-fourth of cases are caused by a uniparental disomy of the maternal copy of the chromosome. Such abnormalities distinguish the etiology from Angelman syndrome, which results from loss of the maternal copy of this region. As with Angelman syndrome, it is most often a sporadic condition and affects about 1 in 16,000 to 25,000 births (Moldavsky, Len, and Lerman-Sagie, 2001). The effect of the genetic abnormality is thought to cause dysfunction of the hypothalamus (Swaab, 1997).

Typical physical features include almond-shaped palpebral fissures, down-turned mouth, hypopigmentation, obesity, short stature, strabismus, and scoliosis. Individuals with this condition typically have a history of hypotonia in infancy with weak cry and poor reflexes and may have had failure to thrive due to poor feeding. They also may have had reduced motor activity and excessive daytime somnolence as children, and some time between 1 and 6 years of age became hyperphagic due to a lack of satiety, which led to obesity. The hyperphagia is associated with hoarding, foraging, stealing food or money to buy food, aggression, and temper tantrums. Individuals often develop medical complications from obesity, including diabetes, hypertension, and obstructive sleep apnea. Additionally, they have hypogonadism and lack a pubertal growth spurt. A small percentage meets the criteria for attention deficit hyperactivity disorder. About half develop obsessive-compulsive disorder, and skin-picking is common. They are typically stubborn, irritable, and aggressive and have poor coping and socialization skills (Dykens et al., 1992; Moldavsky, Len, and Lerman-Sagie, 2001).

Cognitively, these individuals have mild-to-moderate MR or borderline intellectual functioning. They generally have good verbal skills and long-term memory and may be particularly skillful with visuospatial integration, such as completing jigsaw puzzles (Dykens et al., 1992).

Smith-Magenis Syndrome

Smith-Magenis syndrome (A. C. Smith et al., 1986) is a rare condition resulting from a deletion of about 1.5 to 9 Mb in the region of 17q11.2, although the size of the deletion generally does not correlate with the severity of symptoms, which is rather variable (Struthers et al., 2002). This condition is associated with relatively mild facial dysmorphism, which may include a tented, fleshy upper lip, midface hypoplasia, and prominent forehead and chin. Up-slanting palpebral fissures and a broad nasal bridge give a slightly Down syndrome–like appearance. Medical problems associated with this condition include cardiac defects, renal impairment, myopia, hearing impairment, hoarseness, short stature, and hypotonia. Affected individuals are usually sociable and good-natured but have moderate MR and language delays, with receptive language usually better then expressive language. Sleep patterns are generally disrupted because of inverted circadian rhythm, corresponding to diurnal elevations in melatonin (Moldavsky, Len, and Lerman-Sagie, 2001; Gropman, Duncan, and Smith, 2006).

Behavioral issues are prominent in Smith-Magenis syndrome. One behavior that typifies this syndrome is an involuntary, spasmodic hugging of the upper body or clasping the hands below the chin while squeezing the arms tightly to the body, which seems to occur when the individual is happy or excited (Moldavsky, Len, and Lerman-Sagie, 2001). Problematic behaviors include temper tantrums, hyperactivity, impulsivity, aggression, and self-mutilatory behaviors. Depending on the study, between 70 and 100 percent of affected individuals engage in self-injurious behaviors, such as head-banging, wrist-biting, pulling out fingernails or toenails, or inserting foreign bodies in orifices. In fact, picking or pulling out one's nails (onychotillomania) and compulsion to insert foreign bodies into one's body orifices (polyembolokoilamania) may be unique to this condition (Gropman, Duncan, and Smith, 2006).

Other Conditions

Many other disorders are being identified as genetic causes of MR, but most are very rare, given the usually sporadic nature of the occurrence of these types of mutations. Two of the more common conditions are Patau (Patau et al., 1960) and Edwards (Edwards et al., 1960) syndromes (trisomy 13 and 18, respectively). Although they occur more commonly than many of the conditions discussed here, they are more than 90 percent fatal within the first year because of failure of vital organ systems. Only rare cases are known to live through childhood, such as one 19-year-old with Edwards syndrome discussed by Petek et al. (2003).

Another example of a syndrome involving MR occurs with deletion of the 22q13 region, which is near the deleted region in velocardiofacial syndrome. This deletion causes moderate-to- severe MR, severely impaired expressive speech, hypotonia, and dysmorphic features, but individuals lack the significant behavioral problems typically seen with such degrees of MR. The loss of a copy of the *SHANK3* gene, which codes for a structural protein in the post-synaptic density, appears to play a major role in the etiology of these signs and symptoms (Wilson et al., 2003).

Many cases of MR occur without "syndromic" features but are likely caused by genetic factors. Although it can be more difficult to identify the etiology in such conditions, some researchers have identified chromosomal regions that may be involved in intelligence. For instance, Higgins et al. (2000) identified the subtelomeric region of chromosome 3p as such a region by linkage analysis in families with nonsyndromic MR.

Management in the Community

Sharkey and colleagues (2005) provide general guidelines for when to request chromosomal analysis to increase the likelihood of identifying genetic conditions. These recommendations include presence of global neurocognitive delay, craniofacial dysmorphisms, a major malformation, unusual behaviors, abnormal skin patterns (dermatoglyphs), poor prenatal growth, and a family history of learning disabilities, malformations, or multiple miscarriages.

Laboratory Work-up

Although many causes of MR are not identifiable, genetic analyses can be useful in determining the etiology of such conditions. Cytogenetic screening is effective at identifying translocations, inversions, deletions, duplications, and structural chromosomal anomalies, such as ring chromosomes or the fragile X site. Thus, standard karyotyping is useful for confirming DS, as well as other trisomy conditions, or identifying DS cases that result from translocations. Fluorescent in situ hybridization (FISH), which provides multiple-image analyses of chromosomes and chromosome fragments, is useful for identifying microdeletions, such as in Angelman, Prader-Willi, Smith-Magenis, velocardiofacial, and Williams syndromes. More specific analysis of methylation patterns for imprinting can be useful in assessing Angelman and Prader-Willi syndromes. Genotyping is useful for clarifying particular gene mutations. For instance, in the case of Rett syndrome, more than 200 mutations have been identified, with more than 60 percent caused by six particular mutations in the methyl binding domain or transcription repression domain (Turner et al., 2003). It is important to note that many mutations do not have a causal link to the developmental disorder (Laccone et al., 2002).

Neuropsychological Evaluation

Evaluation of neuropsychological function is important to determine individual strengths and weaknesses to optimize treatment approaches. Assessment of affected individuals with MR depends on the age of the individual. Some of the more common assessment tools include the Bayley Scales of Infant Development II for infants and very young children, the Stanford Binet and Wechsler Scales after age 2, the Wechsler Preschool and Primary Scale of Intelligence—Fourth Edition for preschoolers, the Wechsler Intelligence Scale for Children—Third Edition for school-age children, and the Wechsler Adult Intelligence Scale—Third Edition for adults (Wecshler, 2003a, 2003b; Wecshler, 2008). Behavior scales are also important for assessing adaptive behaviors.

Approach to Treatment

Management of cases of MR with genetic causes depends on the particular conditions and the variability of phenotypic expression. Many conditions are associated with medical problems that should be appropriately referred for evaluation and treatment. For instance, individuals with DS should have echocardiography for possible ventral septal defects or endocardial cushion defects, neck x-ray to assess atlantoaxial instability (between the first and second vertebrae) if any breathing problems, pain, or motor deficits occur, and sleep studies if obstructive sleep apnea is suspected. They should also have routine assessments of vision, hearing, gluten-sensitive enteropathy, and thyroid function (Tyler, 2004; Benke, 2005). Persons who have fragile X syndrome may require follow-up with ophthalmology or cardiology (de Vries et al., 1998). Individuals with Williams syndrome may require dietary control of calcium and vitamin D for hypercalcemia, monitoring of cardiovascular conditions and blood pressure, and treatment with surgery, if necessary. They may also benefit from filtered ear protection for hyperacuisis and may require special dental care (Fisch, 2005). Individuals with Smith-Magenis syndrome typically require treatment of gastrointestinal problems, such as constipation or acid reflux (Gropman, Duncan, and Smith, 2006). Treatment of epilepsy with medications is important, as commonly seen in Angelman syndrome (A. C. Smith et al., 1996). Appropriate management of vision and hearing impairments will also help improve the person's quality of life.

Management of behavioral issues is essential in these conditions and should be optimized for the individuals' needs. Controlled environments or assisted living situations can be helpful for individuals with moderate levels of MR, and full-time care may be needed for more severe levels of impairment. Behavioral therapy is helpful for managing symptoms, such as attention deficits, hyperactivity, aggression, and self-injurious behaviors, that are seen in many of these conditions. Furthermore, enhancing communication with sign language can also be useful for helping individuals with language deficits express themselves, thus reducing maladaptive behaviors associated with frustration (de Vries et al., 1998; Gropman, Duncan, and Smith, 2006).

Medications can be useful for treating symptoms in these conditions, but generally have mixed results. For instance, SSRIs are often helpful for treating depression in individuals with DS, as well as anxiety and aggression in fragile X syndrome, although some individuals develop increased activation and outbursts (Hagerman, 1997; Smith, 2001). These medications can also be helpful for treating anxiety in persons with Smith-Magenis syndrome, but medications to treat the inverted circadian rhythm have generally not been as useful in this condition. In fact, beta-blockers have been slightly more useful in blocking daytime melatonin secretion than use of melatonin at nighttime or stimulants in the daytime. Mood stabilizers and antipsychotics have been somewhat helpful for behavioral control but are limited by side effects such as weight gain and adverse effects on lipid levels (Gropman, Duncan, and Smith, 2006). More detailed discussion of treatment with medications can be found in the psychopharmacology chapter of this book.

Considerations for Pregnancy

Parents of children with syndromes involving MR often worry about recurrence in another child. With the exception of fragile X syndrome, these conditions are almost invariably sporadic. Even in that case, women can be tested for the degree of permutation of the fragile X expansion to assess their risks of having a child with this condition, given that an estimated 1 in 259 women are carriers for the permutation (Hagerman, 1997). Risk for DS can be estimated by maternal age and adjusted by the triple screen of protein levels during pregnancy and high resolution ultrasound of the fetus. For more definitive diagnosis of trisomic conditions or the fragile X site, DNA in the fetus can be analyzed by amniocentesis or chorionic villus sampling. Thus, genetic counseling is important for women of advancing maternal age, as well as those with a family history of MR.

In addition to healthy parents having variable risks of having a child with a genetic syndrome, individuals affected by these genetic conditions risk passing these mutations on to their own children. In fact, their risk is 50 percent for autosomal dominant (including trisomy) conditions. Thus, genetic counseling is important for high-functioning individuals with such conditions.

CASE EXAMPLES

Henry, a 29-year-old single man, is brought to your office by his parents, who would like to know what could explain his moderate MR and peculiar behaviors, as no one else in the family has such a condition. He lives with his parents and needs reminders to wash and to change his clothes on a daily basis. He repetitively turns on and off light switches, rocks back and forth, hides food in the refrigerator, talks to himself, and prefers to be alone. Despite a normal pregnancy and delivery, he had global developmental delays in infancy and had been in special education classes through the 12th grade. He missed a lot of school because of recurrent bouts of congestive heart failure until surgical correction of a ventricular septal defect at age 7. What is the diagnosis and prognosis?

As the clinician, you are concerned that Henry may have a genetic syndrome, given the lack of known environmental exposures. You refer the family to a geneticist, who performs a high-resolution karyotype, fragile X molecular test, and FISH for 22q11 deletion. The results show a deletion of 22q11, confirming the diagnosis of velocardiofacial syndrome. You discuss the diagnosis with the family and offer follow-up if Henry develops psychotic symptoms or abnormal changes in mood. ▶

Suzanne, a 23-year-old woman with moderate MR, is brought to your office by her parents, who are concerned about her excessive daytime somnolence. She lives with her parents and is generally sociable and well behaved but occasionally has temper tantrums and bangs her head on the wall or tries to pull out her fingernails if her parents do not intervene. Her parents would like her to sleep at night instead of in the daytime to match their schedule of working and caring for her. How do you manage this case?

Given the history of onychotillomania, altered circadian rhythm, and MR, you are concerned that Suzanne has Smith-Magenis syndrome. You refer the family to a geneticist, who confirms a deletion in the 17q11.2 region of FISH. You discuss proper sleep hygiene with the family and offer a trial of beta-blockers to try to reduce the excess daytime melatonin. ▶

Trevor, a 44-year-old man with DS and mild MR, comes to your office at the recommendation of his primary care physician for forgetfulness and a decline in his job performance at the grocery store over the past two months. His medical workup was normal, but his primary care physician is concerned about dementia. How do you proceed?

You obtain a thorough history from Trevor and find out that he has lost interest in his work and has poor sleep and decreased appetite. There is a low risk that he has Alzheimer disease at this point, but it is important to monitor him for continued decline in functioning. Given his depressive symptoms, you begin a trial of an SSRI to improve his mood and cognitive functioning. ▶

Conclusion

MR results from a multitude of factors, many of them genetic. The most common genetic causes of MR are Down and fragile X syndromes, but community clinicians need to be familiar with several less-common syndromes as well, for each has unique characteristics and implications for management.

Researchers continue working on identifying new genes associated with conditions involving MR and seeking to understand how such mutations affect cognitive functioning. As demonstrated by the conditions discussed in this chapter, we are only beginning to understand the exact genes involved in developmental syndromes and how such genes lead to cognitive impairment. We are also in the early stages of understanding the most effective treatments for these conditions. Nevertheless, it is important for clinicians to be aware of current treatments being studied, as treatments will evolve. Moreover, clinicians need to feel comfortable treating the variety of psychiatric symptoms common in this population and to know when to refer individuals for genetic screening and other appropriate medical care.

References

Amir R, Van den Veyver IB, Wan M, et al. 1999. Rett syndrome is caused by mutations in X-linked MECP2, encoding methyl-CpG-binding protein 2. *Nature Genetics* 23: 185–88.

Angelman H. 1965. Puppet children: A report of three cases. *Developmental Medicine and Child Neurology* 7: 681–88.

Benke PJ. 2005. Down syndrome. In *Griffith's 5-Minute Clinical Consult*. Philadelphia: Lippincott Williams & Wilkins.

Chelly J. 1999. Breakthroughs in molecular and cellular mechanisms underlying X-linked mental retardation. *Human Molecular Genetics* 8(10): 1833–8.

Coppus A, Evenhuis H, Verberne GJ, et al. 2006. Dementia and mortality in persons with Down's syndrome. *Journal of Intellectual Disability Research* 50(10): 768–77.

de Vries BB, Halley DJ, Oostra BA, Niermeijer MF. 1998. The fragile X syndrome. *Journal of Medical Genetics* 35(7): 579–89.

Down JLH. 1887. On some of the mental affections of childhood and youth. London: J & A Churchill.

Dykens EM, Hodapp RM, Walsh K, Nash LJ. 1992. Profiles, correlates and trajectories of intelligence in individuals with Prader-Willi syndrome. *Journal of the American Academy of Child and Adolescent Psychiatry* 31: 1125–30.

Edwards JH, Harnden D, Cameron A, et al. 1960. A new trisomic syndrome. *Lancet* 1: 787–90.

Fisch GS. 2005. Williams syndrome. In *Griffith's 5-Minute Clinical Consult*. Philadelphia: Lippincott Williams & Wilkins.

Gropman A, Duncan W, Smith A. 2006. Neurologic and developmental features of the Smith-Magenis syndrome (del 17p11.2). *Pediatric Neurology* 4: 337–50.

Hagerman RJ. 1997. Fragile X syndrome: Molecular and clinical insights and treatment issues. *Western Journal of Medicine* 66: 129–37.

Higgins JJ, Rosen DR, Loveless JM, Clyman JC, Grau MJ. 2000. A gene for nonsyndromic mental retardation maps to chromosome 3p25-pter. *Neurology* 55: 335–40.

Laccone F, Zoll B, Huppke P, et al. 2002. MECP2 gene nucleotide changes and their pathogenicity in males: Proceed with caution. *Journal of Medical Genetics* 39: 586–88.

Moldavsky M, Lev D, Lerman-Sagie T. 2001. Behavioral phenotypes of genetic syndromes: a reference guide for psychiatrists. *Journal of the American Academy of Child and Adolescent Psychiatry* 40(7): 749–61.

Patau K, Smith DW, Therman E, etal. 1960. Multiple congenital anomaly caused by an extra autosome. *Lancet* 1: 790–93.

Petek E, Pertl B, Tschernigg M, et al. 2003. Characterization of a 19–year-old "long-term survivor" with Edwards syndrome. *Genetic Counseling* 14(2): 239–44.

Prader A, Labhart A, Willi H, Fanconi G. *Ein Syndrom von Adipositas, Kleinwuchs, Kryptorchismus und Idiotie bei Kindern und Erwachsenen, die als Neugeborene ein myotonieartiges Bild geboten haben.* 1956. VIII International Congress of Pediatrics, Copenhagen.

Raynham H, Gibbons R, Flint J, Higgs D. 1996. The genetic basis for mental retardation. *Quarterly Journal of Medicine* 89(3): 169–75.

Rett A. 1966. Über ein eigenartiges hirnatrophisches Syndrom bei Hyperammonämie im Kindesalter. *Wiener klinische Wochenschrift* 76: 609–13.

Sharkey FH, Maher E, Fitzpatrick DR. 2005. Chromosome analysis: What and when to request. *Archives of Disease in Childhood* 90(12): 1264–69.

Shprintzen RJ, Goldberg RB, Young D, Wolford L. 1981. The velo-cardiofacial syndrome: A clinical and genetic analysis. *Pediatrics* 67: 167–72.

Smith A, Wiles C, Haan E, et al. 1996. Clinical features in 27 patients with Angelman syndrome resulting from DNA deletion. *Journal of Medical Genetics* 33(2): 107–12.

Smith AC, McGavran L., Robinson J, et al. 1986. Interstitial deletion of (17)(p11.2p11.2) in nine patients. *American Journal of Medical Genetics* 24(3): 393–414.

Smith DS. 2001. Health care management of adults with Down syndrome. *American Family Physician* 64(6): 1031–38.

Struthers JL, Carson N, McGill M, Khalifa MM. 2002. Molecular screening for Smith-Magenis syndrome among patients with mental retardation of unknown cause. *Journal of Medical Genetics* 39: e59.

Swaab DF. 1997. Prader-Willi syndrome and the hypothalamus. *Acta Paediatrica* Suppl. 423: 50–54.

Swillen A, Devriendt K, Legius E, et al. 1997. Intelligence and psychosocial adjustment in velocardiofacial syndrome: A study of 37 children and adolescents with VCFS. *Journal of Medical Genetics* 34(6): 453–58.

Turner H, MacDonald F, Warburton S, Latif F, Webb T. 2003. Developmental delay and the methyl binding genes. *Journal of Medical Genetics* 40: e13.

Tyler C, Edman JC. 2004. Down syndrome, Turner syndrome, and Klinefelter syndrome: primary care throughout the life span. *Primary Care: Clinics in Office Practice* 31(3): 627–48, x–xi.

Verkerk AJ, Pieretti M, Sutcliffe JS. 1991. Identification of a gene (FMR-1) containing a CGG repeat coincident with a breakpoint cluster region exhibiting length variation in fragile X syndrome. *Cell* 65: 905–14.

Wecshler D. 2003. Wecshler Intelligence Scale for Children, 4th ed. San Francisco: Psychological Corporation.

Wecshler D. 2008. Wecshler Adult Intelligence Scale, 4th ed. San Francisco: Psychological Corporation.

Williams JCP, Barrett-Boyes BG, Lowe JB. 1961. Supravalvular aortic stenosis. *Circulation* 24: 1311.

Wilson HL, Wong AC, Shaw SR, et al. 2003. Molecular characterization of the 22q13 deletion syndrome supports the role of haploinsufficiency of SHANK3/ PROSAP2 in the major neurological symptoms. *Journal of Medical Genetics* 40(8): 575–84.

6

Prenatal Exposure to Toxic Substances

Roxanne C. Dryden-Edwards, M.D.

Given the frequency, preventability, and potentially devastating effects associated with prenatal exposure to toxic substances of any kind, it behooves the general psychiatrist to have a working knowledge of the special issues associated with those conditions and how to manage them. More than 40,000 babies born in the United States every year have problems as a result of exposure to alcohol in utero, and 1 to 2 in 1,000 have full-blown fetal alcohol syndrome (MayoClinic.com, 2008). Cytomegalovirus, the most common congenital infection, affects up to 2 percent of live births worldwide (Lipitz et al., 2002). Some surveys indicate that 20 percent of pregnant women acknowledge smoking during pregnancy (Cornelius and Day, 2000).

By the time many individuals who have suffered the developmental sequelae of exposure to prenatal drugs or other toxicants are assessed by a general psychiatrist, the window for providing acute medical treatment during infancy and childhood is long past. This chapter focuses on interventions that would more likely have an impact on these individuals if they come to the attention of mental health professionals, particularly the general psychiatrist. Although developmental disabilities (DDs) of any cause put individuals who have them at higher risk for exposures to toxicants such as lead throughout their lifetime (Graft et al., 2007), such risks are beyond the already considerable scope of prenatal drug exposures and therefore will not be addressed here.

Fetal Alcohol Spectrum Disorders

Fetal alcohol spectrum disorders (FASDs) are considered the most preventable cause of DD. They are also the most common known cause of mental retardation (MR) in the United States. Some estimate that 40,000 babies born per year in the United States experience some kind of problem related to alcohol intake by the mother during pregnancy, including everything from cognitive limitations and behavioral problems to low birth weight and heart problems (MayoClinic.com, 2008). The incidence of infants who show signs of prenatal exposure to alcohol is up to 12 per 1,000 live births in the United States (University of South Dakota, 2002; Giarratano and Williams, 2007). These numbers take on new meaning when the number of individuals living with fetal alcohol syndrome (FAS) or FASD is examined. In 1999, it was estimated that nearly 8,000 babies were born with FAS and almost 50,000 had an FASD. Also in 1999, it was estimated that about 340,000 adults aged 19 to 69 years had FAS and more than 2 million adults in that age group had an FASD (University of South Dakota, 2002).

There seems to be increased prevalence of FASD in babies born to mothers over 30 years of age, and there can be a genetic predisposition to the disorder. Once socioeconomic status is controlled for, there does not appear to be any association with FASD based on race. While binge maternal alcohol use apparently increases the risk of the fetus developing an FASD, some studies have described an increase in the number and severity of symptoms associated with fetal exposure to alcohol even when the mother has as little as one drink per week.

Although the syndrome associated with prenatal exposure to alcohol was first described by Paul Lemoine in 1968 in France, there are biblical references to mothers being advised to avoid drinking alcohol during pregnancy (O'Leary, 2002). Greek philosopher Aristotle made reference to women who drank while pregnant and then gave birth to disabled children, and in the eighteenth century, reference was made to the children whose mothers were affected by the "gin epidemic" that was the result of exceedingly low gin prices at that time (University of South Dakota, 2002).

Alcohol may cause negative effects for the fetus by acting directly on fetal tissue, arresting or changing cell development, or it may act indirectly as a result of the by-products of alcohol metabolism. Acetaldehyde is one such toxic product of alcohol metabolism that can accumulate in the fetal brain.

Alcohol also has been shown to interfere with nutritional and hormonal factors that are necessary for normal development of the fetus. As a result of these negative effects, children who were exposed to alcohol prenatally often have cognitive and behavioral problems. Overall head size is decreased in children with FAS, with structural changes observed in areas such as the parietal lobes, cerebellum, hippocampus, basal ganglia, and corpus callosum. Individuals with FAS are therefore vulnerable to compromised intellectual functioning, motor abilities, memory, and executive functioning (higher-level cognitive functions involved in planning behavior to achieve goals, solving problems, thinking abstractly, and being flexible).

In addition to affecting brain development, FAS or FASD may place individuals at risk for having a reduction in birth weight, as well as continued growth restriction and muscle weakness. The developing fetus is also at risk for developing a number of heart defects, such as atrial and ventricular septal defects, tetralogy of Fallot, and pulmonary artery stenosis.

To meet diagnostic criteria for FAS, the Centers for Disease Control and Prevention recognize specific assessment criteria. These include documentation of three facial abnormalities (smooth philtrum, thin vermilion border, small palpebral fissures), growth deficits, and central nervous system abnormalities (structural, neurological or functional, or a combination). At birth, newborns with FAS exhibit some combination of head and facial deformities that include long thin upper lips, small eyes, flattened maxilla, and small head. If these deformities are not obvious at birth, the syndrome may be identified later when the infant displays poor sucking, irritability, excess growth of body hair (hirsutism), and failure to thrive. Growth retardation with weight, length, or head circumference below the 10th percentile is another common assessment finding in FAS.

One of the challenges of diagnosing FAS in teens and adults is that many of the physical characteristics of the syndrome fade with age. Unfortunately, most of the myriad cognitive, behavioral, emotional, and social problems brought on by the disorder remain throughout the life cycle (O'Leary, 2002). Functionally, individuals with FAS or FASD often exhibit abnormalities displayed in delayed motor abilities, hyperactivity, and developmental deficits which may unfold over time. Parents may have difficulty bonding and providing appropriate care because of the infant's being easily overstimulated and crying inconsolably. Language, motor, memory, growth, and other developmental milestones are delayed.

By the time the child reaches school age, decreased cognitive functioning, school failure, social problems, and difficulties managing anger and stress may occur. In adolescence and adulthood, difficulties often continue in the form of secondary disabilities, including mental health problems, delinquency, difficulty in maintaining employment or other independent living skills, as well as abuse of alcohol or illicit drugs (Giarratano and Williams, 2007). Adults with FASD tend to have difficulty with abstract reasoning, recognizing the likely consequences of their behaviors, remembering, maintaining good judgment and good self esteem, and managing their impulses. The impulsivity often presents as lying, stealing, and defiant behavior. Emotionally, lifelong risks of FASD include anxiety, attachment problems, attention deficit hyperactivity disorder, conduct disorder, depression, eating disorders, oppositional defiant disorder, suicidality, psychosis, and inappropriate sexual behaviors (University of South Dakota, 2002).

The effects of alcohol on a fetus seem to increase with increasing age of the mother. Although binge drinking is associated with worse outcome than regular alcohol intake in general, no amount of alcohol intake during pregnancy should be considered safe, given the individualized nature of the amount of alcohol that can result in FASD (Williams and Ross, 2007).

Exposure to Other Drugs of Abuse

Research presents somewhat conflicting results regarding the effects of prenatal exposure to cocaine. Some studies indicate few long-term effects of cocaine once the effects of low birth weight, other drugs, and environmental influences are factored in (Frank et al., 2001; Messinger et al., 2004). Other studies show a significantly negative behavioral impact of cocaine on children (Bada et al., 2007). There is also research that finds that cocaine can have a specifically negative impact on language development (Morrow et al., 2003) and that it predisposes children to developing learning disabilities in general. In fact, some research indicates that children who have been exposed to cocaine prenatally may be almost three times as likely to develop a learning disability as children who have not been exposed (Morrow et al., 2006). However, those effects tend to decrease with age and are decreased or increased by positive or negative psychosocial factors, respectively (Singer, Minnes, and Short, 2004; Williams and Ross, 2007).

Marijuana tends to have its primary impact on the attentional abilities of the individual who was exposed prenatally (Williams and Ross, 2007). Although children who are exposed to opiates in utero tend to have slower cognitive and physical development initially, those difficulties tend to resolve by the time they are toddlers as long as other risks for delayed development are ameliorated (Handelsman et al., 2003; Davies and Bledsoe, 2005).

Although a legal toxicant, nicotine has been shown to have a significantly negative effect on language and reading abilities in children up to at least 12 years of age in the absence of exposure to other toxicants. These effects may take place at nicotine levels that are lower than the levels that cause growth retardation. Further, children exposed to nicotine in utero have been found to be at increased risk for becoming oppositional, hyperactive, and aggressive (Cornelius and Day, 2000).

Congenital Infections

A number of congenital viral infections, such as congenital rubella and cytomegalovirus (CMV), can produce microcephaly as a result of intrauterine growth restriction. Herpes simplex virus can result in encephalitis (Laartz et al., 2006). Prenatal infection with herpes viruses, Epstein Barr virus, or CMV has been associated with cerebral palsy (Gibson et al., 2006). Children who are born infected with HIV are at higher risk of developmental delays than are their unexposed counterparts (Handelsman et al., 2003).

CMV is the most common congenital infection in the world (Lipitz et al., 2002). Some 400 to 4,000 cases of congenital toxoplasmosis occur in the United States every year. In addition to the risk of MR, blindness, epilepsy, or death during infancy, some individuals who have this infection first develop seizures when they are 20 to 30 years old (Jones, Lopez, and Wilson, 2003).

Environmental Toxicants

Concerns about in utero exposure to environmental toxicants stem from both the known effects of such exposure and the fact that few of the top 3,000 environmental toxicants have been studied in relation to their effects on a developing fetus (Stein et al., 2002). Of the few that have been studied, the effects of lead, mercury, and polychlorinated biphenyls (PCBs) have been researched the most extensively.

Sources of lead are most commonly lead dust in paint and soil that has been contaminated with lead dust and car emissions. Research describes prenatal exposure to lead as being associated a multitude of problems. Specifically, it appears to increase the risk of MR, reading disability, aggression, hyperactivity, distractability, and antisocial behaviors (Graft et al., 2006). Individuals who were exposed to lead in utero are also more likely to develop more destructive and withdrawn behaviors in preschool (Wasserman et al., 1998), as well as schizophrenia and obesity in adulthood (Opler et al., 2004; *Medical News Today*, 2008). It is noteworthy, however, that the magnitude of the many developmental consequences of prenatal exposure to lead tend to be smaller than those associated with the socioeconomic factors that often accompany such exposure (Wasserman and Factor-Litvak, 2001).

By far, emissions from coal-burning power plants are the most common source of mercury in the atmosphere. That contaminant then falls to the earth and is found in high concentrations in large fish, such as tuna or swordfish, and in whales; it is also found in bass and pike. A high amount of maternal consumption of contaminated fish is the primary source of exposure to mercury in utero. Such exposure increases the risk of MR, attention problems, irritability, cerebral palsy, seizures, blindness, deafness, speech and memory problems, and shyness in exposed children (Graft et al., 2006).

PCBs are primarily found in pesticides and are stored in animal tissues, particularly fat tissue. Therefore, maternal exposure directly to pesticides and indirectly to meat or dairy products that come from animals exposed to pesticides is the primary source of fetal PCBs. Such exposure can result in permanent learning and memory problems as well as hearing loss and behavioral problems (Szpir, 2006).

The Role of the Psychiatrist

Psychiatrists can make a significant contribution both in preventing prenatal drug exposure experienced by the children of their patients and in ensuring that the individuals they treat who have DDs resulting from prenatal exposure to toxicants receive optimal care. While conducting a thorough history and examination of patients may be taken for granted, it is the hallmark of good care and often results in discovering a history of toxic exposure. In addition to referring back to the assessment chapter of this book, the general psychiatrist should ask specific questions that will elicit a history of prenatal exposure to toxicants. For example, asking family members about how much alcohol, tobacco, or other substances may have been taken in by the mother during pregnancy and infections or other illnesses that may have occurred at that time can prove invaluable to identifying individuals with DDs who may have been affected by a prenatal insult. Questions that may not readily occur to the practitioner should be posed as well, including maternal occupations that may have resulted in exposure to toxicants (e.g., working on a farm, in fishing, or in an industrial plant), as well as home and family conditions that may have put the person with DD at risk for exposure to toxicants in utero (e.g., secondhand smoke from smoking family members, the age of the house the family lived in during the pregnancy, the proximity of the home to industrial plants; Graft et al., 2006).

By encouraging both male and female patients to fully participate in their medical and mental health treatment; to avoid exposure to nicotine, alcohol, illicit drugs, and other toxicants; to address any medical or substance abuse issues they may have; and to maintain the highest level of general health before a pregnancy, the general psychiatrist, like any other physician, can reduce the risk of their patients' children's being exposed to prenatal toxicants of all kinds. The psychiatrist can positively affect the outcome of a patient's pregnancy by encouraging good prenatal care and self-care such that the risk of exposure to infection, drugs, or other environmental toxicants is minimized (Durkin et al., 2000; Brosco, Mattingly, and Sanders, 2006). In this regard, patient education is a key factor, given how little awareness the general public has about alcohol intake during pregnancy and its effects on the fetus. For example, some studies indicate that 30 percent of women believe it to be safe to drink during pregnancy and as little as 22 percent of women are even aware of the existence of FAS (O'Leary, 2002).

For patients whose children incur a DD as a result of exposure to a toxic substance, the psychiatrist can play a pivotal role in counseling parents and other caregivers in how to minimize the impact of the exposure and in helping the person with DD to achieve the highest quality of life. For example, the approach that educators take to teaching individuals with DD has been shown to improve when teachers are educated about the students who had prenatal exposure to a toxicant (Watson and Westby, 2003). Knowing which individuals have toxic exposure–based DDs can greatly improve outcomes. For example, interactions that persons with DDs and their families have with social service agencies can lead to behavior- and stress-management training and to respite services, both of which have been shown to improve the quality of life of all involved. A case in point involves an 18-year-old man whose ability to remain in a group home setting rather than in a more restrictive placement was greatly improved once the staff at the group home were educated about the FAS with which he lives. Promoting a household and surrounding community that is high on structure and absent any violence can also have positive effects on the life of the person with DD who was prenatally exposed to a toxic substance (University of South Dakota, 2002).

Understanding the specific challenges individuals and their families face depending on the kind of toxic exposure that occurred can provide psychiatrists important knowledge about specific approaches to the individual with a DD. For example, individuals with FASDs and their families can greatly benefit from knowing that the severe difficulties that the affected individual can have with maintaining emotional structure and consistent behaviors is a result of the condition rather than being purposeful. Psychiatrists can therefore guide persons with FASD and their loved ones to emphasize the need for the individual with FASD to receive information and instructions that are brief, consistent, and repeated, and for the individual to be in home, school, or work environments that are safe, predictable, supportive, and well structured (Chambers and Vaux, 2006).

Conclusion

General psychiatrists will better serve and likely improve the lives of their patients by having at least a cursory knowledge of the tremendous impact that toxic prenatal exposure may have on those they treat. As in nearly all psychiatric work, knowing which questions to ask and then asking them and acting on the answers is almost more important than having the "correct" answers. Knowing how to guide, educate, and learn from individuals with DDs who had prenatal exposure to a toxicant can go a long way to being an effective practitioner and therefore health advocate for the people being cared for.

REFERENCES

Bada HS, Das A, Bauer CR, et al. 2007. Impact of prenatal cocaine exposure on child behavior problems through school age. *Pediatrics* 119(2): 348–59.
Brosco JP, Mattingly M, Sanders LM. 2006. Impact of specific medical interven-

tions on reducing the prevalence of mental retardation. *Archives of Pediatric Adolescent Medicine* 160: 302–9.

Chambers C, Vaux K. 2006. Fetal alcohol syndrome. Available at http://emedicine.medscape.com/article/974016-overview.

Cornelius MD, Day NL. 2000. The effects of tobacco use during and after pregnancy on exposed children. *Alcohol Research and Health* 24(4).

Davies J, Bledsoe J. 2005. Prenatal alcohol and drug exposures in adoption. *Pediatric Clinics of North America* 52(5): 1369–93.

Durkin MS, Khan NZ, Davidson LL, et al. 2000. Prenatal and postnatal risk factors for mental retardation among children in Bangladesh. *American Journal of Epidemiology* 152(11): 1024–33.

Frank DA, Augustyn M, Knight WG, Pell T, Zuckerman B. 2001. Growth, development and behavior in early childhood following prenatal cocaine exposure: A systematic review. *JAMA* 285(12): 1613–25.

Giarratano G, Williams AW. 2007. Gene-environment influences on fetal alcohol syndrome: State of the science. Available at http://journal.hsmc.org/ijnidd 3(2):1.

Gibson CS, MacLennan AH, Goldwater PN, et al. 2006. Neurotropic viruses and cerebral palsy: population based case-control study. *British Journal of Medicine* 332: 76–80.

Graft CJ, Murphy L, Ekvall S, Gagnon M. 2006. In-home toxic chemical exposures and children with intellectual and developmental disabilities. *Pediatric Nursing* Nov–Dec.

Handelsman E, Thompson B, Li D, et al. 2003. Long-term growth and developmental outcomes in children with in utero cocaine and opiate exposure born to HIV-infected women. 10th Conference on Retroviral Opportunistic Infections, Hynes Convention Center, Boston, Feb. 10–14, 10: Abstract no. 770.

Jones J, Lopez A, Wilson M. 2003. Congenital toxoplasmosis. *American Family Physician* May 13.

Laartz B, Gompf SG, Allaboun K, Marinez J, Logan JL. 2006. Viral infections and pregnancy. Available at www.emedicine.medscape.com.

Lipitz S, Achiron R, Zalel Y, et al. 2002. Outcome of pregnancies with vertical transmission of primary cytomegalovirus infection. *Obstetrics and Gynecology* 100: 428–33.

MayoClinic.com. 2008. Fetal alcohol syndrome. Available at www.mayoclinic.com/health/fetal-alcohol-syndrome/ds00184.

Medical News Today. 2008. Unexpected link found between prenatal lead exposure and obesity in males. February.

Messinger DS, Bauer CR, Das Λ, et al. 2004. The maternal lifestyle study: Cognitive, motor, and behavioral outcomes of cocaine-exposed and opiate-exposed infants through three years of age. *Pediatrics* 113(6): 1677–85.

Morrow CE, Bandstra ES, Anthony JC, et al. 2003. Influence of prenatal cocaine exposure on early language development: longitudinal findings from four months to three years of age. *Journal of Developmental and Behavioral Pediatrics* 24(1): 39–50.

Morrow CE, Culbertson JL, Accornero VH, et al. 2006. Learning disabilities and intellectual functioning in school-aged children with prenatal cocaine exposure. *Developmental Neuropsychology* 30(3): 905–31.

O'Leary C. 2002. Fetal Alcohol Syndrome: A Literature Review. Canberra, Australia: Commonwealth Department of Health and Ageing.

Opler MGA, Brown AS, Graziano J, et al. 2004. Prenatal lead exposure, delta-aminolevulinic acid and schizophrenia. *Environmental Health Perspectives* 112(5): 548–52.

Singer, LT, Minnes, S, Short, E. 2004. Cognitive outcomes of preschool children with prenatal cocaine exposure. *JAMA* 291(20): 2448–56.

Stein J, Schettler T, Wallinga D, Valenti M. 2002. In harm's way: Toxic threats to child development. *Journal of Developmental Behavioral Pediatrics* 23(Suppl. 1): 13–22.

Szpir M. 2006. New thinking on neurodevelopment. *Environmental Health Perspectives* February 114(2): A100–107.

University of South Dakota. 2002. *Fetal Alcohol Syndrome Handbook*. Sioux Falls: University of South Dakota School of Medicine and Health Sciences Center for Disabilities.

Wasserman GA, Factor-Litvak P. 2001. Methodology, inference and causation: environmental lead exposure and childhood intelligence. *Archives of Clinical Neuropsychology* 16(4): 343–52.

Wasserman GA, Staghezza-Jaramillo B, Shrout P, Popovac D, Graziano J. 1998. The effect of lead exposure on behavior problems in preschool children. *American Journal of Public Health* 88(3): 481–86.

Watson S, Westby CE. 2003. Prenatal drug exposure: Implications for personnel preparation. *Remedial and Special Education* 24(4): 204–14.

Williams JH, Ross L. 2007. Consequences of prenatal toxin exposure for mental health in children and adolescents. *European Child and Adolescent Psychiatry* 16(4): 243–53.

7

Acquired Brain Injury

Gregory J. O'Shanick, M.D., and
Ronald C. Savage, Ed.D.

Acquired brain injury (ABI) in the developing brain (i.e., infants, children, adolescents, and young adults to about the age of 22 years) is often confusing, both with respect to incidence and prevalence data and to treatment methodologies. ABI is a clinical term that combines populations of individuals who sustained "external physical force injuries" (e.g., blunt trauma to the head, acceleration-deceleration events to the brain, penetrating brain injuries) with those who sustained brain injuries from "internal occurrences" (e.g., birth-related trauma, stroke, infectious diseases, neurotoxic poisonings, anoxia). The former group of ABIs is also referred to as traumatic brain injury (TBI). This chapter describes TBIs and identifies their impact on the developing brain, studies, treatment needs and assessment, and the roles of various caregivers, particularly the psychiatrist. In this chapter, TBI and ABI are used interchangeably.

Traumatic Brain Injury in Children

According to the Centers for Disease Control and Prevention (CDC), TBI is the leading cause of death and disability acquired after birth in children in the United States. CDC data estimate that about 1.7 million children from 2001 to 2004 sustained a TBI serious enough for the child to be referred to an emergency room. The CDC also reports that the annual number of TBI-

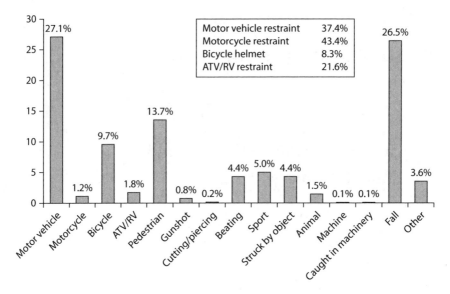

Figure 7.1. Mechanism of injury for traumatic brain injuries in children. Box shows percentage wearing restraints when injured. *Source*: Savage, 1999

related deaths in the 0 to 14 age group is more than six times the number of deaths related to HIV/AIDS, 20 times the number of deaths from asthma, and 38 times the number of deaths from cystic fibrosis. The CDC also reports that among children up to 14 years of age, TBI results annually in an estimated 2,685 deaths, 37,000 hospitalizations, and 435,000 emergency room visits (Langlois, Rutland-Brown, and Thomas, 2004). CDC data do not include children with TBI (e.g., sports-related concussions) who received no medical care or who were seen only in private doctors' offices.

Mechanisms of TBI among children vary by age group. For example, the National Pediatric Trauma Registry reports that children under the age of 5 years are most susceptible to TBI because of falls and assaults (e.g., abuse, shaken baby syndrome). Over the age span of birth to 19 years, the largest cause of TBI was motor vehicle traffic accidents. Children were injured in car crashes as passengers during their younger years or were injured in even greater numbers as drivers when adolescents. Young children are especially vulnerable to being struck by motor vehicles while walking or biking. The trauma registry also found that many of the children and adolescents were not properly restrained (e.g., seatbelts, child safety seats, helmets) in the motor vehicle, which contributed to the severity of the injuries. Figure 7.1 shows a breakdown of the ways in which children receive TBIs (DiScala and Savage, 2003).

The Pathophysiology of Traumatic Brain Injury

The essential microscopic neuropathological finding in TBI, extensively studied in animals and humans, is the widespread and asymmetric disruption of axonal integrity known as diffuse axonal injury (DAI; Strich, 1956). While asymmetric focal cortical contusions and hemorrhaging may also occur as the brain tissue impacts the bony ridges found on the floor of the cranial vault, DAI is the distinguishing feature of TBI. This disconnection, largely random and incomplete, results in a decrease in the speed of interneuronal communication. Classic studies of DAI have centered on the role of acute mechanical shearing of axons at the gray-white interface of the cortex and accompanying microscopic hemorrhaging of adjacent capillaries. As such, the mistaken clinical wisdom that the most severe injury and symptoms occur immediately after the impact has been perpetuated in medical education for decades. More recent studies in humans and other animals (Povlishock and Katz, 2005) define that, in addition to the mechanical tearing of axons (referred to as "cell murder" by some authors), a second etiology of axonal disruption exists. In this process, termed "cell suicide," traumatic mitochondrial damage results in a later loss of the neuronal capacity to sustain its cellular integrity with a subsequent disconnection of the cell body from the axon. This type of DAI may evolve over days to weeks following the initial injury and is not generally accompanied by any hemorrhagic finding. This later "cell suicide," while providing a window of opportunity in the treatment of severe TBI, also explains the often noted and misinterpreted decline in function found in concussive injuries (also known as mild TBI).

The severity of TBI can be defined by several methods, the most commonly used at this time being the Glasgow Coma Score (GCS; Teasdale and Jennett, 1974). A subsequent pediatric version of the GCS was created to address developmental language limitations inherent in applying the adult scale to children. This instrument assesses the patient's acute level of function in three domains (eye movement, verbal response, and motor ability), with scores ranging from 3 to 15. The categories of injury are defined as severe (3–8), moderate (9–12), and mild (13–15). While most researchers view

Table 7.1.   Severity grades of traumatic brain injury

Mild
    Altered or LOC <30 minutes
    With normal CT scan and/or MRI
    GCS 13–15
    PTA <24 hours
Moderate
    LOC <6 hours
    Abnormal CT scan and/or MRI
    GCS 9–12
    PTA <7 days
Severe
    LOC >6 hours
    Abnormal CT scan and/or MRI
    GCS <9
    PTA >7 days

Notes: LOC = loss of consciousness; GCS = Glasgow Coma Score; PTA = posttraumatic amnesia

this as an excellent scale to address moderate and severe injury, its utility in the mild category has been disputed, largely because a score of 15 after the serious event of an impact to the head of acceleration-deceleration event is defined as a mild TBI. Further complicating the GCS' usefulness in mild TBI is the lack of any method to assess short-term memory or attention, two critical changes seen in mild TBI. While sports-related concussion instruments assess these additional domains, the widespread use of such instruments is not prevalent (American Academy of Neurology, 1997). A retrospective means of assessing TBI severity can include measures of length of the period of unconsciousness (if present) or the duration of post-traumatic amnesia, or PTA (the period of time following the TBI from injury to the return of consistent short-term memory functioning). Table 7.1 compares the three different methods of assessing severity.

In 2003, the CDC published and disseminated an education module to physicians that included their case definition of a mild traumatic brain injury:

Injury to the head arising from blunt trauma, acceleration or deceleration forces with one or more of the following conditions attributable to the head injury:

• Transient confusion, disorientation or impaired consciousness;
• Dysfunction of memory around the time of injury; or

- Loss of consciousness lasting less than 30 minutes.
  Any period of observed or self-reported:
- Seizures acutely following injury to the head;
- Irritability, lethargy, or vomiting following head injury, especially among
  infants and very young children; or
- Headache, dizziness, irritability, fatigue, or poor concentration, especially
  among older children and adults.

Acquired Brain Injury from "Internal Occurrences"

Brain injuries as a result of spontaneous vascular insults (e.g. embolic, hemorrhagic, aneurysmal, arteriovenous malformation) are less common causes in children. These result in a focal area of neuronal damage or death that is manifested as a specific neurofunctional deficit governed by the area of injury. While also asymmetric, these lesions do not coexist with a DAI as found in TBI. As such, the recovery of functioning is circumscribed and potentially more amenable to neuroplasticity and a cortical reassignment of those lost functions to either adjacent regions or ipsilateral reassignment. This phenomenon has limits relative to the specialization or certain neuronal populations (e.g., language and age-at-injury vulnerabilities). Studies have defined a poor outcome if such vascular events occur between the ages 6 and 12 months.

The second form of "internal occurrence" ABI occurs in a systemic and symmetrical pattern and includes toxic exposure, infection, anoxic-hypoxic, metabolic, and hypotensive etiologies. Hemispheric symmetry is noted in neuronal damage and can be a function of metabolic rate, as in herpes simplex encephalitis, hypoglycemia, or hypotension (Perlstein and Attala, 1966; Kohl, 1988; Auer, 2004; Alix, 2006; Whitley, 2006) or of vascular supply, as in subcortical "watershed infarcts." This symmetric distribution of damage renders neuroplasticity relying on ipsilateral redistribution of function less effective.

The Developing Brain after Acquired Brain Injury

A child's brain is constantly changing and adapting. Developmental milestones are reached at various ages and stages in children's lives. Therefore, ABI in children needs to be understood within the context of typical brain development, as well as in relationship to the child's age at the time of the injury and the particular regions of the brain that sustained damage. We now understand through long-term studies of children with brain injuries (Max et al., 2006), that neuroplasticity is much more complicated than we previously thought. In addition, as children's brains develop, the world around them also becomes more complex. Learning in school becomes more difficult, social and behavioral expectations increase, and the adult world of competitive work, relationships, and independence looms before them. Thus, TBI needs to be understood as a "developing phenomenon" in children. For example, preschoolers with injuries to the frontotemporal regions of the brain may look medically fine within a few weeks or months after an injury; however, as they age and their brains mature, cognitive and behavioral deficits emerge (Savage and Urbanczyk, 1995).

The conventional thinking about pediatric TBI used to be that the child's brain was resilient to trauma because it was much more "plastic" than the adult brain and could grow new cells and circuits that enabled the child to overcome the effects of TBI. This thinking turned out to be based on little evidence. It was published by Margaret Kennard in 1936 in the *American Journal of Physiology* and is known as the Kennard principle (Kennard, 1936). She took a group of chimpanzees and created lesions (focal damage) in the motor cortex of their brains, the part of the brain responsible for generating skilled voluntary movements. After a period of brief observation, she found that younger chimps were more likely than older ones to recover their ability to perform a skilled action. She attributed this to the fact that the younger chimps were still growing. She developed this into a universal principle that she applied to human children and adults. In retrospect, that research was hardly a solid basis for making the generalization that human children were more likely to overcome the cognitive, motor, emotional, psychosocial, and behavioral consequences of a TBI than were human adults. It turns out that long-term observation of Kennard's chimps showed that the younger chimps that she described as fully recovered developed problems with spasticity and motor control later in their lives as their brains matured and then were required to perform more complex motor tasks (Finger, 1999).

Beginning in the mid-1990s, researchers began accumulating data that directly challenged the validity of the Kennard principle. Marjaleena Koskiniemi, Jeanette White, Barbara Benz, and Cynthia Beaulieu, and others followed the progress of preschoolers and elementary school children who had a TBI of equivalent severity and charted their neurocognitive development over

Table 7.2.   Stages of brain development

Newborn to 6 years
   During this period of overall rapid brain growth, all regions of the brain—those governing
      frontal executive, visuospatial, somatic, and visuoauditory functions—show signs of syn-
      chronous development.
   Children perfect such skills as the ability to form images, use words and place things in serial
      order. They also begin to develop tactics for solving problems.
Ages 7 to 10 years
   The sensory and motor systems continue to mature in random up to about age 7½, when the
      frontal executive system begins accelerated development.
   The maturation of the sensory motor regions that begins at about age 6 peaks just as children
      begin to perform simple operational functions such as determining weight and logical-
      mathematical reasoning.
   By age 10, while visual and auditory regions of the brain mature, children are able to perform
      formal operations such as calculations and perceive new meaning in familiar objects.
Ages 11 to 17 years
   This stage primarily involves the elaboration of the visuospatial functions, but it also includes
      maturation of the visuoauditory regions. Successive maturation of the visuoauditory, visuo-
      spatial and somatic systems reach their maturation peak within 1-year intervals of each
      other.
   Young people enter the stage of dialectic ability.
   Youth in this age range are able to review formal operations, find flaws with them, and create
      new ones.
   Meanwhile, the visuoauditory, visuospatial, and somatic systems of the brain continue
      developing.
Ages 18 to 21 years
   During the final stage of childhood development, which begins around 17 or 18 years, the
      region governing the frontal executive functions matures.
   Young people begin to question information they are given, reconsider it and form new
      hypotheses incorporating ideas of their own.

---

time. One of their studies showed that children younger than 4 years of age did
worse over time than those whose TBI occurred when they were older than 4
and that children younger than 7 years did worse over time than those who suffered a TBI when they were older than 7. The research showed that the younger
the children at the time of the TBI, the more likely they would grow up with
severe, permanent deficits. This is because the developing brain of the toddler
is the foundation of the intellectual house that will be built through preschool,
grades K–12, and college. Significant damage to that foundation will cause big
problems with the house erected on it. The difficult part is that the damage
may not be immediately apparent and will manifest itself sporadically at critical junctures of later life. Time will reveal most wounds (Finger, 1999).

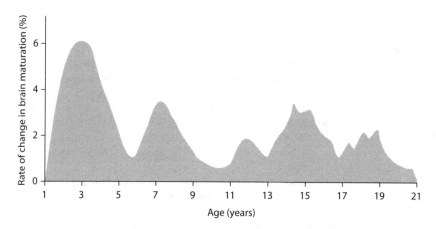

Figure 7.2. Rate of change of maturation increments: All brain regions (in percentages). *Source:* Savage, 1999

Thus, we need to consider the injured brain of a child alongside typical neurological development (i.e., at what age did this injury happen and what regions of the brain were damaged). Individuals normally pass through five developmental stages between birth and 19 years. Table 7.2 summarizes the brain maturation (i.e., brain growth, increased neuroconnections, pruning, and refinement) in typical development and figure 7.2 shows the time at which peaks in neurological development occur (Savage, 1999).

The greatest percentage of brain maturation occurs in the child's early years, birth through age 5. Thus, injury to a child's brain before age 5 may have devastating consequences because the injury occurred at a peak time for neurological maturation. Consider the poor outcomes of infants and toddlers who sustain severe head trauma from being "shaken and impacted" (i.e., shaken baby syndrome). Ewing-Cobbs and colleagues proposed that recovery from severe brain injury may be limited to the skills that were already established at the time of injury. Recovery of previously acquired skills, however, may not necessarily ensure continued development of new and later emerging skills or skills in a rapid state of development at the time of injury (Ewing-Cobbs, Barnes, and Fletcher, 2003; Chapman et al., 2004, 2006).

In addition, because different regions of the brain have varied periods of developmental timing, children who sustain damage early in life to the frontotemporal regions of the brain may continue to see deficits in executive functioning skills. Such behavior challenges can continue to emerge in late adolescence and early adulthood (Figure 7.3).

Last, we are now recognizing that children who have a severe brain injury may be at risk for manifesting what is known as *neurocognitive stall* during the second phase of brain recovery. This neurocognitive stall is a halting or slowing in later stages of cognition and social and motor development beyond a year after brain injury. Thus, despite remarkable recovery during the

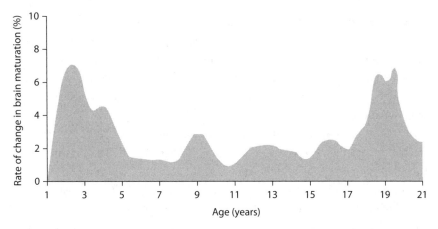

Figure 7.3. Rate of change of maturation increments: Frontotemporal region (in percentages). *Source*: Savage, 1999

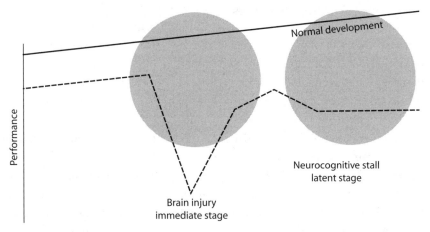

Figure 7.4. Two stages of recovery of pediatric traumatic brain injury. Slope of top of graph shows normal development. Circled dips show decline in growth that occurs at the time of the injury and in the aftermath of the injury. *Source*: Chapman, 2007

first year after a traumatic brain injury, children may appear to "hit a wall" and not meet developmental milestones in their continued cognitive growth. This neurocognitive stall may emerge despite the child's seeming to have recovered cognitive abilities commensurate to the preinjury level (Chapman, 2006; see Figure 7.4).

Optimizing Health and Functioning of Children with a TBI

Nonrestorative sleep is a critical and correctable independent cause of neurocognitive dysfunction across the age spectrum. Two fundamental forms of the problem exist: inefficient and insufficient sleep. To be optimally restorative, one needs to proceed sequentially through the five stages of sleep (stages 1 through 4 and rapid eye movement, or REM, sleep) several times each night. Stages 3 and 4, also known as slow-wave sleep, appear to have significant import in the consolidation of memory and in the overall sense of being refreshed on arising. These stages are vulnerable to the effects of reduced nocturnal oxygen levels (as in sleep apnea, significant gastroesophageal reflux, or severe upper respiratory disturbance) with the effect being excessive sleepiness during the day. Inefficient sleep can also occur in the context of nocturnal pain states that may require the use of antispasticity agents, anti-inflammatory drugs, or, in serious situations, narcotic analgesia.

Nutritional status must also be stable to ensure appropriate recovery from ABI. Deficiencies of vitamin cofactors (B12 and folic acid) involved in neurotransmitter functioning may present as mood, balance, and cognitive dysfunction that will impede progress in recovery after injury. Anemia and dehydration contribute to fatigue and impaired initiation independently of damage to the frontal lobe. Malnourishment, especially protein deprivation, is well recognized as a contributor to impaired neurological development and will delay neurological recovery as well.

Trauma-related pain states adversely affect attention, concentration, and cognitive functioning, both directly and by interfering with sleep efficiency. Optimizing nocturnal pain control is essential to minimizing daytime pain distraction and fatigue. Further, adequate nocturnal pain control decreases the need for excessive daytime analgesia, which directly compromises alertness and learning potential. Spasticity and contractures of muscles influence attention due to localized pain, skin irritation, and pressure sores associated with positioning problems in severely injured children. As the use of oral antispasticity agents is associated with cognitive clouding, reservoir delivery systems (e.g., baclofen pumps) offer an alternative to the need for higher circulating levels of medication through a more focused region of delivery. Spasticity intervention with either botulinum toxin or phenol ablation eliminates central neurocognitive side effects in severe spasticity management (Alexander and Moore, 2001).

Neurological recovery requires the consistent exposure to meaningful sensory stimulation in a graduated manner. When sensory processing is impaired as in visual field cuts, visuospatial/visuointegration deficits, hemi-inattention, auditory processing disorders, and olfactory deficits, recovery is compromised if appropriate adaptations are not used to compensate for these difficulties. In children with neurovestibular damage, tactile defensiveness and kinesthetic learning is altered by faulty postural sensorimotor input. Agitation and inattention may result (Allison, 1992).

While overt seizures obviously impact awareness and rehabilitation efforts, episodic inattention states due to subclinical seizures must be corrected. Lapse-like episodes or abnormal sensory experiences such as micropsia or macropsia, olfactory hallucinations, or unprecipitated vertigo or tinnitus are associated with partial seizure states that may not be detected by routine EEG, whether the result of sleep deprivation or not. An interview-based instrument, the Iowa Interview for Partial Seizure Symptoms, identifies those individuals who display epilepsy spectrum disorders (Hines et al., 1995) and may preferentially respond to anticonvulsant intervention for these phenomena.

While pharmacological intervention is often mandated for the above-noted issues, side effects of medication therapy may compromise sensory awareness, motor skills, and alertness. Critical reviews of these phenomena are available for further reference (O'Shanick, 1997).

Changes Resulting from Brain Injury

Brain injuries can result in a number of changes, some appearing soon after the injury and others appearing as the brain develops. Below are some common changes that are found after a TBI, some indications about how they might manifest themselves in a classroom setting, and some suggestions for teachers in optimizing the learning experience for students with TBIs.

Changes in Attention

The most obvious signs of changes in a child's attention after a brain injury are sleepiness and fatigue. But students may have difficulty with the following:

- paying attention
- filtering out distractions
- dividing attention between two or more topics or activities

In the classroom, students may

- have difficulty following the teacher's instruction or understand a lesson because of an inability to filter out distractions in the classroom or internal feelings or thoughts.
- have difficulties with attention may result in the student talking out of turn, introducing irrelevant topics, or responding inappropriately.

To offset changes in attention, teachers can

- connect new learning to prior knowledge.
- use clearly defined objectives that are meaningful for the student.
- use short and concise instructions and assignments.
- reward on-task behavior.
- use novel, unusual, relevant, and stimulating activities.
- monitor time of day for effects of medications and increased fatigue and arrange rest periods, breaks, or physical activity to minimize fatigue.
- talk with physician about effects of medication on alertness and attention.
- watch for wandering attention and redirect the student to the task when necessary.
- explore many cueing systems (e.g. verbal cues, gesture cues, or written notes to remind the student to stay on task).
- remove unnecessary distractions in the classroom and suggest that parents do so at home where homework is done.
- use verbal cues, such as inserting questions within a lesson and directing attention to the task.

Changes in Perception

Signs that a child has changes in perception include difficulty with the following:

- seeing objects in a part of the visual field
- perceiving spatial orientation of objects
- separating objects from background stimuli
- recognizing objects if too much is presented at once or too rapidly
- scanning and visually searching in an organized manner
- summarizing narrative information
- giving specific information about verbally presented info
- auditory learning
- integrating tactile with visual and auditory information

In the classroom, students may

- be unable to do even easy math problems if they are on a worksheet filled with other math problems.
- be overwhelmed by classrooms with lots of pictures on the wall or lots of noise.
- appear to have weak reading comprehension unless he or she uses a line marker or enlarged print.

To offset changes in perception, teachers can

- move the student's seat closer to the teacher and blackboard and other learning materials.
- describe the visual instructional material in concrete terms.
- limit the amount of visual information on a page.
- give longer viewing times or repeat viewing when using visual instructional materials.
- suggest covering parts of the page to facilitate reading.
- place arrows or cue words, left to right, on the page to orient the student to space.
- teach the student to use the cues systematically to scan left to right.
- provide large print books or use books on tape.
- place materials within the student's best visual field; consult with

an ophthalmologist, optometrist, or occupational therapist about possible visual-perceptual problems.

For students who have greater difficulty with auditory than with visual perception, teachers can offset changes in perception in the following ways:

- limit the amount of information presented
- give instructions or other verbal information in small units
- present verbal information at a relatively slow pace with pauses for processing time and repetition if necessary
- state information in concrete terms; use pictures or visual symbols if necessary
- have the student sit close to the teacher with an unobstructed view
- teach the student to ask questions to ensure comprehension
- teach the student to request slower or repeated presentation if given too rapidly

Changes in Memory

Signs that a child has changes in memory include difficulty with the following:

- recalling events from earlier in the day or from previous days
- following a schedule or keeping track of activities
- registering new information or words recently learned, particularly when under stress
- searching memory in an organized way
- retrieving stored information and words

In the classroom, students may

- fail to complete assignments unless given written reminders or repeated instructions.
- miss classes or do assignments incorrectly.
- need an unexpectedly large number of repetitions to learn simple motor sequences, classroom routines and rules, and textbook information.
- need reminders to repeat information over and over to place something in memory.

- need to search memory to find information that has been previously learned.
- require compensatory strategies to improve memory.

To offset these changes in memory, teachers can

- make the material to be learned significant and relevant to the student.
- match the student's learning style (e.g., visual learner) with the instructional method.
- give meaning to rote data to enhance comprehension and learning.
- summarize information regularly as it is being taught.
- give multisensory presentations.
- control the amount of information given at one time.
- couple new information with previously learned information.
- teach note-taking techniques.
- teach the student to use a datebook for appointments, assignments, and other important information.
- teach one or more of the following techniques: visual imagery, "chunking" techniques (organizing information into easily retrieved segments), association techniques, mnemonic devices such as acronyms, repetition and rehearsal techniques or adaptive devices such as appointment books, calendars, alarm watches, and tape recorders.

Changes in Organization

Signs that a child has changes in organization include difficulty with the following:

- breaking a task into steps or parts
- seeing relationships among things
- organizing objects into groups or events into sequences
- organizing information into larger units
- grasping a major concept from detailed information.

In the classroom, students may

- be unable to decide what to do first when given a task such as getting ready for gym class.
- be able to read sections but be unable put information together and

identify the main ideas to write a short summary for high school English class.

- jump from topic to topic in conversation and appear socially awkward.

To offset changes in memory, teachers can

- make an organizing template for the student to use and add information.
- limit the number of steps in a task.
- provide part of a sequence and have the student finish it.
- give cues, such as "Good, now what would you do?"
- structure thinking by using timelines, outlines, flow charts, graphs.
- use categories to focus on one topic at a time.
- identify the main idea and supporting details.
- categorize details using who, what, when, where, and why questions.
- teach the student to look for these types of details when reading or listening to lecture material.
- ask parents to help students practice organizational skills at home.
- have the student use a checklist to keep on task.

Changes in Reasoning, Abstract Thinking, and Problem Solving

Signs that a child has challenges with reasoning, abstract thinking, and problem solving include difficulty with the following:

- understanding abstract levels of meaning
- drawing conclusions from facts
- considering hypothetical explanations for events
- determining the exact nature of the problem
- considering information relevant to solving the problems
- considering a variety of possible solutions
- weighing the relative merits of alternative solutions.

In the classroom, students may

- do well with basic math calculations; may have great difficulty with solving word problems or with the more abstract relationships in algebra.
- lose the train of conversation when a figure of speech is used.

- forget the locker combination and become upset rather than considering carefully who can help.
- fail to understand a text after one or two readings and still not use strategies to help with comprehension.

To offset changes in reasoning, abstract thinking, and problem solving, teachers can

- clearly and repeatedly define abstract concepts using concrete terms.
- give specific strategies for drawing conclusions from sets of facts
- give specific and repeated instructions on how to connect word math problems to calculations and equations.
- avoid using figures of speech and, when used, define concretely and repeatedly.
- develop a guide to help students through the stages of problem solving (e.g., identify the problem, gather information for solving the problem, create a plan of action, evaluate the effectiveness of the plan).
- ask questions about alternatives and consequences.
- use real-life problems for group discussion.
- promote brainstorming for alternative solutions and their usefulness.
- introduce roadblocks and complications to encourage flexibility.
- give ongoing nonjudgmental feedback.
- break large tasks into sequences of smaller tasks.

Conclusion

Acquired brain injuries in the developing brain adversely affect function not only in the short term but also over the course of the child's life. While differences exist between focal and diffuse tissue damage regarding initial presentation and diagnostic studies, strategies for maximizing success in academic, social, and community endeavors are largely targeted toward specific behavioral challenges that reflect damage to frontal control systems, speed of processing, and acquisition and memory. Comprehensive intervention requires assessment and stabilization of nutritional, neuromedical, pharmacological, and environmental factors to achieve positive outcomes and maximal community independence.

REFERENCES

Alexander J, Moore D. 2001. Primary care for children with brain injury. *North Carolina Medical Journal* 62(6): 349–53.

Alix JJP. 2006. The pathophysiology of ischemic injury to developing white matter. *McGill Journal of Medicine* 9(2): 134–40.

Allison M. 1992. The effects of neurologic injury on the maturing brain. *Headlines* October/November 2–10.

American Academy of Neurology. 1997. Special report: practice parameter: the management of concussion in sports (summary statement). *Neurology* 48: 581–85.

Anderson VA, Catroppa C, Morse SA, Haritou F. 1999. Functional memory skills following traumatic brain injury in young children. *Pediatric Rehabilitation* 3(4): 159–66.

Auer RN. 2004. Hypoglycemic brain damage. *Metabolic Brain Disorders* 19(3–4): 169–75.

Chapman SB. 2006. Neurocognitive stall: A paradox in long-term recovery from pediatric brain injury. *Brain Injury Professional* 3(4): 10–13.

Chapman SB, Gamino JF, Cook LG et al. 2006. Impaired discourse gist and working memory in children after brain injury. *Brain and Language* 97(2): 178–88.

Chapman SB, McKinnon L, Levin HS. 2001. Longitudinal outcome of verbal discourse in children with traumatic brain injury: Three-year follow up. *Journal of Head Trauma Rehabilitation* 16: 441–45.

Chapman SB, Sparks G, Levin HS. 2004. Discourse macrolevel processing after severe pediatric traumatic brain injury. *Developmental Neuropsychology* 25: 37–61.

DiScala C, Savage RC. 2003. Epidemiology of children hospitalized with TBI. *Brain Injury Source* 6(3): 8–13.

Ewing-Cobbs L, Barnes MA, Fletcher JM. 2003. Early brain injury in children: Development and reorganization of cognitive function. *Developmental Neuropsychology* 24: 669–704.

Finger S. 1999. Margaret Kennard on sparing and recovery of function: A tribute on the 100th anniversary of her birth. *Journal of Historical Neuroscience* 8(3): 269–285.

Hines ME, Kubu CS, Roberts RJ, Varney NR. 1995. Characteristics and mechanisms of epilepsy spectrum disorder: an explanatory model. *Applied Neuropsychology* 2(1): 1–6.

Kennard M. 1936. Age and other factors in motor recovery from precentral lesions in monkeys. *American Journal of Physiology* 115: 138–46.

Kohl S. 1988. Herpes simplex virus encephalitis in children. *Pediatric Clinics of North America* 35(3): 465–83.

Langlois J, Rutland-Brown W, Thomas K. 2004. Traumatic brain injury in the United States: Emergency department visits, hospitalizations and deaths. Available at www.cdc.gov/ncipc/pub-res/TBI_in_US_04/TBI-USA_Book-Oct1.pdf.

Max JE, Levin HS, Schachar RJ, et al. 2006. Predictors of personality change due to traumatic brain injury and adolescents six to twenty-four months after injury. *Journal of Neuropsychiatry and Clinical Neuroscience* 18(1): 21–32.

O'Shanick GJ. 1998. Pharmacologic intervention in children and adolescents with traumatic brain injury. In M Ylvisaker (ed.), *Rehabilitation Following Traumatic Brain Injury in Children and Adolescents*, 53–59. Newton, MA: Butterworth-Heinemann.

Perlstein MA, Attala R. 1966. Neurologic sequela of plumbism in children. *Clinical Pediatrics* 5: 292–98.

Povlishock JT, Katz DI. 2005. Update of neuropathology and neurological recovery after traumatic brain injury. *Journal of Head Trauma Rehabilitation* 20(1): 76–94.

Savage RC. 1999. *The Child's Brain: Injury and Development*. Wake Forest, NC: Lash and Associates Publishing.

Savage RC, Urbanczyk B. 1995. Developmental milestones: The impact of brain injury on neurodevelopment. The Perspectives Network.

Strich SJ. 1956. Diffuse degeneration of the cerebral white matter in severe dementia following head injury. *Journal of Neurology, Neurosurgery and Psychiatry* 19(3): 163–85.

Teasdale G, Jennett B. 1974. Assessment of coma and impaired consciousness: A practical scale. *Lancet* 2: 81–84.

Tyler J, Savage R. 2003. Students with traumatic brain injury. In FE Obiakor, CA Utley, AF Rotatori (eds.), *Effective Education for Learners with Exceptionalities*, 299–323. Boston: JAI Publishers/Elsevier Science.

Whitley RJ. 2006. Herpes simplex encephalitis: Adolescents and adults. *Antiviral Research* 71(2–3): 141–48.

8

Assessment of Developmental Disabilities

Stephanie Hamarman, M.D.

The Challenge of Meaningful Diagnosis

Developmental disabilities (DDs) often include mental retardation, autistic spectrum disorders, seizure disorders, and sensory impairments such as deafness and blindness. The term *dual diagnosis* in this context refers to mental retardation plus a psychiatric diagnosis.

What Is Mental Retardation?

Mental retardation (MR) is important to identify and is often missed. MR should be in the differential of every child being examined for DDs. Since the 1960s, there has been increased emphasis on mainstreaming and caring for persons in the community versus institutionalization. Thus, persons with MR are in the community and may present to primary care physicians. Identifying a child with MR can have important consequences for the child's development later, because once he or she has been identified, the mandate from the federal government Americans with Disabilities Act and Individuals with Disabilities Education Act entitles him or her to services.

The definition of MR includes not only an IQ of less than 70 but also difficulties in adaptive functioning (see the *Diagnostic and Statistical Manual of Mental Disorders,* 4th edition, DSM-IV-TR; American Psychiatric Association, 2000). Deficits in adaptive skills can be measured on instruments such as the revised Vineland Adaptive Behavior Scales (Sparrow, Balla, and Cicchetti, 1984). Various levels of MR are specified in the DSM-IV: mild (IQ of 50–70), moderate (IQ of 35–49), severe (IQ of 20–34), and profound MR (IQ < 20). Borderline MR can be noted as a V code. The determination of IQ level is important, as it has consequences for knowing what other comorbid conditions to look for, for treatment, and for prognosis.

Adaptive skills refer to a capacity for personal self-sufficiency on a day-to-day basis. The requirement of adaptive skills in the DSM-IV-TR definition of MR is key because some persons with an IQ below 70 may, when they grow to be adolescents or adults, have learned sufficient adaptive skills that they are able to function totally or largely independently and thus would not technically meet the criteria for MR. This is more typical of persons who as children score in the mild mentally retarded range (Egerton, Bollinger, and Herr, 1984). This DSM-IV-TR definition of MR appears to have better utility than the American Association of Mental Retardation (AAMR; 1992) definition, which disregards the use of IQ in favor of a "needs based assessment relative to 10 different areas of functioning." How IQ is computed dates to 1911 when Dr. Lewis Terman adapted the IQ test by taking the mental age and dividing it by the child's chronological age, then multiplying this equation by 100 to yield the individual's IQ (Reference.com, 2009). It is important to note that adaptive skills can be developed, in contrast to IQ.

The Problem of Diagnostic Overshadowing

Somewhat paradoxically, for many years, the diagnosis of MR tended to cause clinicians and researchers to overlook the presence of associated psychiatric and behavioral problems. That is, many conditions comorbid with MR, when they were noted at all, were assumed to be a function of MR. It was as if the diagnosis of MR overshadowed other psychiatric issues. As Dykens and Volkmar (1997) wrote, the stressors of having a significant intellectual and adaptive deficit should, if anything, make a person more likely to have problems. This *diagnostic overshadowing* originally described by Reiss et al. in 1982 remains a problem in clinical practice (White et al., 1995). Also, there is a separation of MR and mental health services in many states, which is an obstacle to appropriate identification and treatment of mental disorders.

Studies of dual diagnosis (i.e., the presence of both MR and mental illness) typically find prevalence three to six times that in the general population (Bruininks et al., 1996). Others (Rutter et al., 1976) have found the rate of behavioral problems in children with MR to be several times higher: 30 to 42 percent versus children with normal IQ (5.4%). Persons with MR may have a variety of associated clinical features, depending most importantly on their level of retardation. Persons with mild MR have psychiatric difficulties that are fundamentally similar to, but generally more frequent than, those seen in the general population. This is not true for individuals with severe impairment (Dykens, 1999a). Specific medical conditions associated with MR are more likely in a group with an IQ lower than 50, whereas lower socioeconomic status is more frequent in the group with mild MR (Szymanski and King, 1999). People with severe-to-profound MR come to diagnosis at a younger age and are more likely to exhibit related medical conditions, exhibit dysmorphic features, and have a range of behavioral and psychiatric disturbances (Mundy, Seibert, and Hogan, 1984). In contrast, persons with mild MR often come to diagnosis much later, typically when academic demands become more prominent in school, are less likely to have medical conditions that could account for the MR, and usually are of normal appearance without dysmorphic features (Dykens, 1999b). In this latter group, although rates of psychopathology are increased relative to nondisabled populations, the range and nature of problems seen are fundamentally similar to those in normative samples (Syzmanski and King, 1999). Persons with moderate levels of MR are intermediate between these two extremes, and the nature of associated psychiatric and behavioral disorders undergoes a marked shift between the mild and more severe levels of MR (Sovner, 1986).

Patterns of psychopathology and prevalence of specific disorders also differ in persons with or without MR. For example, relative to the general population, some researchers believe that people with MR are more likely to show psychosis, autism, and behavioral disorders and are less likely to be diagnosed with substance abuse and affective disorders (Moss et al., 1997). Others, for example, feel that affective disorders are prevalent in those with MR (Gualteri, 2002).

Genetic Causes and Behavioral Phenotypes

Volkmar and Dykens (2002) discuss psychiatric and behavioral problems that are associated with MR and that a growing body of work focuses on psychiatric and behavioral difficulties relative to specific genetic causes (Hodapp and Dykens, 2001). Features have been identified that are unique or highly frequent to specific syndromes and in some cases to specific genetic or biological processes, such as hyperphagia coinciding with Prader-Willi syndrome (Holm, Cassidy, and Butler, 1993), attention and social problems with fragile X syndrome (Hagerman et al., 1986), inappropriate laughter with Angelman syndrome (Williams et al., 1995), the unusual cry with cri-du-chat syndrome (Gersh et al., 1995), and the self-hug with Smith-Magenis syndrome (Finucane et al., 1994). In some instances, features are relatively syndrome specific, such as the unusual hand-washing stereotypes of Rett syndrome (Van Acker, 1997). More frequently, features are shared in various conditions, such as attention problems are frequent in fragile X, Williams, and cri-du-chat syndromes (Baumgardner et al., 1995; Dykens and Clarke, 1997; Einfeld, Tonge, and Florio, 1997). Opitz (2000) identified more than 750 known genetic causes of MR, and as many as one-third of all people with MR have already been diagnosed with a known genetic disorder (Mononen, Lauriala, and Kaariainen, 1995). With these advances, research regarding behavioral phenotypes is gaining momentum. Examples of some particular phenotypes or syndromes that have unique psychiatric vulnerabilities include increased rates of obsessive-compulsive symptoms in cases of Prader-Willi syndrome (Dykens, 1999b) and anxiety, fears, and phobias in cases of Williams syndrome (Dykens, Hodapp, and Finucane, 2000).

Inherent Difficulties in Assessing Persons with Mental Retardation

A major problem in the assessment of psychiatric disorders in the population with MR is the applicability of traditional DSM or International Classification of Diseases (ICD) diagnoses for persons with MR (Sovner, 1986). Many of these concerns relate to the psychiatric interview itself, including acquiescence, bias, and the limited abilities of many persons with MR to answer questions about the onset, duration, frequency, and severity of symptoms (Moss, 1999).

A comprehensive model of dual diagnosis is lacking in part because existing risk factors for psychopathology in the general population cannot simply be applied to the population with MR because those with MR have unique characteristics. As the severity of MR increases, the presence of psychiatric conditions becomes increasingly difficult to recognize and to distinguish.

This population has difficulty introspecting as well as communicating feelings and thoughts. Self-report is essential for the diagnosis of depressive disorders, anxiety disorders, and schizophrenia (Aman et al., 2003). Clinicians can try to attend to physical manifestations of mental illness (Szymanski, King, and Goldberg, 1998). Extreme cheerfulness, altered sleep and eating patterns, reduction in psychomotor skills, and agitation can be important physical clues for diagnosing a mood disorder. Severe intellectual disability may preclude the presence of certain psychiatric disorders; for example, is it possible for individuals with no expressive or receptive language to communicate that they are experiencing delusions or hallucinations?

Psychiatric illness may change in persons with MR. In the Expert Consensus Survey (Rush and Francis, 2000), experienced workers were asked how confident they were that they could diagnose various psychiatric disorders among a population with MR reliably. Workers were confident in diagnosing autistic disorder much of the time, followed by obsessive-compulsive disorder and major depressive disorder. Some researchers found that conduct disorder and attention deficit hyperactivity disorder (ADHD) seem to be diagnosed with high reliability. Panic disorder, PTSD, and schizophrenia were seen as among the most difficult to diagnose among persons with MR (Aman et al., 2003).

It is not necessarily true that some form of developmental adjustment needs to be made when considering the significance of other ratings of children with MR, because parents and teachers may already make some allowance when rating such children. Mental age is also not a good indicator of what an individual aspires to socially. For example, a teenager with an IQ of 55 usually does not desire to associate with an 8-year-old but rather wishes to be with other teenagers. Some behaviors are not seen in children with typical development, such as pica, stereotypies, and self-injury.

Biopsychosocial Factors

There has been an increased link of persons with MR to have psychopathology based on specific biological problems. These include increased rates of seizure disorders (Bird, 1997; R. Kaplan, Arbelle, and Magharious, 1998); abnormal neurological functioning that is, in most cases, undetected (Peterson, 1995; Robertson and Murphy, 1999); high rates of sensory or motor impairment (Hodapp, 1998); biochemical or neurologic abnormalities associated with unusual behavior, such as self-injury (King, 1993); and genetic causes that carry higher than usual risks of certain maladaptive psychiatric vulnerabilities (Dykens, 1999a).

Psychological risk factors include aberrant personality styles, including an outer-directed orientation and being too wary or disinhibited with others (Zigler and Bennett-Gates, 1999; Dykens, 1999b); atypical motivational styles or abnormal levels of sensitivity to basic human drive, such as the need for attention, the increased risk of negative experiences, which may lead to learned helplessness, low expectancies for success, and depression (Zigler and Bennett-Gates, 1999); negative evaluations of the self instead of not just liking one aspect of the self (Evans, 1998), and the reinforcement of negative behaviors leading to more entrenched maladaptive behavior interactions (Reiss and Havercamp, 1997).

Specific social risk factors include poor communication or assertiveness skills, increased frustration, and acting out behavior (Nezu and Nezu, 1994); social strain, low levels of social support (Lungsky and Havercamp, 1999); social stigma with a subsequent negative impact on daily living, adjustment, and esteem (Edgerton and Gaston, 1991); peer rejection and ostracism (Siperstein, Leffert, and Wenz-Gross, 1997); inappropriate responses to social cues, which may exacerbate stigma and isolation from others (Greenspan and Granfield, 1992); increased risk of exploitation and abuse, which may worsen behavioral and emotional problems (Ammerman et al., 1994); and family stress, including low levels of financial and emotional support (Saloviita, Italinna, and Leoinonen, 2003).

Clearly, there needs to be an assessment of cognitive abilities and adaptive skills, clinical assessment, including a careful developmental and family history, physical examination, and laboratory studies. For example, a strong family history of certain dysmorphic features should raise the possibility of an inherited condition. A history of significant birth trauma, exposure to environmental toxicants, or exposure to marked psychosocial adversity are some factors that should be also considered as part of the assessment of people with developmental disabilities.

Focus on Symptoms, Especially Those That Respond to Medication

Issues often of concern in the developmentally disabled population include hyperactivity, inattention, symptoms of irritability, and aggression toward self and others. In the presentation of autism, some aspects of social behavior can be improved with a reduction in the targeted symptoms of hyperactivity, inattention, irritability, and aggression, although the core symptoms of social impairment may not be treated with medication. In any case, it is important to figure out which symptom is most troubling to the individual. Differential diagnosis can be difficult (for example, telling Asperger disorder from obsessive-compulsive personality disorder). In persons with Asperger disorder, there is a more restrictive pattern of interests and activities and in social relatedness.

The symptoms of motor hyperactivity and inattention occur frequently in people with pervasive developmental disorders (PDD), particularly younger individuals. While the diagnosis of comorbid ADHD is not made if symptoms occur exclusively during the course of PDD, core symptoms of ADHD are often present in persons in the autistic spectrum. It is helpful to think of symptoms that may be responsive to pharmacotherapy. Below are some ways that pharmacotherapy can ameliorate symptoms: (AAMR, 1992):

- reduction of arousal symptoms, such as irritability, aggressiveness, or psychomotor excitement
- improvement in mood symptoms, like labile affect, flat affect and social withdrawal
- improvement in perceptual functioning, like hallucinations
- improvement in cognitive processes, for example, looseness of association or delusions
- improvement in verbal communication as in incoherence; echolalia or mutism
- improvement in behavioral symptoms such as mannerism; stereotypies, echopraxia, negativism, catalepsy, and deteriorated manners
- decrease in rituals and preoccupations

An improvement in the features of ADHD includes reducing excessive motor activity, attention difficulties, the inability to sit still, impulsivity, poorly organized activity, and disruption of others (American Association on Mental Retardation, 1992).

Diagnostic Instruments and Scales

IQ: Psychological Workup

IQ is measured by the Wechsler Intelligence Scale for Children—Fourth Edition (WICS-IV; Weschler, 2003) or Leiter International Test of Intelligence Revised (Ford and Milner, 1997). If the Leiter is not feasible, then the Mullen Scale of Early Development (Mullen, 1995) can be used. Because these tests have different standard deviations and identical scores are not strictly comparable, there are difficulties. The WISC-IV assesses verbal IQ, performance IQ, and full-scale IQ, while the Leiter emphasizes performance IQ. These tests are performed by psychologists as opposed to physicians.

Autism Instruments: ADIR and CHAT

The Autism Diagnostic Interview—Revised (ADIR) is a clinically administered, semistructured instrument designed to aid in the diagnosis of children, adolescents, and adults when autism or another PDD is being considered. ADIR incorporates the clinically oriented DSM-IV and the more research-oriented ICD-10 assessments of autism spectrum disorders (World Health Organization, 1993). ADIR consists of 111 detailed items and usually takes 2 to 4 hours to complete using a parent or other primary caregiver as a principal informant. Because of its length, it is usually used for research purposes only. It addresses three primary areas: social interaction, communication, and repetitive behaviors. It is useful for confirming the clinical diagnosis of autistic disorder, not for measuring change or outcome.

The Checklist for Autism in Toddlers (CHAT) may be helpful (Baird et al., 2001). Included here are the five key items on the CHAT screen: Does your child ever pretend or pretend with other things? Does your child ever use an index finger to point to indicate interest in something? If you point to something, does the child look across to see what you are pointing at? Gain the child's attention and then give the child a toy cup and teapot and say, "Can you make me a cup of tea?" Does the child pretend to pour tea, drink it, and so on? Say to the child, "Where is the light, or show me the light." Does the child point with an index finger at the light? To record yes on this item, the child must look up at your face around the time of pointing.

Some have tried to design instruments to capture unique aspects of dually diagnosed persons that the DSM-IV and ICD-10 and other sources miss. Two of these are the Nisonger Child Behavioral Rating Form (NCBRF) and the Psychiatric Assessment Schedule for Adults with Developmental Disability, Revised (PAS-ADD; Moss et al., 2000). The NCBRF was designed specifically for children with DDs (Aman et al., 1996). It has been noted that, although there are many good standardized instruments for assessing behavioral problems in children of average ability (Aman et al., 1992), it may not be satisfactory simply to use them unchanged for assessing children with MR. This is because the structure and expression of psychopathology may change with cognitive disability (Aman and Singh, 1994).

The NCBRF has 10 social competence scales and 55 items addressing acting out and internalizing behavior, for a total of 65 items. Another scale used is the Aberrant Behavior Checklist (ABC; Aman and Singh, 1994). The ABC was derived by factor analysis, and it has 58 items resolved onto five subscales: (1) Irritability, Agitation, and Crying; (2) Lethargy and Social Withdrawal; (3) Stereotypic Behavior; (4) Hyperactivity and Noncompliance; and (5) Inappropriate Speech.

Aman and his group (Aman et al., 1996) conclude that the NCBRF is an additional tool that will strengthen the set of options available to workers in the MR/DD area and that it appears to be consistent with other research and to provide good coverage for both acting out and internalizing problems.

The PAS-ADD checklist contains 29 items concerning symptoms of psychiatric disorder split into five scales. These five scales are combined to produce three total scores: (1) affective/neurotic disorder, (2) possible organic disorder, and (3) psychotic disorder (Sturmey et al., 2005).

Other Scales That May Be Helpful

There is heterogeneity in clinical presentation among individuals with PDD, so it is important to identify at baseline the predominant symptoms that are the target of treatment, particularly ones that are amendable to pharmacologic intervention. The ABC Irritability subscale encompasses such targets as tantrums, aggression, and self-injury. For changes in repetitive behavior, the compulsion subscale from the Children's Yale Brown Obsessive Compulsive Scale can be useful (Scahill et al., 1997).

To date, there is no comprehensive scale for assessing change in developmentally disabled individuals. The measurement of subtle changes and social behavior is difficult. Until a more comprehensive scale is developed, clinicians and researchers will continue to use rating scales that measure change in particular symptoms clusters of target behaviors.

Visual and Hearing Impairments

Carville (2001) says that research indicates that sensory impairments are more common in persons with intellectual disability. Psychiatric disorders are believed to be more common in children with visual impairment when associated with other disabilities. Some authors believe that hearing impairment can result in personality disorders. Studies have also shown a higher prevalence of psychiatric disorders in children with hearing impairment and higher incidence of deaf people in psychiatric hospitals compared with the general population. Psychiatric disorders in children with hearing impairment are particularly associated with low IQ and low communication ability, especially in those with multiple disabilities. There is little evidence for higher incidence of schizophrenia with hearing impairment. People with visual impairment can demonstrate many autism-like features. Individuals with hearing impairment may also demonstrate some features similar to those persons with autism, but an association with autism has not been conclusively made. Persons with both visual and hearing impairments commonly demonstrate problem behavior (for example, self-injury). Usher syndrome, which is the most common cause of deafness and blindness, is associated with psychiatric disorders, particularly psychosis. The need for assessment of sensory functioning in people with intellectual disabilities, the difficulties inherent in conducting such an assessment, and the need for special services are particularly important. Intellectual disability can coexist with other disabilities (for example, cerebral palsy, epilepsy, psychiatric illness, and sensory impairment; Carville, 2001).

Medical Conditions

Medical conditions vary depending on the cause of the MR (for example, cardiac problems in Down and Williams syndromes and the risk of Alzheimer dementia in adults with Down syndrome). Ryan and Sunada (1997) report that up to 75 percent of persons with MR who were referred for psychiatric assessment have undiagnosed or untreated medical conditions and that nearly 50 percent receive nonpsychotropic medications that could have behavioral side effects. The presence of associated difficulties (for example, seizures, motor impairments, and sensory problems) may further complicate accurate psychiatric diagnosis.

Medical Work-Up

To determine medical conditions that occur with MR, the following medical workup should be completed:

1. A physical examination should be conducted.
2. If psychoneurological signs are found, an MRI of the brain should be considered.
3. If there is evidence of seizures, sleep-deprived EEG (electroencephalogram) should be pursued.

4. All children should have adequate hearing and vision screening.
5. A blood test to rule out fragile X syndrome and urine testing to rule out abnormalities in amino acids or organic acid metabolism should be performed.
6. If there is any learning or cognitive delay, blood lead levels should be considered.
7. Baseline measures of vital signs, height, and weight should be made and monitored.

The physical examination should also include assessment of growth and developmental status and observation for facial features or other physical findings that could suggest a specific medical condition. Persons with MR may be at increased risk of certain medical conditions (Ryan and Sunada, 1997). In a review of a cohort of cases, Mullen (1995) noted that at least 15 percent of patients develop epilepsy by adulthood, and the risk was increased when associated disabilities were present or when there was a history of postnatal injury.

Ryan and Sunada (1997) discuss that medical comorbidity was about double that of people referred to mental health assessment without MR. If there is any atypical feature in a primary psychiatric presentation, an MRI scan of the brain should be done, unless other information suggests investigation for microcalcifications, in which case CT would be used. For example, if there was tremor or liver function abnormalities, copper ceruloplasm may be obtained to rule out Wilson disease. Ryan and Sunada (1997) discuss the importance of analyzing incidents or events that are clearly not generalized tonic, or absence seizures with a videotape of the episodic event. They also state that most incidents are found to be related to anxiety disorder, such as posttraumatic stress disorder or tic disorder. However, if features are atypical or treatment ineffective, tests such as EEG, EKG, and pulse oximetry should be performed. Ryan and Sunada also emphasized the importance of addressing intermittent fatigue with an MRI of the brain or lumbar puncture to assess multiple sclerosis. Intermittent joint swelling and arthralgia should be addressed by testing antinuclear antibodies, erythrocyte sedimentation rate, and rheumatoid factors. Paresthesias warrant that levels of vitamins B1, B2, B6, B12, folate, and niacin be analyzed. If unrevealing, proceed with EMG and full metabolic screen.

Snoring and a history of airway obstruction or brain injury should prompt a sleep study to assess for sleep apnea or other dyssomnia. Flushing rash or other autonomic symptoms should prompt tests to rule out pheochromocytoma, carcinoid tumors, porphyria, autoimmune disorders, Lyme disease, tuberculosis, syphilis, or HIV or other viral problems. Splinting, guarding, and targeted self-injury may be signals regarding pain, and thus the specific site should be evaluated regarding possible pain. An example is peptic ulcer disease detected in a person who is referred for "inappropriate scratching of the stomach area." There should be follow-up of obvious physical signs; for example, a person with hirsutism, rounded face, accumulation of fat between the shoulder blades, centripetal weight gain, and pigmenti stria should be evaluated for Cushing syndrome.

It was interesting that in the Ryan and Sunada study almost all of the people in the sample with MR had no other diagnosis. The most common psychiatric diagnoses were anxiety disorders (including post-traumatic stress disorder and depression). This is in contrast to Aman's study of experts. The physical symptoms found by Ryan and Sunada were rarely part of the patient's chief complaint. The most common conditions that Ryan and Sunada identified were epilepsy (untreated or underdiagnosed in 45.8% of the cases), hypothyroidism (12.7%), Tourette syndrome (11.5%), gastroesophageal reflux (9.7%), severe gross head trauma (8.8%), chronic pain (8.7%), cerebral palsy complicated (6.5%), penetrating brain injury (6.3%), abnormal spike in wave EEG (5.4%), and arthritis autoimmune disorders (5%). Ryan and Sunada examined a total of 1,135 people with MR referred for a mental health assessment. They particularly note that the more commonly seen and undiagnosed or untreated medical problems in these individuals were seizure disorders and endocrine conditions. Ryan and Sunada state that the most common mechanisms by which medical problems influence behavior are indirect. They confer a nonspecific stress on the person's system that interferes with the effectiveness of other treatments and programming the person is receiving. Ryan and Sunada said listening to the individual who can describe events is primary. Nonverbal individuals often will respond in revealing and significant ways using other means of communication (for example, facial expression, body movements, hand movements, drawing, and the use of paper and pencil). This study advocates for unstructured observation time.

What to Make of Speech Delay

Speech delay may be present in persons with DDs. A delay in speech development may be a symptom of many different disorders, including MR, hearing loss, expressive language disorder, psychosocial deprivation, autism, selective mutism, receptive dysphagia, and cerebral palsy (Leung and Kao, 1999). Hearing loss may be conductive or sensory neural. Conductive loss is commonly caused by otitis media with diffusion. Such hearing loss is intermittent and averages losses below 15 to 20 decibels. Sensory neural hearing loss may result from intrauterine infection, kernicterus, ototoxic drugs, bacterial meningitis, hypoxia, intracranial hemorrhage, certain syndromes (such as Pendred, Wartenberg, and Usher syndromes), and chromosomal abnormalities. Sensory neural hearing loss is typically most severe in higher frequencies of sound (Leung and Kao, 1999).

Children with an expressive language disorder fail to develop use of speech at the usual age. These children have normal intelligence, normal hearing, good emotional relationships, and normal articulation skills. The primary deficit appears to be a brain dysfunction that results in an inability to translate ideas into speech. Comprehension of speech is appropriate to the age of the child. These children may use gestures to supplement their limited verbal expression. While a late bloomer will eventually develop normal speech, the child with an expressive language disorder will not do so without intervention (Whitman and Schwartz, 1985). A child with expressive language disorder is at risk for language-based learning disabilities such as dyslexia. Bilingualism is also in the differential of a child with speech delay, and it is an important consideration. A bilingual home environment may cause a temporary delay in the onset of both languages. The bilingual child's comprehension of the two languages is normal for a child of the same age, however, and the child usually becomes proficient in both languages before the age of 5 years.

Receptive aphasia is a deficit in the comprehension of spoken language. Production difficulties in speech delay stem from this disability in comprehension. Children with receptive aphasia show normal responses to nonverbal auditory stimuli. Their parents often describe such children as not listening, rather than not hearing (Leung and Kao, 1999). Most children with receptive aphasia gradually acquire a language on their own, understood only by those who are familiar with them.

How Some Specific Psychiatric Symptoms Present in Mental Retardation

Autism

In their article, "Autism: A Medical Primer," Prater and Zylstra (2002) discuss autism and indicate that there are certain things to look for, such as echolalia, deficiencies in symbolic thinking, self-stimulation, self-injurious behavior, and seizures.

Lecavlier et al. (2004) address behavioral and emotional problems in young people with PDD. They state that ample evidence indicates that young people with PDD present a wide range of behavior and emotional problems, with symptoms of anxiety, depression, and ADHD being the most frequently reported (Gillberg and Billstedt, 2000). The authors also state that an important barrier to the study of behavioral and emotional problems is the heterogeneity of symptoms presented by individuals with PDD. Such individuals often differ significantly in cognitive and adaptive functioning. Also, the nature and severity of autistic behaviors vary and change with development.

Comparisons across studies and generalizations of findings have been hampered by the fact that many studies contain small or clinically referred samples or did not use standardized instruments. There are noteworthy exceptions (Tonge and Einfeld, 2003; Gadow, DeVincent, and Azizian, 2004). There are also studies that compared the severity and prevalence of DSM-IV symptoms in preschoolers and elementary school children to clinic controls and community-based samples. In both studies, the preschoolers with PDD (N = 182) presented with more severe DSM-IV psychiatric symptoms than did their peers in regular and special education and to some extent to non-PDD psychiatric referrals. School-age children with PDDs (N = 301) exhibited a pattern of psychiatric symptoms highly similar to non-PDD clinic referrals. Thus, symptoms in preschoolers were more severe, but those of school-age children were highly similar to non-PDD clinic referrals (Gadow et al., 2004, 2005). The highest screening prevalence in the school-age children was found for ADHD, oppositional defiant disorder, and generalized anxiety disorder (Lecavalier et al., 2004).

Mental retardation is not a diagnostic criterion for PDDs but is frequently present. There should be a high index of suspicion for the diagnosis of MR in any child with or without a PDD showing delayed speech, dysmorphic features (minor abnormalities, hypertonia generally or of the extremities, and general inability to do things for self). There should be an assessment of the maternal pregnancy with the involved child including questions regarding mother's use of tobacco and alcohol, her lifestyle or other risks for sexually transmitted diseases, and weight gain or weight loss, signs of infection, surgery, or hospitalization during pregnancy.

Often extremes in infant temperament are present. Common syndromes to be aware of include Down syndrome, fetal alcohol syndrome, fragile X syndrome, and velocardiofacial syndrome. Also, according to Daily, Ardinger, and Holmes (2000), if the child with MR has a head circumference below the 5th percentile or above the 95th percentile, an MRI scan of the brain should be considered.

Seizure Medications

Treatments for epilepsy and other medical conditions may carry some behavioral toxicity, which can increase the likelihood of diagnosed mental illness in persons with MR. Phenobarbital has been widely reported to increase the risk of motoric hyperactivity and disinhibition in children and individuals with developmental disorders, and phenytoin may cause cognitive toxicity, as is the case for essentially any of the medications used for the management of epilepsy (B. J. Kaplan and Sadock, 1995).

ADHD

For persons with MR, the diagnosis of ADHD is qualified as being excessive for the individual's mental age. In the context of profound MR, attention span, distractibility, or on-task behavior are predictably variable, thus making the diagnosis of ADHD difficult if not impossible (B. J. Kaplan and Sadock, 1995).

Impulse-Control Disorders

Another set of disorders include the impulse-control disorders of self-injury and aggression. Self-injurious behavior and aggression are common in MR and increase with the severity of the cognitive disability. Self-injurious behavior typically takes the form of chronic repetitive and frequently stereotypic behavior causing trauma. It may occur in the context of specific genetic syndromes, such as the self-biting in Lesch-Nyhan syndrome and finger and nail pulling in the Smith-Magenis syndrome, but more commonly occurs in persons with unknown or nonspecific causes for the MR. Self-injurious behavior was specifically cited as a reason for referral in 36 percent of 251 cases examined. Self-injurious behavior as a presenting syndrome is generally not helpful in predicting the ultimate psychiatric diagnosis. The single exception may be the diagnosis of stereotypic movement disorder, which was specifically created to capture persons who engage in self-injurious behavior in the absence of another psychopathologic diagnosis. Because self-injurious behavior and aggression are nonspecific symptoms, it is recommended that the clinician take into account the presence or absence of a variety of factors to arrive at a presumptive diagnosis (B. J. Kaplan and Sadock, 1995). Among these factors are the chronicity of the behavior, whether it may serve a communicative function, whether it is invariant, whether it occurs in context with regression from a previous level of function, and whether associated neurovegetative signs correlate with it.

Anxiety Disorders

Some individuals who are clearly avoidant, who exhibit autonomic arousal in the face of stimuli that most of their peers would not find aversive, and who present with other features of anxiety but cannot articulate their subjective state, might be given a diagnosis of anxiety disorder, not otherwise specified (NOS). An individual with MR may not be able to identify suggestive anxiety as an underlying cause of distress and an individual's aggression or agitation may be suggestive of a disorder of impulse control rather than reflective of underlying anxiety. Indeed, common symptoms of anxiety in the population with MR include aggression, agitation, compulsive or repetitive behavior, self-injury, and insomnia. Panic may be expressed as agitation, screaming, crying, or clinging that might even pass as delusional or paranoid behavior. Phobias may also occur in this population and may be even more common in persons with DDs. Ryan and Sunada (1997) noted that persons with DDs are at high risk for abuse, thus placing this population at a greater risk for posttraumatic stress disorder, making this disorder an important diagnosis to consider in individuals with MR (B. J. Kaplan and Sadock, 1995).

Eating Disorders

The diagnoses of anorexia and bulimia are precluded for individuals with severe or profound retardation. Rather, it appears that pica is the most common eating disorder among persons with MR.

Psychosis

The diagnosis of schizophrenia requires that a person relate the experience of delusions or hallucinations, so, as Leung and Kao (1999) suggested, in individuals with profound MR and limited communicative ability, the diagnosis of classic schizophrenia is arguably impossible. Nonetheless, some individuals display presumptive evidence of response to hallucinations (for example, striking or shouting at empty space or throwing imaginary peers from furniture) or may adapt catatonic postures that appear to be psychotic in origin. In these persons, the diagnosis of psychosis, NOS, should be considered.

Learning problems, social skill deficits, and low self-esteem are often associated with DDs and are risk factors for the development of mood disorders. Differences may emerge among persons with severe-to-profound disability but equivalents of mood disturbance are easily recognizable, including irritability, crying, problems in sleep and appetite, regulation, agitation, social withdrawal, and isolation. Aggression or self-injurious behavior may be seen as a behavioral manifestation of dysphoria, regardless of developmental level. These symptoms for the diagnosis of depression were codified in a manual giving criteria for use with adults with MR (B. J. Kaplan and Sadock, 1995; Royal College of Psychiatrists, 2001).

Sleep disorders ultimately require the subjective input of the patient regarding adequacy of rest, recurrence of nightmares, and so on.

It may be difficult to distinguish between an impulse-control disorder, NOS, perhaps characterized by an individual's engaging in impulsive or aggressive acts, and an anxiety disorder, NOS, perhaps suggested by an individual who strikes out in the context of a stressor that most people would not notice. One suggested approach to maladaptive behavior that because of a lack of diagnostic specificity for each of these symptoms, the diagnostic decision tree can not be constructed; it is more useful to ask a series of questions about the expression of a particular behavior. If the behavior is of recent onset, one is more likely to consider an acute medical or psychiatric cause. If the behavior is highly situational, occurring primarily in the context of a stress of task demands, the likelihood of a psychosis or mood disorder is probably reduced. If attempts are made to avoid the behavior by self-restraint, it may be that some ego dystonic features are present (B. J. Kaplan and Sadock, 1995).

Conclusion

Assessing persons with developmental disabilities has many challenges. One challenge is knowledge of mental retardation and how individuals with mental retardation may present psychiatrically, because psychiatric symptoms are often more difficult to identify in this population. Diagnostic overshadowing (i.e., misattributing all of a patient's psychiatric symptoms to mental retardation and thus completely missing the psychiatric symptoms) is also a problem. It is important to be aware of specific genetic causes and particular behavioral phenotypes in the developmentally disabled population. Biological, psychological, and social factors are important to consider in the assessment and formulation of a treatment plan. It is key to focus on symptoms that may respond to medication. A variety of diagnostic instruments and scales can be helpful: IQ testing, particular autism assessment instruments (ADIR and CHAT), the ABC, and the Children's Yale Brown Obsessive Compulsive Scale. Visual and hearing impairments are important comorbid conditions that must be identified and addressed. A good medical workup to identify and treat co-occurring medical conditions is also vital, as is an assessment of any speech delay.

References

Aman MG, Lindsay RL, Nash PL, et al. 2003. Individuals with mental retardation. In A Martin, L Scahill, and DS Charney (eds.), *Psycho-pharmacology: Principles and Practice*, 617–30. New York: Oxford.

Aman MG, Singh NN. 1994. *Aberrant Behavior Checklist: Community Supplementary Manual*. East Aurora, NY: Slosson Educational Publications.

Aman MG, Singh NN, Stewart, Field CJ. 1992. Psychometric characteristics of the aberrant behavior checklist. *American Journal of Mental Deficiency* 89: 492–502.

Aman MG, Tasse MJ, Rojahn J, Hammer D. 1996. The Nisonger CBRF: A child behavior rating form for children with developmental disabilities. *Research in Developmental Disabilities* 17(1): 41–57.

American Association on Mental Retardation. 1992. *Mental Retardation: Definition, Classification and Systems of Support*, 9th ed. Washington, DC: American Association of Mental Retardation.

American Psychiatric Association. 2000. *Diagnostic and Statistical Manual of Mental Disorders*, 4th ed., text rev. Washington, DC: American Psychiatric Association.

Ammerman RT, Hersen M, Van Hasselt VB, Lubetszky MJ, Sieck WR. 1994. Maltreatment in psychiatrically hospitalized children and adolescents with developmental disabilities: Prevalence and correlates. *Journal of the American Academy of Child and Adolescent Psychiatry* 33: 567–76.

Baird G, Charmin T, Cox A, et al. 2001. Current topics: Screening and surveillance for autism and pervasive developmental disorders. *Archives of Disease in Childhood* 84: 471.

Baumgardner TL, Reiss AL, Freund LS, Abrams M. 1995. Specification of the neurobehavioral phenotype in males with fragile X syndrome. *Pediatrics* 95: 744–52.

Bird J. 1997. Epilepsy and learning disabilities. In O Russell (ed.), *Seminars in the Psychiatry of Learning Disabilities*, 1st ed., 223–44. London: Gaskell Publishers.

Bruininks RH, Woodcock RW, Weatherman FR, Hill BK. 1996. *Scales of Independent Behavior,* rev. ed. Boston: Riverside Publishing.

Carville S. 2001. Sensory impairments, intellectual disability and psychiatry. *Journal of Intellectual Disability Research* 45(6): 467–83.

Daily DK, Ardinger HH, Holmes GE. 2000. Identification and evaluation of mental retardation. *American Family Physician* 61(4): 1059–67.

Dykens EM. 1999a. Direct effects of genetic mental retardation syndromes: Maladaptive behavior and psychopathology. *Review of Research in Mental Retardation* 22: 1–26.

Dykens EM. 1999b. Personality-motivation: New ties to psychopathology, etiology, and intervention. In E Zigler and D Bennett-Gates (eds.), *Personality Development in Individuals with Mental Retardation,* 249–70. Cambridge: Cambridge University Press.

Dykens EM, Clarke DI. 1997. Correlates of maladaptive behavior in individuals with 5p- (cri du chat) syndrome. *Developmental Medicine and Child Neurology* 39: 752–56.

Dykens EM, Hodapp RM, Finucane BM. 2000. *Genetics and Mental Retardation Syndromes: A New Look at Behavior and Interventions.* Baltimore: Paul H. Brookes.

Dykens EM, Volkmar FR. 1997. Medical conditions associated with autism. In DJ Cohen and FR Volkmar (eds.), *Handbook of Autism and Pervasive Developmental Disorders,* 2nd ed., 388–407. Hoboken, NJ: Wiley.

Edgerton RB, Bollinger M, Herr B. 1984. The cloak of competence after two decades. *American Journal of Mental Deficiency* 88: 384–51.

Edgerton RB, Gaston MA. 1991. *I've Seen It All: Lives of Older Persons with Mental Retardation Living in the Community.* Baltimore: Paul H. Brookes.

Einfeld SL, Tonge TB, Florio T. 1997. Behavioral and emotional disturbance in individuals with Williams syndrome. *American Journal of Mental Retardation* 102: 45–53.

Evans DW. 1998. Development of the self-concept in children with mental retardation: Organismic and contextual factors. In I Burack, RM Hodapp, E Zigler (eds.), *Handbook of Mental Retardation and Development,* 462–80. Cambridge: Cambridge University Press.

Finucane BM, Konar D, Haas-Givler B, Kurtz M, Scott CI. 1994. The spasmodic upper body squeeze: A characteristic behavior in Smith-Magenis syndrome. *Developmental Medicine and Child Neurology* 36: 78–83.

Ford L., Milner B. 1997. Leiter International Performance Scale—Revised (Leiter-R). Wood Dale, IL: Stoelting.

Gadow KD, Devincent CJ, Azizian A. 2004. Psychiatric symptoms in preschool children with PDD and clinic comparison samples. *Journal of Autism and Developmental Disorders* 34: 379–93.

Gadow KD, Devincent CJ, Pomeroy J, Azizian A. 2005. Comparison of DSM-IV symptoms in elementary school aged children with PDD versus clinic and community samples. *Autism* 9(4): 392–415.

Gersh M, Goodard SA, Pasztor LM, et al. 1995. Evidence for a distinct region causing a cat-cry in patients with 5p deletions. *American Journal of Human Genetics* 56: 1404–10.

Gillberg C, Billstedt E. 2000. Autism and Asperger syndrome: Coexistence with other clinical disorders. *Acta Psychiatrica Scandinavica* 102: 321–30.

Greenspan S, Granfield M. 1992. Reconsidering the construct of mental retardation: Implications of a model of social competence. *American Journal of Mental Retardation* 96: 442–53.

Gualteri CT. 2002. *Brain Injury and Mental Retardation: Psychopharmacology and Neuropsychiatry.* Baltimore: Lippincott, Williams & Wilkins.

Hagerman RI, Jackson AW, Levitas A, Rimland B, Brandon M. 1986. An analysis of autism in 50 males with the fragile X syndrome. *American Journal of Medical Genetics* 23: 359–74.

Hodapp RM. 1998. *Development and Disabilities: Intellectual, Sensory and Motor Impairments.* Cambridge: Cambridge University Press.

Hodapp RM, Dykens EM. 2001. Strengthening behavioral research on genetic mental retardation syndromes. *American Journal of Mental Retardation* 160: 4–15.

Holm VA, Cassidy SB, Butler MG. 19993. Prader-Willi syndrome: Consensus diagnostic criteria. *Pediatrics* 91: 398–402.

Kaplan BJ, Sadock, VA. 1995. Psychopathology and mental retardation. In BJ Kaplan, VA Sadock (eds.), *Comprehensive Textbook of Psychiatry*, 6th ed., 2207–41. Baltimore: Lippincott Williams & Wilkins.

Kaplan R, Arbelle S, Magharious W. 1998. Psychopathology in pediatric complex partial and primary generalized epilepsy. *Developmental Medicine and Child Neurology* 40: 805–11.

King BH. 1993. Self-injury by people with mental retardation: A compulsive behavior hypothesis. *American Journal of Mental Retardation* 98: 93–112.

Lecavalier L, Aman MG, Hammer D, Stoica W, Matthews GL. 2004. Factor analysis of Nisonger Child Behavior Rating Form in children with autism spectrum disorders. *Journal of Autism and Developmental Disorders* 34: 709–21.

Leung A, Kao C. 1999. Evaluation and management of the child with speech delay. *American Family Physician* 59(11): 3121–8, 3135.

Lunsky Y, Havercamp SM. 1999. Distinguishing low level of social support and social strain: Implications for dual diagnosis. *American Journal of Mental Retardation* 104: 200–204.

Mononen T, Lauriala K, Kaaiainen RA. 1995. A population-based study on the causes of severe and profound mental retardation. *Acta Pediatrica* 84: 261–66.

Moss SC. 1999. Assessment: Conceptual issues. In N Bouras (ed.), *Psychiatric and Behavioural Disorders in Developmental Disabilities and Mental Retardation*, 18–37. Cambridge: Cambridge University Press.

Moss SC, Emerson E, Bouras N, Holland A. 1997. Mental disorders and problematic behaviors in people with intellectual disability: Future directions for research. *Journal of Intellectual Disability Research* 41: 440–47.

Moss SC, Emerson E, Kiernan C, et al. 2000. The PAS-ADD Checklist, rev. ed. Brighton, UK: Pavillion.

Mullen EM. 1995. Mullen Scales of Early Learning. Circle Pines, MN: American Guidance Service.

Mundy P, Seibert S, Hogan A. 1984. Relationship between sensorimotor and early communication abilities in developmentally delayed children. *Merrill-Palmer Quarterly* 30: 33–48.

Nezu CM, Nezu AM. 1994. Outpatient psychotherapy for adults with mental retardation and concomitant Psychopathology: Research and clinical imperatives. *Journal of Consulting and Clinical Psychology* 62: 34–42.

Opitz JM. 2000. Vision in the search for gene mutations causing mental deficiency. *Neurology* 55: 335–40.

Peterson BS. 1995. Neuroimaging in child and adolescent neuropsychiatric disorders. *Journal of the American Academy of Child and Adolescent Psychiatry* 34: 1560–76.

Prater C, Zylstra R. 2002. Autism: A medical primer. *American Family Physician* 66(9): 1667–74.

Reference.com. 2009. Lewis Terman. Available at www.reference.com.

Reiss S, Havercamp SH. 1997. The sensitivity theory of motivation: Why functional analysis is not enough. *American Journal of Mental Retardation* 101: 553–66.

Reiss S, Levitan GW, Szyszkoj. 1982. Emotional disturbances and mental retardation: Diagnostic overshadowing. *American Journal of Mental Deficiency* 86: 567–74.

Robertson D, Murphy D. 1999. Brain imaging and behavior. In N Bouras (ed.), *Psychiatric and Behavioural Disorders in Developmental Disabilities and Mental Retardation*, 49–70. Cambridge: Cambridge University Press.

Royal College of Psychiatrists. 2001. *Diagnostic Criteria for Psychiatric Disorders for Use in Mental Retardation*. London: Gaskell Publishers.

Rush AJ, Frances A. 2000. The expert consensus guideline series: Treatment of psychiatric and behavior problems in mental retardation. *American Journal of Mental Retardation* 105: 159–228.

Rutter M, Tizard I, Yule W, Graham P, Whitmore K. 1976. Research report: Isle of Wight studies, 1964–1974. *Psychology and Medicine* 6: 313–32.

Ryan R, Sunada K. 1997. Medical evaluation of persons with mental retardation referred for psychiatric assessment. *General Hospital Psychiatry* 19(4): 274–80.

Saloviita T, Italinna M, Leoinonen E. 2003. Explaining the parental stress of fathers and mothers caring for a child with intellectual disabilities: A double ABCX model. *Journal of Intellectual Disability Research* 47(4–5): 300–312.

Scahill L, McDougle CJ, Williams SK, et al. 1997. Children's Yale-Brown Obsessive Compulsive Scale modified for pervasive developmental disorders. *Journal of the American Academy of Child and Adolescent Psychiatry* 45: 1114–23.

Siperstein GH, Leffert IS, Wenz-Gross M. 1997. The quality of friendships between children with and without learning problems. *American Journal of Mental Retardation* 102: 111–25.

Sovner R. 1986. Limiting factors in the use of DSM-III with mentally ill/mentally retarded persons. *Psychopharmacological Bulletin* 22:1055–59.

Sparrow S, Balla D, Cicchetti D. 1984. Vineland Adaptive Behavior Scales. Circle Pines, MN: American Guidance Service.

Sturmey P, Newton JT, Cowley A, Bouras N, Holt G. 2005. The PAS-ADD checklist: Independent replication of its psychometric properties in a community sample. *British Journal of Psychiatry* 186: 319–23.

Szymanski L, King BH. 1999. Practice parameters for mental retardation and co-morbid mental disorders. *Journal of the American Academy of Child and Adolescent Psychiatry* 38 5S–31.

Szymanski LS, King BH, Goldberg B. 1998. Diagnosis of mental disorders in people with mental retardation. In S Reiss and MG Aman (eds.), *Psychotropic Medications and Developmental Disabilities: The International Consensus Handbook*, 3–17. Columbus: Ohio State University Press.

Tonge BJ, Einfeld SL. 2003. *Psychopathology and Intellectual Disability: The Australian Child to Adult Longitudinal Study*. San Diego: Academic Press.

Van Acker R. 1997. Rett's syndrome. In DI Cohen and FR Volkmar (eds.), *Handbook of Autism and Pervasive Developmental Disorders*, 2nd ed., 60–93. Hoboken, NJ: Wiley.

Volkmar FR, Dykens E. 2002. Mental retardation. In M Rutter, E Taylor (eds.), *Child and Adolescent Psychiatry*, 4th ed., 697–710. Oxford: Blackwell Science.

Wecshler D. 2003. Wecshler Intelligence Scale for Children: Technical and Interpretative Manual, 4th ed. San Antonio, TX: Psychological Corporation.

White MJ, Nichols CN, Cook RS, et al. 1995. Diagnostic overshadowing in mental retardation: A meta-analysis. *American Journal of Mental Retardation* 100: 293–98.

Whitman RL, Schwartz ER. 1985. The pediatrician's approach to the preschool child with language delay. *Clinical Pediatrics* 24: 26–31.

Williams CA, Zori RT, Hendrickson I, et al. 1995. Angelman syndrome. *Current Problems in Pediatrics* 25: 216–31.

World Health Organization. 1993. *The ICD-10 Classification of Mental and Behavioral Disorders: Clinical Descriptions and Diagnostic Guidelines*. Geneva: World Health Organization.

Zigler E, Bennett-Gates D (eds.). 1999. *Personality Development in Individuals with Mental Retardation*. Cambridge: Cambridge University Press.

PART III •

COMMUNITY
LIVING

9

Community Integration, Living Alternatives, and Employment

Ramakrishnan S. Shenoy, M.D.

In the past thirty years, the concept of community living for individuals with developmental disabilities (DD) has undergone a radical and dramatic change. In 1967, state-operated centers and "training schools" dominated long-term care and served 195,000 residents. In 2003, these numbers shrank to 48,000, and there is evidence that this number is still shrinking rapidly (Braddock and Hemp, 2003). The reasons for this shift are many, including improved understanding of long-term care methods, advocacy by groups that see institutional care as less than desirable, legal remedies such as the Americans with Disabilities Act (ADA; 1990) political pressures to reduce state budgets for long-term care institutions, and the availability of federal programs such as the Medicaid 1915(c) home and community-based waiver program (Miller, Ramsland, and Harrington, 1999). In this chapter, the terms *developmental disabilities* and *mental retardation* (MR) are used synonymously. Even though DD can exist without MR, the issues and problems are similar, as are approaches to evaluation, treatment, and placement.

Living Arrangements

The home and community-based waiver program has given an impetus to the efforts to relocate individuals with DD into community group homes and intermediate care facilities for the mentally retarded (ICFMRs). The waiver program provides funds for community supports for persons who carry a diagnosis of MR and have significant deficiencies in their health status and skill levels, communication, task-learning, self-care, mobility, behavior, and community living. States may have slight variations in this list, but they follow similar evaluations to determine eligibility for the funds. The waiver program is considered "the payer of last resort," which means that individuals cannot be eligible for other or public funding to support their needs.

Of historic interest is the *Olmstead* decision (*Olmstead v. L.C.*, 1999), in which the Supreme Court gave individuals with DDs a right to community placement if professionals concur that such placement would be beneficial and if the state can reasonably accommodate those services. In *Olmstead*, the Supreme Court stated, "recognition and unjustified institutional isolation of persons with disabilities is a form of discrimination and reflects two evident judgments": (1) "institutional placements of people with disabilities who can live in, and benefit from, community settings perpetuates the unwarranted assumptions that persons so isolated are incapable or unworthy of participating in community life" and (2) "confinement in an institution severely diminishes everyday life activities of individuals, including family relations, social contacts, work options, economic independence, educational advancement and cultural enrichment." This decision covers not only people in institutions but also people with disabilities who are at risk of institutionalization, including people with disabilities on waiting lists to receive community-based services and support. The Court indicated that one way states can show they are meeting their obligations under the ADA and the *Olmstead* decision is to develop a "comprehensive, effectively working plan for placing qualified people with mental disabilities in less restrictive settings." Based on this, almost all states have developed or are in the process of developing such plans. In support of these state efforts, President George W. Bush issued Executive Order 1317: Community-Based Alternatives for Individuals with Disabilities (the Olmstead Executive Order) on June 18, 2001, in which he extended application of the Supreme Court *Olmstead* decision to all Americans with disabilities and called on selected federal agencies, including the U.S. Department of Labor, to support governors in their implementation of the *Olmstead* decision.

Humanitarian movements and empirical studies have emphasized the positive results of moving developmentally disabled individuals to community homes (Conroy and Bradley, 1985; Dagnan et al., 1995). A comprehensive study done in Oklahoma by Spreat and Convoy in 2001, using 346 individuals with MR of ages ranging from 15 to 69, compared community living with life in two different institutions. Using objective measures of adaptive behavior, community integration, service provision, and health care indicators, the authors found better community integration and adaptive behavior in the individuals who were moved to the community. Some negative factors were noted with community placement, including unmet needs in the technology area (e.g., communication devices, motorized wheelchairs). This was later remedied when the Assistive Technology Act was passed into law in 1998. This act provided funding to all states to support and promote public awareness of assistive technology, to improve access to technological devices, to rewrite state laws and policies to promote better and quicker access, and to provide outreach support. The other deficiency in community placement was and continues to be the fact that persons with MR residing in the community have more difficulty accessing medical care than those who live in institutions. A study (Golding, Emerson, and Thornton, 2005) confirmed the long-held belief that individuals placed in special community-based residences showed a significant increase in domestic skill activity, a decrease in observed occurrence of problem behaviors, an increase in the quality of life, and an increase in engagement and staff contact.

In the Developmental Disabilities Assistance and Bill of Rights Act of 2000, Congress found that "disability . . . does not diminish the right of individuals with DDs to live independently, to exert control and choice over their own lives, and to fully participate in and contribute to their communities through full integration and inclusion in the mainstream of the economic, political, social, cultural and educational mainstream of United States society" (Section 101(a)(1)) and that "the goals of the Nation properly include the goal of providing individuals with developmental disabilities with the information, skills, opportunities and support to . . . live in homes and communities in which such individuals can exercise their full rights and responsibilities as citizens" (Section 101(a)(16)(B)) and "achieve full integration and inclusion in society in an individual manner, consistent with unique strengths, resources, priorities, concerns, abilities and capabilities of each individual" (Section 101(a)(16)(E)).

In the field of MR, experts believed that individuals became disturbed as a result of learned responses, such as environmental conditioning and caregiver management (Bouras, 1995). The idea was that if individuals with MR were integrated into the community, the presence of behavioral and psychiatric symptoms would disappear. This proved to be a fallacy, because once community integration started, the need for behavioral and mental health services increased because of changing the definitions of acceptable behavior. Behaviors that were tolerated in institutions were viewed as abnormal in the context of mainstream society (Cutler, 2001). The consequence of this shift in populations was that behavioral issues that had been addressed in institutions then had to be addressed in community settings (Menolascino, 1983).

The process of the move from institutional to community-based settings was itself fraught with hurdles. The individuals who were shifted had been accustomed to the same routines of care, feeding, and day programs or workshops for many years. The disruption of this routine led to placement failures and return to the institution in the early days of deinstitutionalization. In more recent times, health care professionals have recommended and have had greater success with gradual transitions and by emulating the structure of the institution for a longer period of time. The individual is then weaned off of his or her previous way of life by gradual exposure to the community.

Community residences are either ICFMRs or group homes. ICFMRs must comply with Title XIX of the Social Security Act and provide health and rehabilitative services and active treatment for individuals receiving services toward the achievement of a more independent level of functioning or an improved quality of life. ICFMRs generally serve individuals that have significant physical limitations and MR but do not need full-time nursing care. The individuals they serve need more intensive training and supervision than may be available in a group home. In addition, the individuals being served are not able to self-administer medications or respond to emergency situations such as fire or natural disasters. In contrast, group homes are a congregate residential service providing 24-hour supervision in a community-based, homelike dwelling. These services are provided for individuals with MR needing assistance, counseling, and training in activities of daily living or whose service plan identifies the need for a specific type of supervision or counseling available in this setting.

In most states, group homes admit six to eight residents. These individuals are more mobile and functional than those in ICFMRs and participate in community activities and day programs and make decisions with the help of their legally authorized representatives. Some states have crisis stabilization services that include temporary intensive services and support that avert emergency psychiatric hospitalization or institutional placement or prevent out-of-home placement. The aim is to stabilize the recipients and strengthen the current living situation so that the person with a DD can be maintained in the community during and after the crisis (Virginia Department of Mental Health, Mental Retardation and Substance Abuse Services, 2000).

Community residences use programs such as day support, behavioral support, habilitative services in the field of activities of daily living (hygiene, improved behavioral functioning and effectiveness, improved eating habits, etc.), and behavior-management programs for more disruptive behaviors. Most programs use clubhouse programs to allow persons with DDs to make decisions about activities and improve social and vocational functioning through skills training, peer support, vocational rehabilitation, and community resource development (Virginia Department of Mental Health, Mental Retardation and Substance Abuse Services, 2000). All clients receive case-management services and access to timely medical and dental services. In the initial phases of deinstitutionalization, obtaining adequate services in the community for medical and dental disorders lagged behind the institutional facilities. This has been ameliorated to a certain degree because of better training of newer physicians. Some institutions, such as the Northern Virginia Training Center in Fairfax County, Virginia, have created novel programs to address this issue by using institutional resources to offer services such as dental care, occupational therapy, and behavioral intervention to the community.

Most communities have a shortage of psychiatrists experienced or trained to deal with the mental health problems of the mentally retarded / developmentally delayed population. MR is frequently comorbid with mental illness, and prevalence estimates range from 30 to 70 percent. The data have not been accurately assessed, primarily because health care providers may not be properly trained to diagnose mental health disorders in this population. Kerker et al. (2004) suggested in an article summarizing 52 articles on this subject that methodological limitations of previous research inhibit confidence in study results. To have accurate estimates of prevalence, the curricula of all health care providers should be reviewed and updated to incorporate classroom and clinical experience in MR. Diagnostic approaches have to be modified, depending on the cognitive level of the individual. The presence of communication deficits adds to the complexity of the diagnostic evaluation that is essential before a treatment regimen is suggested. Interview times are longer than with an individual who does not have MR, and medical insurance carriers frequently do not reimburse for this extra time. The psychiatrist's role is complex but can be manageable and rewarding, given some creativity. The role of the psychiatrist as a part of a team of individuals that assist developmentally disabled persons in their community is further discussed in the next chapter on systems management. The psychiatrist has to act as coordinator of medical and behavioral care.

Individuals with MR/DD may have significant health problems. Studies have shown that older adults with MR/DD often die at an earlier age than do adults in the general population. In one survey of 2,752 adults 40 or older, the average age at death was 66.1 years, though many adults with MR/DD live as long as their peers in the general population (Janicki et al., 1999). Many of the disorders that affected this group were the same as those of the average general older population, including cardiovascular, respiratory, and neoplastic disease. The communication problems and cognitive difficulties of the MR/DD population can sometimes cause the diagnosis to be missed or made late. With the emphasis on preventive measures, this trend of earlier death is certain to reverse. Greater emphasis on training of primary care physicians and gerontologists in how to examine and treat clients with MR/DD will also help the situation.

In the community, psychiatrists who work with persons with MR/DD are located in clinics run by community service boards (CSBs) or work in private practice. The CSBs employ psychiatrists, case managers, therapists, and nurses who work as a team to deliver comprehensive mental health services. Some CSBs have specialized MR teams that deal with the more complex cases. The case managers act as liaison between the family homes or the community group homes and the treatment providers. The case manager can also help in crisis situations by arranging for respite care or hospitalization in cases of acute exacerbations of psychotic behavior or severe aggression. The psychiatrist generally works with medication prescription and adjustment, monitoring side effects. Clinics vary in their effectiveness in treating the mentally ill MR population. The biggest obstacle in this type of system is the shortage of mental health professionals who have the background or training to deal with complexity of diagnosis and treatment of clients with MR/DD who also have a mental illness.

The psychiatrist in private practice faces a number of hurdles in dealing with the mentally ill MR/DD population. This is a relatively new field, and few medical schools or graduate programs train students in this field. Most private practitioners work without the assistance of a team. In these circumstances, the most effective method of evaluation and treatment of individuals with MR/DD is by the practitioner making group home visits. In this way, he or she would be able to assess the clients in their natural settings. Training of group home staff to recognize symptoms of mental illness and to distinguish those symptoms from those of physical discomfort is essential. The psychiatrist should participate in team meetings in the group home, where direct care staff, managers, behavioral therapists, and other professionals (e.g., nutritionists) gather to make or revise treatment plans. The psychiatrist can also serve to alert the primary care physicians about unusual symptoms or departures from established behaviors that may be a harbinger of physical illness.

CASE EXAMPLE

Julie, a 35-year-old female with pervasive developmental disorder, autism, and moderate MR, was evaluated by a psychiatrist. She demonstrated numerous behaviors, including screaming, self-injury, stripping clothes off her body, and stereotypical rocking and crawling. With adjustment of her medications, her symptoms improved considerably. She, however, had persistent symptoms of loss of weight, clutching her abdomen, and grimacing with occasional screaming. Her direct care staff complained that she had frequent bulky stools. The psychiatrist brought the matter to the attention of her primary care physician, who ordered a series of tests and discovered that she had gluten sensitivity. With a gluten-free diet, all her symptoms disappeared and she gained weight. ▶

With the advance in knowledge of genetic syndromes and their associated behaviors, psychiatrists are in the best position to pick up clients in their workload who could benefit from genetic testing. Privacy laws should be strictly adhered to in these cases and informed consent obtained from parents or legally authorized representatives so that they could be referred to a center for genetic testing. If a genetic syndrome is discovered, the psychiatrist can play a major role in counseling the parents or other caregivers about the repercussions and also modify the treatment plan to accommodate or modify the genetic aspects of the client's behavior.

Former U.S. Surgeon General Dr. David Satcher held a conference on "Health Disparities and Mental Retardation" in Washington, D.C., in 2001, which included parents, providers and persons with MR. A report, "Closing the Gap: A National Blueprint to Improve the Health of Persons with Mental Retardation," was published in 2002 and contained the recommendations of the conference (Alexander, 2002). The goals of closing the gap were ambitious and are summarized as follows:

1. Integrate health promotion into the community environment of people with MR. This includes improving education of individuals with MR in self-care and wellness, supporting families and direct support persons, and protecting people with MR from occupational hazards.
2. Increase knowledge of health and MR. Identify research priorities, establish a national research agenda, and understand and use research findings.
3. Improve the quality of health care for people with MR by addressing standards of care and the role of practice and by improving the organization and financing of health care to persons with MR.
4. Train health care providers in the care of adults and children with MR. This includes basic and specialized training of health care providers, continuing education for established providers, interdisciplinary education and training, and provider competencies.
5. Ensure that health care financing produces good health outcomes for adults and children with MR.
6. Increase sources of health care services for adults and children, ensuring that health care is easily accessible for them

A few existing programs address the special medical and psychiatric needs of individuals with MR/DD. Third-year students at the Boston University School of Medicine participate in a program in which they are invited to select volunteer family homes of children with special needs. The project, named Operation House Call, helps the medical student in the formative years of his or her career to understand the needs of the families who have children with a DD. In addition, students receive didactic education that covers legal rights, special education, and community resources among other topics of interest in the field of MR/DD. The effect of the program is to sensitize students to the issues of individuals with MR/DD and to train them to be able to listen to patients of all types. The goal of the program was that, with appropriate training, especially before they enter practice, health professionals could learn to see and value the person rather than just perceiving the disabling condition.

The Southern Illinois School of Medicine Division of Developmental Disabilities offers a Technical Assistance Program to enhance psychiatric services to individuals with MR/DD. It assists individuals with MR/DD whose psychiatric disorder and challenging behavior interfere with their ability to function and place individuals at risk for losing their living or work environment, which would prevent them from achieving their maximum potential. It is implemented in collaboration between the Southern Illinois University School of Medicine's Division of Developmental Studies and the Illinois Department of Human Services, Division of Developmental Disabilities. The program does approximately 40 interventions a year. Interventions are done by personal interviews with staff or families or by teleconference. The aim is to help the staff or caregivers understand the cause and remedy for the maladaptive behavior (Southern Illinois University School of Medicine, 2007).

Examples of innovative programs like the ones mentioned abound. Unfortunately, there seems to be little evidence of widespread coordination of resources to enable a unified provision of services to people with MR/DD with concomitant mental illness and to their families or caregivers. Though academic educational and psychology programs have curricula to train professionals to deal with individuals with MR/DD and their families, medical schools have not, in general, contributed to filling the void. Reimbursement for services and lack of grant support may be factors in this matter.

In the United Kingdom, MR has been a recognized psychiatric subspecialty for more than 150 years and there are more than 200 consultant psychiatrists in the field who undergo 3 to 4 years of additional training after a basic psychiatry residency. Increasingly, the subject of DDs is being introduced into the undergraduate curriculum of medical students and general practitioners. British nurses working in the field of MR have received specialized training and qualifications since 1919 and this training is being extended to social workers and psychologists (Day, 1993). The United Kingdom is also working toward different service models like subregional units, community-based services with a small admission facility, integrated services, and spe-

cialty teams for individuals who have MR/DD and severe behavioral problems. Offenders with both mental illness and MR/DD are treated in a three-
level service system. The majority of individuals are treated in semisecure
units in local MR hospitals. Those requiring a higher degree of security are
served in medium security units. Special hospitals provide the highest level of
security for those convicted of the more serious crimes.

Learning to deal with a person with MR/DD can be daunting to the neo-
phyte, even to the experienced psychiatrist. The tools that psychiatrists use
to diagnose and treat mental illness, such as history and mental status examination, are not practical in assisting persons with MR/DD. In these individuals, language, if present, is often difficult to understand because of speech
problems. Cognitive deficits prevent the obtaining of a comprehensive history. Parents or relatives can give accurate developmental and childhood histories, but they are often unavailable or no longer in the custody of the individual in question. The best practice in this situation is to obtain and read all
available material about the individual, including the history of the mother's
pregnancy, developmental milestones, childhood illnesses, behavior problems in infancy and childhood, school issues and behavior in school. In the
southern states, special education programs were not available until relatively recently in rural and poor school districts. School records should be interpreted with caution in these cases. The psychiatrist should be aware of
the cultural and socioeconomic status of the client and take that into consideration during the evaluation. Parents who are educated, are urban, and have
a higher socioeconomic status often pursue diagnostic testing earlier than
those who are poor and uneducated. No evaluation should be carried out
without obtaining adequate documents from the caregiver if at all possible.
These include previous childhood medical and psychological evaluations,
documented changes in behavior, major illnesses or head injuries, genetic
testing, history of seizure disorders, and records of all medications taken. In
a comprehensive official action paper, the American Academy of Child and
Adolescent Psychiatry (1999) published detailed practice parameters for the
assessment and treatment of children, adolescents, and adults with MR and
comorbid mental disorders. This is a comprehensive summary of what a psychiatrist needs to know in the field of MR/DD and should be required reading for all practitioners in the field.

In the community, individuals who have dual diagnosis of MR/DD and
mental illness pose the greatest challenge to successful community place-

ment. These individuals tend to have high-intensity, low-frequency behaviors (such as physical aggression, arson, suicidal threats, and severe self-injury) or low-intensity, high-frequency behaviors (such as public masturbation, refusals to attend day programs, food grabbing, or stereotypic behaviors like biting of fingernails). The former set of behaviors pose a threat to the safety of the resident and others, while the latter can compromise the comfort of the other residents or offend community norms of behavior. In case of the high-intensity behaviors, the community provider frequently requests acute hospitalization and occasionally that the individual return to the institution. Despite the rapid deinstitutionalization of the MR/DD population, community treatment resources have lagged behind because of the limited number of professionals with clinical expertise who can provide effective mental health treatment for this population. Bird and colleagues describe a small study of 10 individuals who failed in their community placements because of aggression, property destruction, and suicidal ideation. In their study these individuals were provided an environment emphasizing a network of mental health and DD services (Bird, Sperry, and Carrevio, 1998). The program focused on application of psychiatric rehabilitation principles that included intensive case management services, staff training, and social-interpersonal skill development. Emphasis was placed on minimizing environmental factors that often set the occasion for and maintained challenging behaviors by developing functional communication systems that enabled individuals to adaptively identify emotions, needs and wants. Plans were tailored to meet the individual needs of each person in the study. Other components of the study were competency-based skills training, community skills acquisition, medication services, and medication self-management. The program model also acknowledged and incorporated the culture of the participant into the diagnosis, treatment, and support services.

Environmental determinants of outcome of community placement are not fully understood. There is no international consensus about the important variables that can determine the relationship between environmental characteristics and outcome of placement. Broad conclusions can be cited from the evidence available: Higher-functioning individuals tend to be more involved in household and community activities. When at all possible, individuals should reside in normal houses with access to various functional spaces. Staffing levels need to be matched to the support needs of residents. Overstaffing and understaffing can be detrimental to outcome. Attention should be placed on staff orientation. The amount and nature of staff attention residents receive can have a significant effect on the residents (Felee and Emerson, 2001).

A variable that has not been explored fully has been the quality of the staff in community-based group homes and other residential settings. Working with a client who has MR/DD as well as behavioral or psychiatric problems can be challenging and demanding for the direct care staff involved with the implementation of behavior and recreational programs. Unfortunately, most programs do not offer pay commensurate with the amount of stress involved in the work. As a result, staff turnover is high, and retaining competent staff people for long periods of time is a challenge. Physical or mental abuse of clients, though not frequent, can and does happen in these situations. In many cases, the psychiatrist is the person who detects the incident of abuse.

CASE EXAMPLE

Angelo is a 40-year-old man who lived in a group home in the community. He came from an abusive background, and his mother had been terminated from guardianship. He was mildly mentally retarded and had bipolar disorder, mixed. He was progressing fairly well until recently, when he became more withdrawn, mute, and almost catatonic. He refused to participate in community activities, withdrew from the day program, and even tried to run away. There seemed to be no precipitant to this new behavior. There was no evidence of noncompliance with medication or any physical ailments that could be detected. After several weeks, the psychiatrist asked him whether any untoward events had occurred in the group home. He described an incident of abuse from a staff member. This person had been terminated because of another complaint. It was suspected that he had post-traumatic stress disorder. Following exploration of this incident and reassurance, Angelo started to improve.

It was estimated in the 1990s that about 60 percent of individuals with MR/DD lived with their families (Fujiura, 1998). Since the increase in Medicaid waiver funding for community group homes, the percentage is probably smaller. Unlike a situation where someone is taking care of an elderly person, the parents' caregiving role in taking care of a child with MR/DD is long. If the individual had maladaptive behavior and had good health, the families tended to request placement in community homes. An additional variable that tended toward placement was the family in which the mother had greater education. A study of parental stress by the same authors concluded that parents reported more stress when the young adult with MR/DD was male and had behavior or mental health problems (McIntyre, Blacher, and Baker, 2002). A study of 105 families (Hayden and Goldman, 1996) indicated that the marital status of the caregiver, the level of retardation and health status of the adult family member with MR/DD, the frequency of maladaptive behaviors, and the number and level of services needed were factors in the stress experienced by families.

The funding for residential care in the community is from different sources, the largest one being the Medicaid waiver program. Policy makers have, in the past few years acknowledged the importance of providing specific support to families that take care of their relatives who have MR/DD (e.g., in the Developmental Disabilities Assistance and Bill of Rights Act of 2000). In 2000, states spent about $69 million to provide cash subsidies to 25,800 families and an estimated $980 million in family support services. This did not include the Supplemental Security Income (SSI) program, which is the single most important family support program. Several states have tried family subsidies to meet the needs of individuals with MR/DD who live with them. This has led to the move toward a budget that is tailored to the need of each individual to enable him or her to achieve the lifestyle desired. Some foundations have picked up on these initiatives and have nurtured these projects (Bernet, 2003).

The psychiatrist plays a crucial role in supporting parents, siblings, and relatives who take care of their relatives with MR/DD. The birth of a child with MR/DD can be profoundly traumatic to the caregivers. Diagnosis is often made at birth or early childhood. The psychiatrist should play a role in counseling the family and by encouraging genetic testing if appropriate. Behavior problems and mental illness usually have a later onset, around adolescence or later. The psychiatrist can evaluate and diagnose the condition and can treat the mental illness and coordinate behavioral interventions as necessary. If the parents or caregivers are unable to care for the individual because of parental health or the individual's behavior problems, the psychiatrist can recommend an appropriate community or institutional placement.

CASE EXAMPLE

Randall, a 40-year-old man with mild MR secondary to perinatal complications, had no behavior problems until about 3 years ago. He had increasingly become irascible with behavior problems and indulged in impulsive
erratic behavior, such as compulsive drinking of fluids, and in verbal aggression. There was no family history of mental illness. He was psychiatrically
hospitalized six times in the course of the year. He was diagnosed with
obsessive-compulsive disorder and treated with clomipramine. This made
him more aggressive. Adding antipsychotic medications did not help. The
parents who were the caregivers were not involved in the treatment by the
treating psychiatrist. The father, who was the guardian, requested a second
opinion from another psychiatrist, who made the diagnosis of bipolar affective disorder, mixed, withdrew the clomipramine and added a mood stabilizer valproic acid. Within days, Randall improved dramatically. The psychiatrist helped to refer him to a suitable community group with the support of
the parents. ▶

This case illustrates how the psychiatrist trained in evaluating and treating
individuals with MR/DD can play a major role in dealing with the families
of these individuals. Understanding the phenomenology of disorders such as
bipolar disorder and how it varies in individuals with MR/DD was essential
in understanding and establishing an accurate diagnosis. Contacts with community resources helped speed up the placement of this individual.

The question of whether the adult with MR/DD who lives with the family
enjoys "quality of life" has been researched. The strong and close family
bonds add to the quality of life of those who live at home. In spite of this,
families' experiences vary widely. Many studies predict a high quality of life,
but some show cause for concern. Some of these factors include severe behavior problems that make it more difficult for the adult MR/DD to have a
close relationship with his or her parents and siblings. Siblings then become
less willing to be the successor caregivers. Nonparticipation in a day program
makes it less likely for the individual to receive other nonresidential services
and less likely for the parent to know about service system options. These individuals also are at risk for emergency placement not consistent with the
wishes of the parents. Men with MR/DD are less likely than their female counterparts to have friends. Women, in contrast, are less likely to have a sibling

be willing to become the successor caregiver. These risk factors should be taken into consideration by the case manager and other staff who deal with these families (Seltzer and Krauss, 2001).

Several factors that have come into play in the past decade have affected care of individuals with MR/DD. These factors include aging of the caregivers, the increasing longevity of people with MR/DD, the growing waiting lists for services in states, the Olmstead Act and access to Medicaid services litigation and the budgetary constraints the states are facing. Community residential services were being provided to 460,455 persons in the states in 2002. Private and nonprofit service providers mostly operated these residential homes. The residential care capacity doubled between 1986 and 2002, an average of 5 percent per year (Rizoll et al., 2004). State-by-state estimates of the size of the aging cohorts in each state are not available but the total number in residential care was estimated to be 707,549 persons in 2002. The psychiatrist should work with the family to ensure that a successor caregiver is designated before the parents get too feeble or incapacitated to make a clear decision. States vary in the way a legal authorized representative can be designated. The psychiatrist should be familiar with the laws governing the procedure in his or her state.

A study of death rates in persons with MR found that in children the highest death rates occurred in skilled nursing facilities, large institutions, and community residences (Eyman, Borthwick-Duffy, and Call, 1988). This seems logical because these children were mostly nonmobile or tube fed and had acute illnesses. In contrast, residents in this category living in their own homes, foster homes, or a health facility had a much lower death rate. In the older age categories, the highest mortalities occurred in skilled nursing facilities. The mortality rate was two to three times higher than that found in other placements. Compared with large institutions, skilled facilities are privately run and have smaller and less-trained staff.

Employment and Leisure

In the 1990s two historic legal happenings, the Olmstead Act and the ADA, changed the employment landscape for individuals with MR/DD. Both of these legal milestones emphasized community integration for people with MR/DD and supported the philosophy of self-determination with the strategy of individual support (ADA of 1990). Nordic researchers espoused the "normalization principle" in the 1960s. It refers to ideas, methods, and experiences expressed in practice in the Scandinavian countries, as well as in other parts of the world. This principle underlies demands for standards, facilities, and programs for the MR/DD population as expressed by the Scandinavian parent movement. Normalization means allowing a normal rhythm of day for people with MR/DD. This applies to eating under normal circumstances and to exercise choice, enjoying rest, harmony, and satisfaction. It involves being able to sleep at a time that is convenient to the client and not the staff. The individual should be given an opportunity to break away from the pattern occasionally. In the area of work, it involves being able to go outside the "home" to participate in vocational activities. Leisure-time activities after work or on the weekend should be as normal as possible. Individuals with DDs should be allowed to experience the normal rhythms of the year, including celebrating holidays and going on vacation. In addition, children should be guided and taught by a few significant adults; school-age individuals should have opportunities to build self-confidence and understanding of themselves; adults should be allowed to experience successes and failures so that they can be more self-reliant; older adults should be allowed to "retire" to places close to where they worked so that they could keep in touch with familiar people and areas.

Other principles of normalization include mixing of the sexes in a manner as free as is common to the culture with normal restraints, not only in day centers and workshops, but also in leisure-time activities. Persons with mild MR should be allowed to marry if they want to. All individuals with MR/DD who work in competitive employment should be paid according to the relative worth of their jobs. Others should have access to allowances or pocket money (Nirje, 1966).

The acceptance of the principle of normalization led to a novel way of looking at issues such as work, leisure, and socialization in the population of people with MR/DD. Residents of group homes and those involved in day programs were introduced to a new perspective of being integrated with the community. They were able to choose their leisure activities, to go on vacation, and to earn money. This was a sea change from the era when individuals with MR/DD were placed in rigid center-based day programs. There have been numerous hurdles overcome since this progress occurred. Some of the issues are yet to be solved. In spite of all the social and legal advances that have been made, including the fact that the Rehabilitation Services Administration of the U.S. Department of Education amended the regulations governing the State Vocational Rehabilitation Program to redefine the term "employment outcome" to mean "an individual with disability working in an integrated setting" (*Federal Register*, 2001), the majority of individuals with MR/DD have not attained this goal.

To be able to work, to earn a livelihood, to obtain benefits (which are tied to a job in the United States), and to retire are the goals of most citizens of this country. Being able to work is highly valued in American society, and doing so allows the individual with MR/DD to feel that he or she is a meaningful contributor to society and integrated with the community. In a review, Wehman and colleagues stated the core values of supported employment. These include job benefits and dignity for the individual employee (Wehman, Revell, and Brooke, 2002). The employer gets a good worker and specialized support to train and maintain the individual. Relatives can see their family member in a fully competent role in the workplace. Society benefits from the fact that it costs less to maintain employment supports than to support the individual in a segregated day program. The teamwork required to make this possible includes trained employment specialists, informed coworkers, mentors, and technological support. The number of people who participate in supported employment nationally had risen to more than 140,000 as of the late 1990s and is likely higher now (Wehman, Revell, and Kregel, 1998).

The American Association on Mental Retardation on its Web page defines supported employment as "paid, competitive employment for people who have severe disabilities and a demonstrated inability to gain and maintain traditional employment." Supported employment occurs in a variety of normal, integrated business environments. The fact sheet estimates that supported employment participants earn nearly $600 million annually and pay more than $100 million each year in federal, state, and local taxes. This reduces the percentage of people on public assistance or disability. As a result, 52 percent of participants' primary income is from a paycheck rather than from public assistance or disability benefits. In their survey they found that individuals with disabilities who participated in supported employment increased their hourly earnings from an average of $0.84 to $4.13, an increase of 490 percent. The average cost of supported employment to the federal rehabilitation program is $4,000; half of all placements cost less than $3,000. The cost of placing an individual in supported employment with support is $4,200 compared with the $7,400 annual cost of maintaining an individual in a day program. Across the states, the costs for supported employment are 40 to 80 percent of the costs of other day services including sheltered workshops and activity centers (Cone, 2009).

Psychiatric Hospitalization

Psychiatrists who practice in the field of mental illness that occurs in the MR/DD population have to overcome several obstacles in making an impact on their patients' mental health issues. Many universities have shied away from this field because of its lack of glamour, the paucity of research funds from foundations, and the lack of interest by the drug companies in working with a population that has complicated issues not readily treatable with medications alone. This leaves the public sector consisting of the community service boards (CSBs) and a few state hospitals along with a smattering of dedicated private psychiatrists to tackle the issue.

One institution that has effected a change in the way that the mental illness aspect of individuals with MR/DD is dealt with is Central State Hospital, in Petersburg, Virginia. The hospital organized an MR/DD team in 2000. The primary aim of the team was to serve as additional resources for the treatment teams on the civil and forensic units. The MR/DD team is mandated by hospital policy to see all patients who are diagnosed with or suspected to have MR/DD. The team then retrieves background data on the patient, does psychological testing, and helps in formulating a treatment plan. The plan includes, but is not confined to, medication evaluation, behavior and aggression management plans, transitions from forensic to civil units, and eventual discharge to the community. In the last phase, the team closely works with the local CSB to ensure a seamless transfer into the community and follows the patient for up to 6 months following discharge. The author has been with the team since its inception. The team has, in its 7 years of existence, evaluated more than 200 cases and has helped in creating treatment plans, in determining appropriate and rational psychopharmacology of patients with co-occurring mental illness and MR/DD, and in formulating behavior support and behavior modification plans for most of the patients served. More than 80 percent of the patients served have been discharged to appropriate group homes in the community. The team follows up the discharged patients for 6 months to ensure smooth transition and to prevent recidivism.

In the private sector, similar arrangements are more difficult to implement. Most individuals with MR/DD are covered by Medicaid, Medicare, or a combination of both. With the cutbacks in these programs, the reimbursement for psychiatric services is abysmally low. The few practitioners who take on patients with MR/DD survive on volume of care and therefore cannot dispense appropriate care in many cases. Several suggestions have been made to emulate the team concept in the treatment of patients who have MR/DD with mental illnesses currently used in the Central State Hospital in Petersburg, Virginia, and this idea is being addressed by that state's General Assembly.

Conclusion

The practice of treating individuals with MR/DD in community settings is evolving. While the transition to the community solves the problem of chronic institutionalization and provides a more natural environment for individuals with MR/DD, it spawns new issues like finding adequate housing and community employment and integrating individuals with MR/DD into the community. With the budget constraints that have plagued our society in recent years, this movement faces major challenges. The psychiatrist who chooses to work with individuals who have MR/DD and mental illness is in a unique situation. The field itself is new in most countries and affords ample opportunities for clinical and systems research. Until recently, research in this field was done by experts in educational and behavioral treatments. The psychiatrist's perspective is unique. He or she has an opportunity to mold the field in the future and make substantial contributions to the medical treatment, community placements, and work programs and to participate in advocacy and legislative efforts to better the living condition of all people with MR/DD.

References

Alexander D. 2002. The surgeon general focuses the nation on health and mental retardation. *Exceptional Parent* 32(5): 28–34.

American Academy of Child and Adolescent Psychiatry. 1999. Practice parameters for the assessment and treatment of children, adolescents, and adults with mental retardation and co-morbid mental disorders. *Journal of the American Academy of Child and Adolescent Psychiatry* 38(12): 1–4S.

Americans with Disabilities Act of 1990. P.L. 101-336, 42 U.S.C. §12101 et seq.

Assistive Technology Act of 1998. P.L. 105-394, 29 U.S.C. §2201.

Bernet W. 2003. Access to support for community lives, homes and social roles: A review of national goals, current knowledge and recommendations for a future research agenda to assist in achieving our national goal. Paper presented at the Invitational Conference on National Goals, the State-of-Knowledge and a Future Research Agenda on Intellectual and Developmental Disabilities, Washington, D.C., January 6–8.

Bird FL, Sperry SM, Carrevio HC. 1998. Community habilitation and integration of adults with psychiatric disorders and mental retardation. *Journal of Developmental and Physical Disabilities* 10(4): 332–48.

Bouras N. 1995. The Frank J. Menolascino lecture: Dual diagnosis towards the year 2000. In RJ Fletcher (ed.), *The NADD Newsletter Book*, 89–92. Kingston, NY: National Association for the Dually Diagnosed.

Braddock D, Hemp R. 2003. *The 2003 Report: Regional and National Perspectives of Developmental Disabilities Services in New Hampshire*. Boulder: University of Colorado School of Medicine, Department of Psychiatry, State of the State in Developmental Disabilities Project.

Cone A. 2009. Supported employment. Available at www.aamr.org.

Conroy J, Bradley V. 1985. *The Pennhurst Longitudinal Study: Combined report of five years of research and analysis*. Philadelphia: Temple University Developmental Disability. Boston: Philadelphia; Human Sciences Research Institute.

Cutler LA. 2001. Mental health services for persons with mental retardation: Role of the advanced practice nurse. *Issues in Mental Health Nursing* 22(6): 607–20.

Dagnan D, Look R, Ruddick L, Jones J. 1995. Changes in the quality of life of people with learning disabilities who move from hospitals to live in community homes. *International Journal of Rehabilitation Research* 18(2): 115–22.

Day KA. 1993. Mental health services for people with mental retardation: A framework for the future. *Journal of Intellectual Disability Research* 37 (suppl. 1): 7–16.

Developmental Disabilities Assistance and Bill of Rights Act of 2000. P.L. 106-402, 42 U.S.C. §6001 et seq.

Eyman RK, Borthwick-Duffy SA, Call TL. 1988. Prediction of mortality in community and institutional settings. *Journal of Mental Deficiency Research* 32(3): 203–13.

Federal Register, January 22, 2001. 66(14), 7249–7258. 34 CFR 361.

Felee D, Emerson D. 2001. Living with support in a home in the community: Predictors of behavioral development and household and community activity. *Mental Retardation and Developmental Disabilities Research Review* 7(2): 75–83.

Fujiura JT. 1998. Demography of family households. *American Journal on Mental Retardation* 103(3): 225–35.

Golding L, Emerson E, Thornton A. 2005. An evaluation of specialized community based residential supports for people with challenging behaviors. *Journal of Intellectual Disabilities* 9(2): 145–54.

Hayden MF, Goldman J. 1996. Families of adults with mental retardation: Stress levels and need for services. *Social Work* 41(6): 656–67.

Janicki MP, Dalton AJ, Henderson CM, Davidson PW. 1999. Mortality and morbidity among older adults with intellectual disability: Health service considerations. *Disability and Rehabilitation* 21(5): 284–94.

Kerker BD, Owens PL, Zigler E, Horwitz SM. 2004. Mental health disorders among individuals with mental retardation: Challenges to accurate prevalence estimates. *Public Health Reports* 119: 409–17.

McIntyre LL, Blacher J, Baker RL. 2002. Behavior/mental health problems in young adults with intellectual disability: The impact on families. *Journal of Intellectual Disability Research* 46(3): 293–99.

Menolascino FJ. 1983. Overview: Bridging the gap between mental retardation and mental illness. In FJ Menolascino and B McCann (eds.), *Mental Health and Mental Retardation*, 3–60. Baltimore: University Park Press.

Miller NA, Ramsland S, Harrington C. 1999. Trends and issues in the Medicaid 1915(C) waiver program. *Health Care Financing Review* 20(4): 139–60.

Nirje B. 1966. The normalization principle and its human management implications: SRV-VRS. *International Social Role Valorization Journal* 1(2): 19–33.

Olmstead v L.C. 1999. P.L. 98-536, 527 U.S. 581.

Rizoll MC, Hemp R, Braddock D, Pomeranz-Essley A. 2004. The State of the States in Developmental Disabilities. Washington, DC: American Association on Mental Retardation.

Seltzer MM, Krauss MW. 2001. Quality of life of adults with mental retardation / developmental disabilities who live with family. *Mental Retardation and Developmental Disabilities Research Reviews* 7(2): 105–14.

Southern Illinois University School of Medicine, Division of Developmental Disabilities. 2007. The technical assistance program. Available at www.siumed.edu.

Spreat S, Conroy JW. 2001. Community placement for persons with significant cognitive challenges: An outcome analysis. *Journal of the Association for Persons with Severe Handicaps* 26(2): 106–13.

Virginia Department of Mental Health. Mental Retardation and Substance Abuse Services. 2000. *Rules and Regulations for the Licensing of Providers of Mental Health, Mental Retardation and Substance Abuse Services* 1: 1–44.

Wehman P, Revell WG, Brooke V. 2002. Competitive employment: Has it become the "first choice" yet? *Journal of Disability Policy Studies* 14(3): 163–73.

Wehman P, Revell WG, Kregel J. 1998. Supported employment: A decade of rapid growth and impact. *American Rehabilitation* 24(1): 31–43.

10

Systems Management

Roxanne C. Dryden-Edwards, M.D.

Having a conceptual understanding of what constitute developmental disabilities (DDs) and of the supports that allow for optimal adjustment of individuals in this population is necessary to help these persons function at the highest level possible in the least-restrictive setting. However, these factors do not work in a vacuum. A review of the management of individuals with DDs shows that care is often provided in a manner that is unplanned and uncoordinated, frequently in inappropriate settings. This chapter will describe an approach to developing and effectively implementing systems of care so that persons with DDs can be as independent and industrious as possible, can contribute to their communities, and can live rich and productive lives. Recommendations will be made to provide psychiatrists in community practice with ideas for how they may participate in the development and improvement of such systems.

Why are care systems for people who have DDs so important in helping these individuals live in the community? Gone are the unfortunate days when persons with DDs were shuttled off to institutions never to be heard from again. Nowadays, three-quarters of recipients of home- and community-based services are individuals with mental retardation (MR) or other DDs (Doty, 2000). Given this information, the most scholarly, current, research-based knowledge of DDs is of little practical use in the absence of appropriate, integrated implementation of support plans. A lack of coordination between care providers and of other mechanisms for ensuring good-quality care invites futile efforts and frustrates caregivers, wastes time and monetary resources, and may result in the compromise or even the complete disintegration of care for and functioning of individuals with DDs. The monetary advantage to keeping persons with DDs within their community is evidenced by the differences in cost between that and the care provided by residential facilities. In fiscal year 2002, states spent an average of $37,816 per recipient of community services paid for by Medicaid Home and Community-Based Services versus $125,746 per resident in placed in a public institution (Roger et al., 2004).

Individuals who are psychiatrically hospitalized and then returned to their previous living arrangement tend to remain hospitalized for a shorter period than those who are discharged elsewhere. That people with DDs seem to be less likely to be discharged to their previous living arrangement than those without a DD is another cause of the increased cost that can result from a lack of planning and coordination among care providers (Saeed et al., 2003).

The potential cost of wasted efforts is considerable when a person with DD must be restricted to residential treatment that could have been prevented by a well-organized, high-quality system of care. Conversely, when service providers work together in a thoughtful, coordinated way that is consumer specific, culturally competent, and predictable although flexible, the benefits can be astounding. A case in point is the example of a woman with mild MR whose sentence and type of confinement after a felony conviction was appropriately adjusted to reflect her DD and, in her case, emotional challenges. Specifically, the victim's family agreed with the prosecutor's recommendation for a shorter sentence and that she be placed in the prison's mental health unit rather than its general population once the victim's family was made aware of these mitigating circumstances. Such an adaptation was possible only as a result of the care and planning her service team took in clearly and methodically assessing and documenting her issues over the course of years of working with her. When systems of care are at odds with or unaware of each other, the outcome can be devastating. When systems work together, the result can greatly enhance the work of art that is the life of the person receiving services. This chapter discusses ways to design, implement, manage, and offer advice about systems on a small or large scale to serve persons with a DD.

What Is a System of Care?

As with other management systems, a system of care for individuals with DDs may be defined by what it is designed to accomplish. Specifically, the system of care should focus on providing for these persons' basic needs (e.g., food, shelter, clothing, and safety), productive activity (e.g., education or work), and recreation (e.g., exercise, social interactions, and the opportunity to develop and engage in individual skills and interests). Funding resources for the system of care must be used for any of these goals to be achieved. Given that the availability of funding depends on how successfully those funds are advocated for, the system of care should also in some way advocate for persons with DDs. Psychiatrists who are involved in the care of this population should therefore remain mindful of those goals for the system of care as they fill a role in the process.

The Planned Lifetime Advocacy Network (PLAN; www.plan.ca) refers to these systems as networks. In addition to the objectives already outlined, this organization is for individuals with DDs and those who care for them and provides links to others in the community, secures and monitors supports and services, provides a forum for network members to support each other, and is a resource for executors and trustees who work with persons with DDs. PLAN also advocates for the interests of this population and feels that assisting with decision making, spending time, and having fun with the individuals with DDs are among the purposes of care systems or networks.

Identifying Members of the Service Team

Once the purposes of a system of care are understood, identifying the members of the service or treatment team is one of the first steps in developing such a system for individuals with DDs. While the person's disability classification, goals for care, and supports needed often influence who are the appropriate members of the service team, the care providers available to the individual are frequently independent of the other factors. The most important of member of the team is always the person receiving the services. Other members of the team often include immediate or extended family members, daily care providers, case managers, job coaches or teachers, physicians and other physical or mental health care providers, clergy members, family friends, and sometimes legal counsel and other legal professionals.

Respecting and facilitating family involvement cannot be underestimated.

When a parent of an adult with DDs was asked by this author what one concept she hoped would be communicated in this book, she responded, "Listen to the parents, listen to the parents, listen to the parents!" Indeed, research on the subject further validates the importance of that sentiment. Family support programs have been found to be associated with participant families' feeling more satisfied with the services received by their adult relative with DDs and less likely to desire out of home placement compared with families who were not recipients of those interventions.

Because about 60 percent of adults with a DD continue to reside with a family member, practitioners who work with this population will often work with their family caregivers as well. Individuals with DDs may achieve increased community integration and monthly wages when their caregiving families receive the help they need through a consumer-directed approach (Heller, Miller, and Hsieh, 1999). No matter what the experiences, training, or degrees of the other members of the care system, the individuals with DD and their family are the principal experts on what it is like to live with a DD or to love and live with someone who has a DD. Caregivers always need to recognize, use, and appreciate that people with DDs and their family member have doctoral-degree equivalent knowledge in that regard.

Rules of Engagement

Once the members of the care team have been identified, it is important to establish the ways in which the group will work, or rules of engagement, as early as possible. Issues such as establishing the goals of the team, determining how to communicate, defining the roles and duties of service team members, building rapport, and promoting motivation are all rules of engagement that are necessary to optimize the functioning of care providers. Establishing these rules lays the foundation for developing the work culture of the group. Any delay of this step encourages individuals to work at odds with the operation of the team and therefore to interfere with the progress of the individual with a DD.

Defining and Achieving Goals

Of paramount importance in the successful operation of any team is determining the objectives that are most likely to lead to achieving the larger goals in cooperation with persons with DDs. Like all aspects of working with this population, determining these objectives will not be effective if it is not done in an integrated manner.

CASE EXAMPLE

Michael, a 21-year-old man with moderate MR, impulsively hit others. His maternal grandmother instructed her daughter to stop giving Michael the clonidine that was being prescribed to address his impulsivity because she read that it is prescribed to treat high blood pressure. Although likely well meaning, the psychiatrist who prescribed the medication had wasted everyone's time by failing to be sure that the Michael's family members had a thorough understanding of why the clonidine was being prescribed, what other conditions it is used to treat, its mechanism of action, and its potential side effects. It would have taken less than 5 minutes to do so and to supplement with written material on the medication. Instead, Michael lost weeks of progress and those who cared for him gained days of frustration and lost hours that could have been spent further enhancing the functioning of this developmentally disabled person. Fortunately, another member of Michael's care team, his primary care physician, took the time to fully explain the treatment, which resulted in resumed compliance with taking the medication and improvement in Michael's symptoms and quality of life. ▶

The preceding example illustrates how psychiatrists often find themselves being initiated into working with persons with DDs as psychopharmacologists for the individual who enters their community practice. The example also shows how ineffective psychiatrists can be when they maintain as their objective merely to "seek and destroy" what is perceived to be abnormal behavior in an individual with a DD. Intricately woven into that illustration is that the grandmother's distrust of the medication may also be the issue of culture, ethnicity, race, and socioeconomic status. The psychiatrist and all other members of the individual's system of care are well advised to learn about, respect, and address the demographics that each team member brings to the work. To do so is far better than to have it acted out unconsciously to the detriment of the person with a DD. Such integration of understanding need not be an overwhelming time commitment. It may involve simply acknowledging the issues, such as that there is an imbalance that the majority in the field of direct care are women and members of minority groups and that the opposite imbalance exists among physicians. Psychiatrists who recognize and address the appropriate distrust that minority group members may have for psychiatry—given the history of medicine in general and psychiatry specifically of assigning pathology to minorities in ways that alternated between at times being excessive and at other times inappropriately minimized depending on the diagnosis and situation—may find other members of the treatment team more receptive to their ideas than to those of the profession who pretend these dynamics do not exist.

These issues understandably extend into the daily decisions made in working with developmentally disabled individuals. All the cultural, ethnic, racial, religious, age-related, socioeconomic, gender, and sexual orientation identifiers that define the members of the care team, as well as each person's individual experiences, are factors in determining each one's view on issues such as what would be the most nurturing living situation, job experience, or effective treatment of any illness for the individual with a DD who is the focus of the care network. It therefore behooves all team members, including the psychiatrist, to be cognizant of their own beliefs and biases, the potential origins of those beliefs and biases, and how to effectively manage them. It is also important for team members to become comfortable with learning about the backgrounds of all the other members of the team, to appreciate the strengths inherent in each person's perspective, and to include those perspectives in the work in a productive and supportive manner.

The seek-and-destroy-pathology approach described previously can also easily lead to a psychiatrist's recommending a medication regimen or other treatment that suppresses the exuberance and even the human essence of the person being served or exposes the individual to other debilitating side effects, rather than the psychiatrist's prescribing medications that would help the individual with DDs.

CASE EXAMPLE

Christina, a 55-year-old woman with cerebral palsy and panic attacks, was taking 14 medications, including six anti-inflammatory medications, three sleep aids, a muscle relaxant, an antianxiety medication, and prescription and herbal hormone replacement medications. While her anxiety was initially significantly increased on hearing the psychiatrist's suggestion that,

rather than increasing the doses of her medication or adding another medication to her current regimen, some of the medications should be weaned
if possible, she experienced rapid and significant relief of anxiety once half
of the medications she was taking were slowly discontinued.

As the above example implies, a more holistic approach that recognizes the
potential side effects of medications and other medical interventions is more
often effective in working with individuals with complex issues, instead of a
disparate approach in which different providers prescribe medications without regard to intervention by others. By frequently assessing the individual
with DDs and having regular communication with the person's caregivers
and job coach, the psychiatrist in the example was able to make suggestions
about the medications the patient was taking that accurately reflected the
patient's progress and ultimately resulted in significant improvement in her
functioning in the community.

Defining Roles of Network Members

Before any working relationships can be formed, trust built, or goals
achieved, the roles of the people who will work with a developmentally disabled person must be established, starting with the person receiving the care
(Hauser, 1997). The importance of this step should not be underestimated.
Besides the consumer of care, other members of the care team often include
parents, siblings and other family members; professional home caregivers;
physicians, nurses, dentists and other health care providers; and teachers
and other members of the community. Community members that can have a
significant impact on consumers of care include clergy, law enforcement offi-
cers, attorneys, employers, coworkers, and job coaches. The cleric who has
known the 19-year-old man with Asperger disorder for his whole life can be
an invaluable counselor to the young man and his family during a time of
crisis. The local police officer who has seen the 35-year-old woman with fragile X syndrome behave bizarrely when stressed can be the difference between the individual's receiving support and treatment rather than incarcer-
ation during times of crisis.

Like the other issues involved in maintaining a functioning care network,
defining roles need not be an excessively time-consuming process to be
highly effective. The psychiatrist may ask that the individual receiving ser-

vices and that person's family members construct a list of everyone involved in his or her care. That list should then be distributed to other care team members so that those supports can be accessed in a timely manner. Any consent forms that are needed to involve each support person should be completed as soon as the list is constructed so that no delays occur in accessing those resources. The team should quickly agree on which of the support systems will be sought for which issue and who will be accessed on a regular versus an as-needed basis, as well as how often certain systems will be routinely involved (e.g., weekly contacts between home care professionals and family members; monthly between the psychiatrist and the consumer and family; quarterly for job performance assessment).

In the process of defining and assigning roles of members of the network, clarity rather than rigidity is in order. While it is inappropriate for a psychiatrist to base the choice of a medication only on the suggestion of another care team member, those colleagues can offer a wealth of information on a daily basis about symptom presentation or the lack thereof in the person with DDs. Recipients of services and family members who bristle in interactions with the psychiatrist and all the real and imagined baggage that entails may be more open to the same feedback when it is reinforced by a family friend, professional caregiver, or trusted member of the clergy. It is therefore advantageous to be part of a system of services that allows for planned, appropriate fluidity among care network members.

Communication

The sheer number of members involved with the care of many persons with DD illustrates the importance of excellent communication among care providers, coordination of services, and quality-assurance mechanisms. Contrary to conventional wisdom, managing the operation of a service team is doable even within the confines of a managed care system. Rather than becoming overwhelmed by trying to maintain weekly contacts with the other members of the team, developing a coherent system of communication can optimize efficiency, decrease the likelihood of burnout by service team members, and result in the best outcome for the person receiving services. Examples of this include the psychiatrist who sends a letter to the staff of a group home where an adult with DDs lives describing any changes made to the person's medication regimen; the job coach who attends meetings with the psychiatrist describing the individual's adjustment to the work setting, and family members meeting with group home staff and attending psychiatric appointments to ensure that both parties are aware of the unique personality, strengths, challenges, likes and dislikes of their loved one. An example of families providing a psychiatrist with a well-rounded picture of their loved one with DDs is a brother who attended all doctors' appointments with his sister and let practitioners know about how much she enjoys and looks forward to seeing a particular television show and about her taste in music. Because of this, practitioners were better able to engage the patient in her own care by expressing interest in those leisure activities.

Good communication may be in the form of maintaining and sharing excellent documentation of service goals, resources provided and progress achieved that is supplemented by more direct contact between service providers when specific difficulties arise. For clearly measurable outcomes, such as the number of self-injurious behaviors, incidents of self-care, and interacting with others, using standardized measures may allow for more specific assessment, interventions, and progress. Although team members will have different styles of exchanging ideas, such exchanges are most effective when done directly versus indirectly. That remains true even when a team member needs to be confronted, as long as a stance of respect among care network providers is maintained.

The 55-year-old woman taking more than 10 medications is an all-too-common example of what can happen in the treatment of persons with DDs: multiple health practitioners making treatment recommendations without finding out what others are doing or without taking the other treatment regimens under consideration when implementing a plan. Each specialist can make the mistake of focusing on just one area of problems, forgetting that all the issues and therefore all the interventions have an impact on one human being. As many psychiatrists work within the restrictive constraints of managed care, maintaining contact with the several professionals, paraprofessionals, and other caregivers of developmentally disabled persons can seem like a daunting task when faced with having to see four or more patients per hour. The good news here is that there are many ways to exchange information with other caregivers even while working within a managed care system. By doing just one thing different to improve such communication, practitioners can see noticeable improvement in the care received and the clinical progress of patients. By simply writing highly descriptive progress notes, improving the legibility of those notes by having them typed, or appointing a support person to relay simple messages (e.g., about scheduling or referral to other specialists as needed), clinicians can improve the lives of individuals with DDs and the lives of those who care for them. Something as easy as ensuring that documents generated are legible, thoughtful, and practical can have an enormous impact on others' ability to understand the treatment that has already been provided and to move forward accordingly. The case of a state prosecutor making the decision not to pursue the death penalty for a mentally retarded defendant with lifelong intermittent explosive disorder based only on reviewing years of medical records that clearly described the defendant's troubles is a striking example of the potential life-and-death impact of excellent communication through documentation. By ensuring good record keeping and appropriately delegating clerical and other administrative duties, the psychiatrist can save time for providing psychiatric care, team participation, and guidance from their professional point of view.

Cultural Issues of Communication

Improving patient care and outcomes and making the work easier to accomplish requires consideration of team members' cultural norms, values, and ways of communicating that cannot and should not be ignored. Poor communication between doctors and patients or ethnic groups that are different from their own is increasingly being suspected as more of an obstacle to effective treatment than even racial bias on the part of the practitioner or preference of the patient (Ashton et al., 2003). The need for culturally effective medical care has been formally recognized by the American Academy of Pediatrics (2004). In one study, African American families using secular professional discourse made use of formal DD services in a manner similar to that of families of European American heritage. Families using the spiritual kin discourse—which is based more on community and family solutions and less on the individual solving his or her own problems—tended to rely on natural or informal supports rather than the DDs service system, as the system did not exemplify the values that these families embraced. It was observed that these two discourses tend to be associated with two distinct worldviews and two distinct ways of using the DD system (Terhune, 2005).

As physicians are all taught as early as the third year of medical school, we cannot expect to gather accurate history from an adult patient who feels judged, demeaned, disrespected, or spoken to inappropriately. Yet, unbeknown to us, patients often walk away from interactions with physicians with those very feelings. The Latino physician who seizes the hand of the hesitant Korean patient may cause that patient to feel her personal space was violated. The well-meaning but misguided African American psychiatrist who speaks Spanish to the Peruvian individual under her care can do great damage to the therapeutic relationship by referring to the patient using the familiar "tu" rather than the more appropriately formal "usted" form of the word *you*. The white doctor can easily and quickly put off an African American patient and family by calling them by their first names before being invited to do so. There are many ways to avoid these pitfalls without feeling a perceived burden at seeking to learn about the cultural background of each person who walks into the office. Doing so will save the psychiatrist time in having to repair rifts in trust or communication in the future. Here are some pointers:

- Err on the side of warm formality with every patient. No adult patient will feel disrespected by a psychiatrist who addresses him or her by title, such as Mr., Mrs., Ms., or Doctor. Making the mistake in the opposite direction, however, can be devastating to forming a therapeutic relationship with a patient and caregivers, particularly when establishing good working relationships with the other members of the care network is fundamental to good outcome with the developmentally disordered population. At the same time, formality should not cross into the realm of the aloof. Inquire about the lives of the patient and caregivers. Doing so humanizes them to the psychiatrist and vice versa (Welch, 2000).
- Simply ask the person who has a DD and the caregivers what they would like to be called. No cultural background dictates what makes each member of the group feel comfortable within this or any other setting.
- Ask the patient and caregivers why they may have changed doctors and what has worked well and not so well in their interactions with other practitioners. That will give the psychiatrist an understanding of the preferences of treatment team members.
- Inquire about any psychiatric or other medical practices they believe to be particular to their culture. Take a respectful stance of interested

inquiry when interacting with all patients, even those who ostensibly
seem to be of the same background that you are.

- Learn about any differences team members may have encountered in
access to or use of health care and mental health care services between
ethnic, racial, religious, socioeconomic, or other groups (U.S. Department of Health and Human Services, 1999).
- Read or otherwise access materials regarding the history of various
ethnic and religious groups and other special populations with health
or mental health providers. Examples of that include the experiments
in torture inflicted on Jewish Holocaust victims, the intentional infection of African American men with syphilis in Tuskegee, Alabama,
psychiatry's history of describing members of ethnic minorities as
being intellectually inferior to members of the majority population,
and the history of forced sterilization of mentally retarded individuals
(Terhune, 2005).
- Remain objective and grounded in the *Diagnostic and Statistical
Manual of Mental Disorders* (DSM), while remaining mindful of how
individuals' normal and symptomatic presentation has a cultural context. It is the author's opinion that there is no more unconscionable
example of the potentially devastating outcome of cultural incompetence than that involving a psychiatrist working in a substance abuse
facility who diagnoses pervasive developmental disorder, not otherwise
specified (PDD, NOS) in any patient who has virtually any language
disorder and fails to engage with that psychiatrist in a cordial manner.
Although that practitioner may point to the necessarily vague criteria
for PDD, NOS, cited in the DSM to justify the diagnosis, this is an example of the importance of keeping the spirit of a mental health detec-
tive in mind along with the specifics of diagnostic criteria. Doing so
can help the practitioner evaluate whether the frequency with which
he or she assigns a particular diagnosis is grossly out of proportion
to that found in the general and clinical populations. This will then
indicate that the professional should consider either a clear and compelling reason to still assign the diagnosis or more likely that their
diagnostic approach may be out of line with accepted standards of
practice.
- Engage culturally specific care providers and organizations as appropriate (Saldana, 2001). The positive impact of having a diverse group

of team members cannot be underestimated. It can simultaneously ease the anxiety of consumers of services and their families while communicating confidence in the value and potential of all groups of people.

Conflict Resolution

Because psychiatrists are trained and experienced at counseling patients and their families in working through conflicts, it is important that skill be used in working with the team of individuals that cares for a person with a DD. Despite the rush of performing assessments and treatment, it behooves the psychiatrist to keep in mind that festering conflict almost invariably leads to undermining all therapeutic interventions. Therefore, preventing and resolving difficulties will make the job of all those who care for the individuals with DDs easier and more effective. Here, the groundwork that has hopefully been laid in team building should minimize problems in the work and make issues between team members easier to solve. Setting the example of understanding and openly discussing the inevitability of differences of opinions and approaches, the impact of festering conflict on the work, the positions and opinions of all involved, as well as formulating appropriate compromise positions wherever possible can lead to rapid resolution of difficulties among team members and ultimately an even more cohesive team than before the conflict occurred.

Education

While psychiatrists may feel used to learning as an ongoing process in connection with licensure requirements, participation in a team process may provide a unique opportunity to learn from as well as to educate other care team members. The psychiatrist either knows or has easy access to technical information pertaining to the diagnosis and the medical and mental health care of people with DDs. Imparting that information in a layperson friendly manner to other team members can arm the service network with the power that is associated with understanding the person with DDs from a phenomenological and technically medical and psychiatric point of view. Although there is wide variability in individual presentations, there may be some commonality of cognition, adaptation, strengths, and weaknesses based on diagnosis. Examples of adaptation include maintaining hygiene; feeding oneself; having adequate speech, language, and motor skills; being able to interact with others; and having or lacking self-injurious behaviors and various medical, dental, and mental health conditions. Such knowledge can therefore have a significantly positive impact on the interventions provided by helping care network members to have realistic goals and expectations and planning for as well as interacting with an individual with DDs in the most productive manner.

The other aspect of education that psychiatrists may find more challenging is receiving the wealth of knowledge that other care network members can offer. Besides the obvious information that other professionals can offer about their particular discipline, individuals with DDs are the best resource for information about themselves, through conversation and observation. Family members are likely the most expert regarding the historical presentation and functioning, past and present care and treatment, as well as family history. Along with hired daily service providers, family members are also uniquely qualified to teach other team members about the daily routines, strengths, challenges, and functioning of the individual seeking services. That information is crucial to developing interventions for challenges, in that the strengths of the person with DDs, like those of any person, should be harnessed to mitigate or alleviate their challenges. By learning from these valuable team members and incorporating their knowledge into how the individual with DDs is understood and assisted, psychiatrists can exponentially enhance the effectiveness of the treatment they provide.

Team Building

The phrase *team building* may evoke in the mind of the psychiatrist nebulous images of rock climbing, hand holding, and self-disclosure with coworkers that is contrary to the dictatorial role that many physicians have been trained to assume. That may be why our profession avoids recognizing the need and implementing this indispensable aspect of working with people with DDs. Without developing and nurturing a cohesive working unit, the opportunities for miscommunication, unresolved conflicts, and inefficient efforts are multiplied.

Be reassured that, while enormously important, creating and maintaining constructive professional relationships among those involved in caring for individuals with developmental disabilities need not be time consuming. Every time one network member meets or otherwise communicates with other care network members is an opportunity to strengthen that relationship. Whether in person, by telephone, electronic mail, or other means of communicating, mentioning the accomplishments of other team members, empathizing with the challenges they face in the work, and encouraging these colleagues to take care of themselves are ways to form and enhance those relationships and take only minutes to implement. Sometimes the psychiatrist is uniquely qualified to suggest interventions by which individuals with DDs, family members, and other caregivers can take daily breaks and regular vacations, appropriately manage their responsibilities, and celebrate their accomplishments. Such mechanisms may be as simple as having team members keep a calendar that indicates break and vacation schedules, thereby facilitating the team's ability to promote timely respite for all members and preventing burnout. For example, review of the literature suggests that respite services are associated with a significant decrease in parental stress for the majority of those who use them (Chan and Sigafoos, 2001).

To promote continuation of the care provided to the individuals with DDs, meticulous contingency planning is in order. Here again, the combination of the psychiatrist's experience with the medical model in the context of team work is invaluable. Specifically, the concept of being responsible for selecting and securing one's own break and vacation coverage rather than leaving it to someone else is the level of commitment that should be brought to the process. Encouraging other team members to see the person covering their responsibilities during any absence as their representative instead of merely someone to take up space until the network member's return is a small but important shift in the mind-set of team members. If all caregivers view the temporary substitute as putting his or her own good professional name on the line, the likelihood that the services provided to the person with DDs will be anything less than excellent at all times will be minimized.

Quality Management

While the best-laid plans are monumentally important in establishing and continuing good team work and care provision, setting up systems to minimize errors, while planning for the inevitable mistakes that all human beings make is just as important. That process is often referred to as quality control or quality assurance management. Here again, it is less important or possible to plan for every kind of mistake that could be made than for team members to agree on a way to prevent mistakes and to address them swiftly, openly, honestly, and effectively. As long as egregious errors are prevented through conscientious education, monitoring, planning, and implementation of care, team members should have no fear of negative consequences involved in making an error. Even the most blatant error should be approached directly, should involve other team members in the resolution of those issues, and should take the approach that learning from a mistake is a valuable part of the work. Advising families of a child with DDs to keep a log of the medications the child receives and to use medication boxes marked with the days of the week are just a couple of examples of how a psychiatrist can make a brief suggestion that prevents potentially life-threatening mistakes from being made.

Contingency Planning

Every life is bound to have episodes of unexpected or urgent circumstances. For people with DDs, their cognitive and sometimes associated physical and mental health vulnerabilities and their need for assistance from others may put them at higher risk for suffering from life crises. Depending on the person and level of disability, a change that is seen by others as minor, like an adjustment in daily routine or the presence of a substitute caregiver due to vacation, can result in a significant challenge to adapt for the individual with DDs. Life events that tend to be difficult for anyone, such as the death of a parent, may be devastating for people living with a DD. It therefore behooves individuals with DDs and those who work with them to develop plans for addressing such issues. PLAN lists the benefits of contingency planning, particularly in planning for the care of persons with DDs following the death of their parents, including the following:

- helping the consumer prepare for the changes that will occur as a result of the crisis
- having supports in place before the change
- advocating for and making decisions with and for the individual with DDs when appropriate
- monitoring the services provided
- providing emotional and other supports necessary for the care recipient to cope with the crisis

In the development of contingency planning, psychiatrists can offer advice on developing mechanisms to manage unexpected circumstances. This advice can range from making simple suggestions—such as having caregivers keep a calendar that indicates when each person involved in caring for a person with DDs plans to be absent from work, thereby providing time to prepare the individual with DDs for the absence—to monitoring stress and helping team members avoid burnout.

To promote smooth continuation of the care provided to the individual with DDs, meticulous contingency planning is in order. The combination of the psychiatrist's experience with the medical model for contingency planning can prove useful. Specifically, the concept of all network members' being responsible for securing their own coverage during absences rather than leaving that planning to someone else is the level of commitment that should be brought to the process. An expression of such commitment to the caregiving process may seem to be a small shift in the stance taken to teamwork but can be an important one, encouraging everyone involved to appropriately see the great value of his or her role.

Care Coordination in Foster Care and Institutional Settings

This discussion of managing care systems for persons who live with DDs would not be complete without addressing the special issues involved in working with those individuals who live in foster care, group homes, or other institutional settings. Despite the efforts to keep people with DDs in community settings, these persons are disproportionately represented in foster care and in institutions. Specifically, up to 50 percent of children in foster care have some form of DD. These out-of-home placements may come about as a result of families becoming economically or emotionally overwhelmed by the needs of the child with DDs or the need to access services through state systems or as a result of abuse or neglect. Likely because of a combination of delays in diagnosis and the increasing challenges that come with entering adolescence, teens make up the age group of people with DDs who are in foster care most often. Because children in this population are more than three times as likely to be abused while in foster care (Sullivan and Knutson, 2000; U.S. Department of Health and Human Services, 2005) and are at disproportionately higher risk for repeated psychiatric hospitalizations (Romansky et al., 2003), the need to improve the education, support, and supervision foster parents of these children receive is clear.

Increasing the number of people involved in caring for the individual with DDs in any setting increases the complexity of the work and makes coordination of services all the more important. While all the issues already described in this chapter hold true when working with a person who is in a foster home or institutional setting, each placement also has unique kinds of challenges as well as strengths. While the best institutional settings can provide well-organized care, problems of impersonal management of the people they serve can easily occur. Therefore, creating and maintaining a cohesive team that uses a well-developed system of quality assurance is of the highest importance when working with persons with DDs who reside either in foster home, a group home, or another institutional setting. Fortunately, programs exist that demonstrate the effectiveness of building cohesive networks of supports for foster children and their families. Such programs use ongoing education of foster families, regular support group meetings, and access to community services to improve the lives of children with DDs who are in foster homes and their families (Cincinnati Children's Hospital Medical Center, 2003).

Foster home placement can and should involve members of the individual's immediate and extended birth family when available, the foster family, case workers and judges, and the numerous professional and community team members addressed in other parts of this chapter. The importance of birth family involvement, whether the child's immediate family or extended family, cannot be underestimated. As foster children become adults and age out of the foster care system, they tend to have better outcomes when they have some kind of connection to their family of origin (Freundlich and Avery, 2005). Maintaining that connection can present unique challenges, particularly when the foster child has a DD. The dynamics between the service recipient's birth family, extended family, and foster family may range from supportive to diametrically opposed and emotionally adversarial. Therefore, the role of the psychiatrist as a member of the foster care team may involve monitoring those dynamics and encouraging all team members to be as supportive as possible to the child with DDs. Birth family members should be commended for making what may have been the difficult decision of placing the person with DDs where he or she may receive the necessary assistance. The foster family or group home staff should be acknowledged for taking that challenge. Establishing and maintaining cooperative relationships among members of this network should be further encouraged by the psychiatrist through this professional's assisting team members in becoming educated about the special needs of the individual with DDs, defining goals that can be agreed on, supporting productive communication, and appreciating the powerful and necessary role of each team member.

People with DDs living in a group home or other institutional setting can also benefit from the expertise of the psychiatrist in encouraging optimal operations of their system of care. Although legal guidelines for providing services to this population are discussed in further detail in chapter 14, ensuring that those guidelines are clearly followed is not always done. Just making well-placed calls to individuals working with the individual in that setting can have significant positive impact on the work that is being done. These communications can send the message that someone who either knows or has facile access to learning what services the individual with DDs should be receiving and the rights he or she has to receiving optimal care is keeping track of what is being provided. By providing resources and suggestions regarding staff trainings, supervision, and other supports, the community psychiatrist can powerfully improve the work being done with consumers of services. The ways in which psychiatrists can effect change in institutional settings are nearly as limitless as the imagination.

Conclusion

Participating in developing and maintaining a highly effective care team is of paramount importance when working with individuals with DDs. Doing so makes the work of the community psychiatrist not just easier but possible. By investing even a small amount of time and energy in advising, supporting, and otherwise communicating with other members of the service network, the community psychiatrist can help ensure that thorough assessments, care plans, living, educational, vocational, and recreational services are completed and appropriately implemented in a timely manner. In teaching and learning from other team members, beginning with the consumer of services and his or her family members, psychiatrists can improve and even save lives.

REFERENCES

American Academy of Pediatrics, Committee on Pediatric Workforce. 2004. Ensuring culturally effective pediatric care: Implications for education and health policy. *Pediatrics* 114(6): 1677–85.

Ashton CM, Haidet P, Paterniti DA, et al. 2003. Racial and ethnic disparities in the use of health services: Bias, preferences or poor communication? *Journal of General Internal Medicine* 18(2): 146–52.

Chan JB, Sigafoos, J. 2001. Does respite care reduce parental stress in families with developmentally disabled children? *Child and Youth Care Forum* 30(5): 253–63.

Cincinnati Children's Hospital Medical Center, Preparation for Parenting Program. 2003. The preparation for parenting program: Final report, 1999–2003. Cincinnati: Cincinnati Children's Hospital Medical Center.

Doty, P. 2000. *Cost-Effectiveness of Home and Community-Based Long-Term Care Services.* Washington, DC: U.S. Department of Health and Human Services / ASPE Office of Disability, Aging and Long-Term Care Policy.

Freundlich M, Avery RJ. 2005. Planning for permanency for youth in congregate care. *Children and Youth Services Review* 27: 115–34.

Hauser M. 1997. The role of the psychiatrist in mental retardation. *Psychiatric Annals, Journal of Continuing Psychiatric Education* 27(3): 170–74.

Heller T, Miller AB, Hsieh K. 1999. Impact of a consumer-directed family support program on adults with developmental disabilities and their family caregivers. *Family Relations, Interventions for Family Caregivers* 48(4): 419–27.

Roger J, Stancliffe K, Lakin C, et al. 2004. Excerpts from the economics of deinstitutionalization. In RJ Stancliffe and K Lakin (eds.), *Cost and Outcomes of Community Services for People with Intellectual Disabilities,* 1–6. Baltimore: Paul H. Brookes Publishing.

Romansky JB, Lyons JS, Lehner RK, West CM. 2003. Factors related to psychiatric hospital readmission among children and adolescents in state custody. *Psychiatric Services* 54: 356–62.

Saeed H, Ouellette-Kuntz H, Stuart, H, Burge P. 2003. Length of stay for psychiatric inpatient services: A comparison of admissions of people with and without developmental disabilities. *Journal of Behavioral Health Services and Research* 30(4): 406–17.

Saldana D. 2001. *Cultural Competency: A Practical Guide for Mental Health Service Providers.* Austin: University of Texas Press.

Sullivan PM, Knutson JF. 2000. Maltreatment and disabilities: A population-based epidemiology study. *Child Abuse and Neglect* 24(10): 1257–73.

Terhune PS. 2005. African American developmental disability discourses: Implications for policy development. *Journal of Policy and Practice in Intellectual Disabilities* 2: 18.

U.S. Department of Health and Human Services. 1999. *Mental Health: Culture, Race and Ethnicity*. Available at www.surgeon-general.gov/library/mentalhealth/cre/execsummary-6.html.

U.S. Department of Health and Human Services. 2005. *Safety, Permanency, Well-Being*. Child Welfare Outcomes Annual Report. Washington DC: U.S. Government Printing Office Available at www.acf.hhs.gov/programs/cb/pubs/cwoo2/index.htm.

Welch T (ed.). 2000. *Culture and the Patient-Physician Relationship: Achieving Cultural Competency in Health Care*: St. Louis: Mosby.

PART IV ◆

INTERVENTIONS

11

Legal and Practical Aspects of Special Education

Robin P. Church, Ed.D., and
Derek Glaaser, Ed.D.

The number of students with disabilities being served in the public schools rose from 4.7 million in 1990 to approximately 6 million in 2004. As reported in the 26th annual report to Congress on the implementation of the Individuals with Disabilities Education Improvement Act (IDEA; 2004; U.S. Department of Education, 2009), graduating rates for students with disabilities are up, dropout rates are falling, and more students with disabilities are being educated in the general education program than ever before (Smith et al., 2008). Against this backdrop, the reauthorization of IDEA in 2004 put into place many new and challenging features that would revolutionize special education and bring it in line with the No Child Left Behind Act of 2002 (NCLB).

But access to education has not always been a guaranteed right for students with disabilities. Public support for free public education began during the early part of the nineteenth century, including, for the first time, a belief in educating certain students, such as those who were middle-class, poor, female, or culturally different, who had previously been excluded. States began enacting compulsory education laws allowing students of different ages and some backgrounds to learn together. In spite of this greater sense of inclusion, until the mid-1970s students with disabilities who did not fit this mold

Table 11.1.   Key legal cases in special education

Case	Provisions

Brown v. Board of Education (1954)	Court determined that
	    segregation of children in public schools solely on the basis of race deprives children of the minority group of equal educational opportunities.
	    racial segregation of students in public schools violates the Equal Protection Clause of the Fourteenth Amendment because separate facilities are inherently unequal.

Diana v. California State Board of Education	Court determined that children for whom English is a second language should be allowed to be tested in their first language.

Parc v. The Commonwealth of Pennsylvania (1972)	Court determined that
	    children with mental retardation could not be denied access to a free appropriate public education.
	    regular classroom placement is preferable to more-restrictive settings.
	    placements cannot change without parents receiving due process.

Larry P. v. Riles (1979)	Court determined that schools could no longer use racially or culturally biased IQ tests to identify students as having mental retardation or determine placements of students in special education classes.

(continued)

of general education classes were ignored, placed in classes by themselves, or transferred to public institutions. Students who had seizures or emotional disturbance or who had mental retardation were excluded from public school and denied the right to an appropriate education.

It wasn't until the civil rights movement of the 1950s and 1960s that attitudes about students with disabilities began to change. With the 1954 passage of *Brown v. Board of Education of Topeka* lending support to the notion that all students had a right to be included in public schools side by side with their peers, advocates began to push for students with disabilities, and the mainstreaming movement was born (Henley, Ramsey, and Algozzine et al., 2006; Smith et al., 2008). This followed on the heels of the deinstitutionalization movement, which advocated for more humane, community-based programming for individuals with disabilities. However, significant challenges, such as the overrepresentation of minority students in special education, re-

Table 11.1. (continued)

Case	Provisions
The Board of Education of the Hendrick Hudson Central SchoolDistrict v. Rowley (1982)	Court determined that schools must provide students with special education needs with sufficient services to benefit educationally from instruction but are not required to maximize the child's potential.

Honig v. Doe (1988)	Court determined that
	    children with disabilities could not have a change in educational placement for actions that are a manifestation of their disability.
	    children with disabilities should "stay put" in their current placement while a determination of appropriate placement is considered.

Olmstead v. L. C. (1999)	Court determined that
	    individuals with developmental disabilities should receive placement in the community rather than in institutional settings when deemed appropriate by the state's treatment professionals.
	    the placement cannot be opposed by the person with developmental disabilities.
	    the placement must be able to be reasonably accommodated given the available resources and the needs of others with developmental disabilities.

mained. In *Diana v. California State Board of Education* (1970) advocates challenged the overrepresentation of minority students in special education, and in the following year the *PARC* decree (*Pennsylvania Association of Retarded Citizens v. Commonwealth of Pennsylvania*) ensured that all students, no matter what level of disability, had a basic right to a "free, appropriate, public education" (FAPE; Turnbull and Turnbull, 1998). Today, improving the educational results for students with disabilities is an essential element of our national policy of ensuring equal opportunity, full participation, independent living, and economic self-sufficiency (IDEA, 2004; Clair, Church, and Batshaw, 2002). Table 11.1 shows key legal cases in education that had an impact on the field of special education.

The first major piece of legislation to ensure the notion of FAPE was Section 504 of the Rehabilitation Act of 1973. This law provided that "no otherwise qualified individual with a disability . . . be excluded from participation

Table 11.2.   Federal legislation related to special education

Legislation	Provisions
Education for All Handicapped Children Act, 1975	Required Free Appropriate Public Education (FAPE)
	Defined disabilities to be covered
	Established assessment guidelines
	Established the individualized education plan (IEP)
Individuals with Disabilities Education Improvement Act (IDEA), 1990	Established use of person's first language
	Replaced use of *handicap* with *disability*
	Established transition planning from high school into postsecondary and adult services
IDEA, 1997	Increased student participation in the general curriculum
	Strengthened the role of parents
	Increased attention to racial and linguistic diversity to prevent mislabeling.
	Ensured school environment was safe and conducive to learning
Elementary and Secondary Education Act (No Child Left Behind / NCLB), 2001	Promoted stronger accountability for results
	Supported more choices for parents
IDEA, 2004	Required equal educational opportunity to students despite economic conditions
	Aligned more closely with NCLB
	Revised the IEP process, due process, and the discipline provisions

in, be denied the benefits of, or be subjected to discrimination under any program or activity receiving Federal financial assistance" (Smith, 2001). The culmination of decades of struggle on behalf of students with disabilities was the passage of the Education for All Handicapped Children's Act of 1975. It provided a number of unprecedented mandates, such as FAPE, procedural rights, due process, and education in the least-restrictive environment (LRE; Wright and Wright, 2007). This single piece of legislation would change forever the process by which students with disabilities receive education in public schools. The 1975 act would be reauthorized many times (1986, 1990, 1997, 2004), each time expanding and refining the practices, policies, and procedures that govern the inclusion of students with disabilities in our schools. See Table 11.2 for key federal legislation that had an impact on the field of special education.

This chapter is designed for professionals in the health field who advocate on behalf of their patients with disabilities and their families and who may need to interact with schools on a regular basis. It will also assist practitioners in understanding the educational and vocational considerations with which their adult patients may have had to contend. By increasing this understanding, practitioners can enhance their ability to advocate for the individuals they serve and help consumers of services and their families advocate for the rights of people with disabilities.

CASE EXAMPLE

Tom, an 18-year-old student, experienced typical developmental milestones until he was 18 months old, when he was diagnosed with epilepsy. Epileptic seizures continued throughout his childhood. In addition, Tom has been diagnosed with pervasive developmental disorder (PDD), attention deficit hyperactivity disorder (ADHD), sleep apnea, speech and language impairment, and emotional disturbance. He has been tested to have a verbal IQ of 92 and a performance IQ of 68. He reads on the sixth-grade level. His written language is on the third-grade level, and math performance is at the fourth-grade level. In class, Tom has significant deficits in adaptive functioning resulting in disruptive behavior and lack of educational progress. Tom requires the services of a one-to-one assistant for educational, medical, and behavioral purposes.

Tom began receiving speech and language services from an early intervention program at the age of 2 ½ years and special education services in prekindergarten in public school. During the first grade, Tom began to demonstrate aggressive behavior toward peers and adults and was assigned a one-to-one assistant. Following continued difficulty the next year, he was referred to a special education school for more intensive services. Tom's school history is significant for behavior problems including high-level disruption, self-injurious behavior, and aggression.

Tom receives both individual and group therapy services in his school. He struggles with accepting responsibility for his actions and is unable to identify alternative ways to cope with stress. He also has difficulty distinguishing fiction from reality when he is under stress, making grandiose statements regarding his physical and mental abilities during conflicts with others. Tom also receives speech and language services to address receptive, expressive, and pragmatic language skills for success in the classroom, community, and vocational settings. He has a difficult time interpreting non-verbal language. He tends to engage adults and peers only in topics of interest to him, inappropriately disengage from conversations, interrupt with another topic, or walk away. Tom also receives occupational therapy for fine motor, sensory motor, handwriting, and organizational skills.

The goal of transition planning is to assist students with disabilities as they prepare to leave school and move to postsecondary education, vocational training, integrated employment (including supported employment), continuing and adult education, adult services, independent living, and community participation. Tom's transition goals on his individualized education plan (IEP) include working with the Division of Rehabilitative Services, completing a vocational assessment to identify potential job areas, and working in an off-campus internship with the support of his one-to-one aide and a school job coach. ▶

Defining Disability from an Educational Perspective

What Is Special Education?

IDEA defines special education as "specially designed instruction designed to meet the unique needs of a child with a disability" (Batshaw, 2002; Hallahan and Kauffman, 2003; IDEA, 2004). It also defines a range of supplemental aids and services, such as assistive technology, and related services, such as occupational and physical therapy, designed to assist students with disabilities in benefiting from their education. *Supplemental aids and services* means aids, services, and other supports that are provided in regular education classes, other education-related settings, and extracurricular and nonacademic settings to enable children with disabilities to be educated with nondisabled children to the maximum extent appropriate (IDEA, 2004). Examples of supplemental aids and services might be assistive technologies such as a computer or adapted physical education.

Related services means transportation and such developmental, corrective, and other supportive services as are required to assist a child with a disability to benefit from special education, and includes speech-language pathology and audiology services, interpreting services, psychological services, physical and occupational therapy, recreation (including therapeutic recreation), early identification and assessment of disabilities in children, counseling services (including rehabilitation counseling), orientation and mobility services, and medical services for diagnostic or evaluation purposes. *Related services* also include school health services and school nurse services, social work services in schools, and parent counseling and training (IDEA, 2004).

Qualifying for eligibility is a two-part process: determining whether there is an identified disability as defined by IDEA and, if so, determining whether the student needs special education and related services to benefit from the education. Students may need special education because of physical, cognitive, academic, communication, or behavioral reasons. IDEA identifies 14 different categories of disability (see the glossary for definitions of these terms):

- mental retardation
- hearing impairment
- deafness
- speech or language impairment
- visual impairment
- emotional disturbance
- orthopedic impairment
- other health impairment
- specific learning disability
- multiple disabilities
- deaf-blindness
- traumatic brain injury
- autism
- developmental delay (applies only to children ages 3–5)

More than 6 million students with disabilities receive special education in public schools or private settings at public expense. There has been a steady increase in the number of students receiving services since 1975, with learning disabilities continuing to account for more than half the students in special education. Three of the 14 categories warrant specific mention with regard to number of students served: other health impaired, autism, and traumatic brain injury (TBI). Other health impairment includes students with attention deficit disorder with and without comorbid learning disabilities. The number of young children being diagnosed with this disorder continues to grow at a disturbing rate. In 1991, 58,749 students were served under this category; in 2002, more than 390,000 students were served.

Autism represents the most alarming growth in any special education category. Part of the increase in numbers is the result of these students having been previously counted under a different category, such as mental retardation. Only since 1997 has autism been a separate category of disability under IDEA. However, these "code jumpers" cannot account for the astounding increases being experienced in every public school system across the country. In 1991, only 5,415 students were coded for "autism." In 2010, we are serving more than 121,000 students with autism ages 6 through 21. There continues to be considerable debate about the causes for such alarming increases, with the Centers for Disease Control now estimating the incidence rates to be 1 in every 150 births.

Traumatic brain injury, created as a separate category in 1990, is another group experiencing significant increases. As emergency medical treatment has advanced, so has our ability to provide immediate care to children and adolescents sustaining life-threatening head trauma. In 1991, only 245 students with TBI were reported in the Annual Report to Congress. In 2002, more than 21,300 students were reported. This explosion in certain special education categories is putting additional stress on an already expensive and overburdened system.

IDEA: Major Provisions

IDEA is the federal legislation for special education services in the United States. It protects the rights of individuals with disabilities and regulates how states and public agencies provide special education and related services to these individuals.

Screening and Identification

Five major provisions are found in IDEA. The first provision involves the screening and identification process for identifying children in need of special education so that those procedures are as accurate as possible before a student's placement in a special education setting. It also helps ensure an unbiased assessment and decision regarding the type of services to be provided. One significant feature of this provision is Child Find, which provides public awareness, screening, and evaluation designed to identify disabilities and to make referrals as early as possible for young children with disabilities and their families who are in need of Early Intervention Services or Preschool Special Education (IDEA, 2004).

Nondiscriminatory Evaluation

The second provision involves ensuring that evaluations are nondiscriminatory. Nondiscriminatory evaluation refers to the selection and administration of tests that are not racially or culturally biased, so as to accurately identify whether or not a student has a disability and is in need of special education services. IDEA (2004) provides specific requirements about how evaluations should be conducted. First, the tests must have been validated for the specific purpose for which they are used, and evaluators must be knowledgeable and trained in the use of the test materials. Second, a variety of instruments and procedures must be used to gather relevant information. Third, the test results need to accurately reflect the student's aptitude or achievement level, rather than reflecting the student's disability.

Free and Appropriate Public Education and Least-Restrictive Environment

The third major provision involves the provision of a free and appropriate public education (FAPE) in the least-restrictive environment (LRE). FAPE involves schools ensuring that students with disabilities are provided with full educational opportunities required for students to benefit from special education services. Having an LRE requires that the educational opportunities provided occur to the maximum extent possible in the setting most similar to a general education placement, while still able to meet the needs of the individual (IDEA, 2004).

Procedural Safeguards

The fourth major provision involves procedural safeguards to protect the rights of children with disabilities and their parents. Procedural safeguards include protection in notification of procedures to the parents, due process hearings, mediation, the appeals process, and placement (IDEA, 2004; Wright and Wright, 2007).

Due Process

The final provision of IDEA (2004) is that individuals with disabilities and their families are guaranteed the right of due process as established by the Fourteenth Amendment of the U.S. Constitution. IDEA identifies specific requirements for both families and schools and provides impartial hearings when a disagreement occurs involving the identification, evaluation, placement, or service delivery for an individual with a disability.

The Referral Process and Ongoing Assessment

The referral process is the initial step for an individual to receive special education services. Any child suspected to have special needs because of a disability may be referred to a school or agency to be considered for special education or related services. The parents, teachers, physicians, community agencies, other individuals, or organizations that work with the child may make referrals. Referrals may also be the result of district-wide testing or screening. Referrals may be made anytime between birth and 21 years of age, but the processes that apply to school-age and young adult students are the focus of this chapter. Referrals for children ages 3 to 21 occur through the local public school (IDEA, 2004).

The referral process includes specific actions that the school must take during the identification process. First, the school must provide written notification to the parents at the time of referral. This notification must identify the process used to determine whether a student has a disability and is in need of special education services. Following notification, the school gathers information to determine whether assessments are justified for a student to determine if an individual has a disability and may be in need of special education services. If the school personnel determine that assessments are justified, they must inform the parents in writing regarding the assessment process and gain consent for the assessments. Likewise, parents must also be notified if a determination is made that assessments are not justified. Parents maintain the right to challenge the decision of the school not to perform the assessments (Office of Special Education Programs [OSEP], 2007). Once eligibility for special education services is determined, a range of service options become available depending on the age of the individual.

Children ages 3 to 21 who are identified as eligible for special education services receive service delivery through the local public school system. Children with disabilities may receive a variety of services within the public school setting, all designed to address issues that adversely affect the educational process. The amount and frequency of special education support is determined by the IEP team, the members of which are outlined later in this chapter. Supports may include special education instruction, related services including speech or language services, occupational therapy, physical therapy, mental health therapy, medical or nursing supports, or individual assistance.

Once a student is identified as eligible for special education services, he or she will also receive periodic reevaluations. The reevaluation process occurs if the school determines that the educational or related services needs, including improved academic or functional performance of the student warrant a reevaluation or the child's parent or teacher requests a reevaluation. A reevaluation may occur not more than once a year, unless both the parent and the school agree otherwise. A reevaluation must occur at least once every 3 years, unless the parent and the public agency agree that the reevaluation is unnecessary (IDEA, 2004; OSEP, 2007).

Section 504 of the Rehabilitation Act prohibits discrimination against individuals who meet the definition of having a disability due to a physical or mental impairment that substantially limits a major life activity (Council for Exceptional Children, 2002). Such impairments may include ADHD, asthma, allergies, communicable diseases, and significant medical conditions (Rosenfeld, 1999). Section 504 guarantees that a child with a disability has equal access to an appropriate education. Unlike IDEA, Section 504 does not require the school to provide an IEP designed to meet a child's specific educational needs. The child may, however, receive accommodations and modifications to his or her educational program. (For an example of a Section 504 Plan, see the Appendix to this chapter.)

What to Teach Special Education Students?

For many years, it was common practice for schools to place students into special education classrooms based on the category of their disability. With the emphasis shifting to inclusion of students in general education, students are now being placed in a noncategorical fashion with the understanding that greater progress will be made if they are allowed to learn alongside their nondisabled peers. This idea of LRE, where students are educated to "the maximum extent appropriate" in a general education setting is a challenging and often contentious component of the IDEA. Many general education teachers (42%) feel this is unmanageable, because of deficiencies in teacher attitude, teacher preparation, administrative support (Henley, Ramsey, and Algozzine, 2006) and more recently to the demands of No Child Left Behind

Act (2001) for greater accountability and participation of all students in state-wide assessments. With respect to attitude, teachers often feel that students with disabilities present an overwhelming need to provide different instruction and behavioral management, thereby distracting the whole class. While IDEA insures that students with disabilities will have access to a free and appropriate education, Congress did not define what it meant by the term *appropriate*. No one instructional approach is right for everyone, and the process of defining appropriate for one student may be different than for another. The Supreme Court in the case of *Board of Education of the Hendrick Hudson School District v. Rowley* (1982) clarified the term *appropriate* to mean reasonably calculated to insure educational progress but not a guarantee of reaching the maximum potential possible. To assist in the process of determining the appropriate placement in the least-restrictive environment, IDEA requires the development of an IEP for each student.

IEP: The Cornerstone of Special Education

The individualized education plan, or IEP, is the document that identifies the services, educational needs, and goals and objectives for any student ages 3 to 21 with a disability. The IEP team meets annually to determine progress toward the plan and update relevant information. The IEP is comprised of several key components. The components presented here include the participants, present levels of performance, goals and objectives, accommodations and modifications, and a transition plan.

Participants

The participants of an IEP team include the individuals working with any student receiving special education services. The participants must include the parents or guardians of the student, the special education teacher, a general education teacher, any related service providers as indicated by the team, and a qualified representative of the public agency (IDEA, 2004; Center on Positive Behavior and Interventions and Supports, 2004). An administrator or representative of the local school system acts as an IEP chairperson and provides guidance to the team regarding the availability of resources to support the student. The participants may also include individuals who are qualified to interpret the results of any assessments being discussed at the meeting. The parent may also include other individuals who work with the student who have specific knowledge or expertise regarding the child. When appropriate, the student may also participate in the IEP team meeting. The team participants develop the IEP at an annual meeting.

Present Levels of Performance

Another component of the IEP is the present levels of performance (PLPs) on assessments for all areas of service in a child's educational program. The PLPs of each individual student with an IEP are assessed each year as a new IEP is being developed. The PLPs are comprised of formal and informal assessments designed to provide the most recent information regarding the academic functioning of the child and to help identify progress made since the last IEP and administration of assessments. The PLPs also help identify specific areas of strength or weakness for the students in each area of their educational program. The team members developing the goals and objectives for the IEP will use the results of the PLPs to identify appropriate areas to target for development and accurate starting points for the goals and objectives.

Goals and Objectives

The goals and objectives found on the IEP identify the target growth for a student receiving special education services for the academic year at issue. The goals are developed for each area of identified need, including academics and related services, and are based on the results of the PLPs. Goals are developed as annual targets, with supporting objectives to be mastered along the way. IEP goals must be designed to be observable and measurable to allow for the clear assessment of progress. Although IDEA did not mandate specific objectives, it is common for goals to be supported by sequential objectives, or benchmarks, toward the achievement of the goal. Schools are required to provide parents progress updates on the same schedule as parents of peers who do not have a disability. The updates to the IEP indicate progress toward the annual goals and objectives.

Transition Plan

Another key component of the IEP is the transition plan. A transition plan is a set of activities developed for a student with a disability to ensure that their academic and functional progress helps prepare them for movement from school to postschool activities. Postsecondary school activities may include vocational education, employment (including supported employment), continuing and adult education, adult services, independent living, or community participation (IDEA, 2004). Transition plans begin at the age of 14, when a statement of transition needs of an individual is identified. At age 16, specific transition services and activities are included, along with the identification and coordination of postsecondary services. The transition plan is based on the individual child's needs, strengths, and interests and may include classroom-based instruction, community experiences, vocational training, and functional daily living skills.

CASE EXAMPLE

Neil is a 20-year-old student with a disability (Federal Classification Code: 14, Autism). He is currently enrolled in a self-contained program at a private separate day school. He receives specialized instruction from a teacher and a teaching assistant. He also receives counseling, speech and language therapy, occupational therapy, and transition as related services. Neil requires the support of a one-to-one aide and is placed in a classroom with nine other students. He has a verbal IQ of 46, a performance IQ of 46, and a full-scale IQ of 40. Neil is on a second-grade reading level and is working on completing forms that require personal information including name, address, and phone number. Neil is on a first-grade math level and is working on counting money totaling to $5.00. Neil has difficulty properly performing personal hygiene skills independently. He uses a picture schedule, which increases his independence during transitions. Neil has a difficult time staying on task and using appropriate language when he is excited or overstimulated. He receives the following accommodations and adaptations in the classroom: (1) supervision for safety issues, (2) assistance when self-stimulatory behaviors (such as rocking or self-talking) interfere with class, (3) modeling appropriate social cues, (4) redirection to task, (5) immediate feedback, and (6) assistance with note-taking and adaptations to class work.

Neil attends weekly community-based instruction classes. He is able to order and pay for a meal from a fast food restaurant with assistance. He can navigate around a grocery store and utilize the store directory to find items with assistance. Neil's transition plan in his IEP, includes activities to connect him to the Developmental Disabilties Administration (DDA). The DDA manages funding for supports and services for people with developmental disabilities. A person is eligible for DDA if they have a severe, chronic disability caused by a physical or mental condition, other than a single diagnosis of mental illness. Services provided include vocational, supported employment, family support services, individual support services, community residential support services, respite care, and behavioral services. The length of services will be lifelong as needed. Beginning in September, Neil will begin work at the League for Disabilities with a job coach to facilitate successful employment. ▮

Extended School Year

IDEA also contains a component for the provision of Extended School Year (ESY) services. ESY services are individualized instructional programs for students with disabilities, which are provided beyond the length of the regular student school year and usually occur during the summer. ESY is provided for students with disabilities when they require continuous instruction or service to prevent regression or loss of skills acquired during the school year. ESY services may also be provided when skills are emerging and continuous instruction or support is necessary for full skill acquisition.

Accommodations and Modifications

The accommodations and modifications section of the IEP identifies the specific strategies and supports required by a student with a disability. Accommodations are supports provided to individuals to allow them equal opportunity to benefit from the general education curriculum. These supports may include changes to the presentation of material, the nature of responses required, time or schedule changes, or setting changes. Specific accommodations may include checklists, visual cues, use of a calculator, note-taking assistance, extra time for tasks, or alternative locations for testing. The activity or required outcome is the same for the child with a disability as those without.

Modifications alter the nature or outcome of an activity expected by a student with a disability and include shortened assignments or simplified versions of material (see Table 11.3 for examples of accommodations and modifications that might be made for students with disabilities). All accommodations and modifications identified by the IEP team are provided to the student for daily classroom instruction, as well as any test or assessments

Table 11.3.   Sample accommodations and modifications

Organizational strategies	Delivery modifications
extra response and processing time	modified materials
time limits extended for assignments	provide extra drill
reduced length or complexity of	provide advance organizers
assignments	reduce quantity of assigned work
give alternative assignments	individualize spelling lists
ask students to repeat directions	provide curriculum geared to student's
provide homework planner	instructional level
provide a structured daily schedule	Reading strategies
Classroom environment strategies	use multisensory approaches
assign preferential seating	use color coding
use individual study carrels	provide graphic organizers
Equipment modifications	develop individual word bank
Braille materials	develop language experience stories
calculator for mathematics	use sound blending or word analysis
use of electronic devices, such as word	Written strategies
processor, computer, augmentative com-	provide graphic organizers (webbing)
munication device	individualize word lists
Presentation modifications	use vocabulary words
give assignments orally and visually	reduce written copying
tape lessons	provide technology supports
test students orally	Math strategies
provide materials in print format	provide sample problems
correct student errors immediately	use flow charts
repeat directions as needed	use manipulatives
accessibility to closed caption or video	use calculator, number line
material	provide practice, reinforcement, and
sign language interpreter	reteaching opportunities
amplification or visual display of test direc-	
tions and/or teacher directions	
large print material	
verbatim audiotape of directions and	
lessons	
verbatim reading of selected sections of	
test or vocabulary by faculty	
note taker	

taken by the child. As part of NCLB, all students receiving special education services must participate in high-stakes testing. A crucial part of the IEP in regard to this requirement is the section on accommodations and modifications. Any accommodations and modifications provided to a child during daily instruction are required for any type of statewide or district assessment as well.

LRE

One final and crucial aspect of the IEP is the determination of LRE, which requires that, "to the maximum extent appropriate, children with disabilities, including children in public or private institutions or other care facilities, are educated with children who are nondisabled" (IDEA, 2004). Additional LRE considerations include that the placement is reviewed annually, based on the needs indicated in the IEP, as close as possible to the child's home or in the school that he or she would attend if not living with a disability, and free of any potential harmful effect on the child or on the quality of services that he or she needs. It is also required that a child with a disability is not removed from education in age-appropriate regular classrooms solely because of needed modifications in the general education curriculum (IDEA, 2004).

The team participants must agree on all aspects of the IEP. If any member of the IEP team disagrees with the recommendations of the overall team, mediation of the disputes must occur. If mediation is unsuccessful in resolving the differences, either the parent or the school may pursue due process.

Where to Teach Special Education Students?

Once the IEP has been developed, the team determines where it can be implemented. A cascade of services or placement options provides interventions along a continuum from least- to most-restrictive ranging from minimal supports in the general education classroom through part-time special classes, full-time special classes, special schools, homebound instruction, and residential educational settings.

Continuum of Service Delivery

Each child's IEP must include an explanation of why the child with a disability would not participate with children without disabilities in the regular class or in extracurricular activities. That is considered to be consistent with the least-restrictive environment.

Delivery of Service: Teaching Models for Students with Special Needs

With each new reauthorization of IDEA, there have been new provisions that represent major advancements in ensuring that every student with a disability receives a high-quality and individually designed program. A hallmark of the 2004 reauthorization was providing access to a challenging curriculum with high expectations for achievement, which increased the focus of special education from simply ensuring access to education to improving the educational performance of students with disabilities. Schools are now required to align special education services with the larger national school improvement efforts including standards, assessments, and accountability (Nolet and McLaughlin, 2005).

Special education services can be delivered to students in a variety of teaching models ranging from "pull out" services including the traditional resource room model in which students with special needs leave the general education class for specific amounts of time during the day to work with special education teachers to "push in" services that bring special education into the general education classroom. Separate special education classrooms are also available for students who need that structure throughout the day. The key ingredient to all these models is successful collaboration between general educators and special educators.

General education teachers have been considered specialists in content, curriculum, and scope and sequence of instruction, while special educators have been seen as having expertise in learning styles, strategies for differentiation, diagnostic and prescriptive teaching, modifications and accommodations, and behavior management. One instructional model, *co-teaching*, is a unique blend of expertise in "what to teach" and "how to teach." It involves the practice of having two or more professionals deliver substantive instruction to a diverse group of students in the same physical space, usually the general education classroom (Cook and Friend, 1995).

Related Services

Students with disabilities are often at risk for mental health issues. Because of this risk, schools often provide support through a variety of services. Mental health services in a school setting may be delivered in a number of ways. The most common approaches to delivery of mental health services involve individual or group therapy services. Individual therapy services are typically delivered by licensed mental health service providers, including social workers, school psychologists, and counselors, sometimes in consultation with psychiatrists. Group therapy services in special education focus on the development of the skills a student requires to be successful in the classroom and benefit from education. This may involve social skill development, recreational groups, or groups focused on specific deficit areas, such as communication, behavior, managing emotions, cooperative learning, or coping strategies. Additional mental health services in special education may involve expressive therapies such as art, music, or drama. The use of these modalities may occur for students with difficulty with more traditional therapy approaches.

Discipline for Students Receiving Special Education Services

Students receiving special education services are protected by specific disciplinary procedures under IDEA. There are several factors behind the IDEA regulations regarding disciplinary procedures. Students receiving special education services are currently overrepresented in the number of students suspended or expelled in schools (Skiba, 2002). The requirements outlined in IDEA are believed to strike a fair balance between having effective discipline and providing appropriate supports for students with disabilities. They also ensure that the right to a free and appropriate public education is not being impinged and that implementation of disciplinary procedures is consistent with law. The regulations provided by IDEA do not prevent school officials from maintaining a safe school environment conducive to learning, as it is recognized that inappropriate behaviors cannot be allowed to interfere with the education of others or to disrupt the education process. The two main categories of disciplinary action covered by IDEA are suspension and expulsion.

Suspension

Suspension from school is generally characterized as the temporary removal of a student from a school setting for disciplinary reasons. However, in-school suspension is another disciplinary tool and is discussed below. The specific regulations provided by IDEA 2004 for disciplinary procedures limit schools to 10 cumulative days of suspension per year for students in special education. Schools are not required to provide special education services during the first 10 days of a suspension. Suspensions up to 10 days can occur against parental approval if discipline procedures are applied consistently to all students. Suspensions of more than 10 days constitute a change in placement and trigger the procedural protections of IDEA. Students may have protection under IDEA only if they are currently receiving special education services or have been referred for special education services and the school had knowledge of the disability.

In-School Suspension

An in-school suspension is defined as the exclusion within the school build-ing of a student from regular education activities for disciplinary reasons. In-school suspension is often used by schools as a consequence for behaviors that do not reach the level of severity requiring out-of-school suspension or expul-sion. In-school suspensions are counted as part of the cumulative 10 days of suspension per year for special education students. Based on changes in the 2004 reauthorization of IDEA, schools are now required to collect and report data regarding in-school suspension to state departments of education for col-lection by the U.S. Department of Education.

CASE EXAMPLE

Vince is 17 years old and was placed in foster care at birth due to the drug addiction of his biological mother. He was adopted at a year and half by his foster family. Vince's parents adopted another son when he was 3, and he had a difficult time adjusting to this change. Vince's adopted mother died on Christmas Eve when he was 5 years old. Vince continues to identify his foster mother's death as an ongoing source of stress.

Vince has had a long history of school difficulty. During kindergarten, he demonstrated aggression and temper outbursts, hitting peers and teachers and destroying class materials. He was referred to the IEP team in first grade for ongoing behavioral concerns. He was given a disability code of 06, emotionally disturbed. In the second grade, Vince continued to demon-strate behavioral and emotional issues and assaulted a staff member. Fol-lowing ongoing difficulty in school, Vince was put on a half day modified schedule. In third grade he was hospitalized at a child and adolescent psy-chiatric center. He was suspended multiple times from his school in his fourth-grade year for making threats and moved to a self-contained pro-gram. In the fifth grade, a referral was made to a private separate day school placement.

Vince is currently a student at a private day school for students with spe-cial education needs. Academically, he experiences difficulty in all content areas, reading and writing on the second-grade level, and performing math at the third-grade level. He has a verbal IQ of 81, a performance IQ of 75, and a full-scale IQ of 77. Vince also has Axis I diagnoses, including attention deficit hyperactivity disorder, oppositional defiant disorder, and major depressive disorder. He struggles at times to identify positive characteristics about himself. When confronted regarding inappropriate behavior, Vince tends to shut down. He has been able to identify areas that cause anxiety, frustration, and stress but is less able to identify alternative coping mechanisms. He also struggles to have appropriate interactions with peers and staff.

Vince has a job after school as a dishwasher in a local coffee shop. He has been working there for the past year and spends most of his earnings on tennis shoes. He has excellent attendance and has not missed a single day of school this year. Vince was a member of the basketball team this past winter, where he demonstrated leadership abilities and excellent teamwork. He and his family report that he has been compliant with his medications.

Vince's transition plan includes specific goals and objectives to support his goal of obtaining long-term employment following high school. Examples of these include (1) research various jobs of interest to determine qualifications and job requirements, (2) create a list of 5 to 10 job skill requirements needed to obtain desired employment, (3) demonstrate disability awareness by identifying accommodations needed in a variety of workplace settings, (4) participate in a variety of job awareness activities (i.e., presentations, guest speakers, and field trips), (5) complete job-related writing activities (i.e., job applications, business letters, resume), and (6) accept constructive feedback from supervisors. ▶

Alternative Education Settings

Alternative education settings are placements created for specific disciplinary violations (IDEA, 2004). Students engaging in drug or alcohol use or bringing in weapons to school are subject to discipline regardless of disability. If the IEP and placement of a student with a disability are determined to be appropriate, that student is subject to the same disciplinary actions as his or her nondisabled peers. For violations requiring an alternative education setting, a placement will be provided for up to 45 days to evaluate the student and determine future placement.

Expulsion

An expulsion for a student is characterized as the permanent removal of a student from the educational setting. Students with disabilities are afforded specific protections regarding expulsion. Following the recommendation for expulsion of a student receiving special education services, the IEP team must meet for a manifestation determination meeting. This mandatory meeting determines if a relationship exists between the student's behavior subject to discipline and that student's disability. It is required when student exceeds 10 days of suspension or if a recommendation for expulsion is made by the school. The meeting must occur within 10 days of the date of disciplinary action. The team must review the IEP to determine if it is appropriate and revise the IEP as necessary.

Manifestation Determination

According to IDEA 2004, an IEP team must reach a determination that behavior was a manifestation of the child's disability if any of the following is true: (1) the IEP or placement were inappropriate or the IEP was not being implemented, including appropriate behavior intervention strategies; (2) the child does not have the capacity to understand the consequences of his or her behavior as a result of the disability; (3) the child's disability prevented his or her ability to control his or her behavior; or (4) the child is unable to conform to the schools rules because of the disability. If any of the statements is true, then the manifestation meeting ends because a relationship between conduct and disability exists. At this point the IEP team would conduct a functional behavior analysis (FBA) and develop a behavior intervention plan (BIP) to address the conduct and provide the proper supports. The FBA and BIP are described in further detail in the next section. If the action resulting in expulsion is determined to not be the result of the disability, the student can be disciplined in the same manner as a student without a disability.

During proceedings to determine manifestation, the student is either suspended, as long as 10 days have not passed, or he or she must remain in current placement until question is resolved. This is referred to as the "stay put rule" (*Honig v. Doe*, 1988). If the parents of a child with a disability disagree with the outcome of the meeting, they may initiate due process proceedings.

Functional Behavior Analysis / Behavior Intervention Plan

One common approach to both preventing increases in behaviors and addressing the outcome of a manifestation meeting is the development of an FBA and a BIP. An FBA is the process of observing and assessing a problem behavior to determine the function of the behavior. Following the identification of when, where, and why the behavior occurs, a BIP is developed to assist in preventing the future occurrence of the behavior and to encourage the development of appropriate replacement behaviors. The BIP identifies both positive and negative consequences to assist the student in reducing the occurrence of the problem behavior.

Positive Behavior Interventions and Supports

Many schools have developed proactive measures to address the behavioral difficulties faced by students with disabilities. One measure, called positive behavior interventions and supports, or PBIS, identifies three main levels of behavior supports to provide for students with disabilities: school-wide support, specific group supports, and individual supports (Center on Positive Behavioral Interventions and Supports, 2004). School-wide supports are proven, effective behavioral practices, interventions, and system-wide strategies to encourage and assist in the reduction of problem behaviors. Specific group supports are specially designed programs for groups of at-risk students. Individual supports are developed for those students with high levels of at-risk behavior. PBIS represents one of many approaches to developing a strong school-wide climate of prevention and support for students with disabilities, as well as those without (see Table 11.4 for a hierarchy of interventions).

Table 11.4.   Hierarchy of behavior interventions

Setting strategies	Limit setting
physical classroom arrangement	clear, concise, and enforceable
structured activities	state what you want the child to be doing
schedule	instead of calling attention to the nega-
good instruction	tive behavior
Surface management	provide enough time for the child to proc-
redirection	ess and respond appropriately
proximity	Time-out
facial expression	in class
nonverbal cues	out of class
Point sheets	state the behavior
token economy	duration
contracts	location
reinforcement	
consequences	

Restraint and Seclusion

No other issue in special education has had such a sensational airing in the press as that of restraint and seclusion. Several deaths occurring at residential treatment facilities where staff were not properly trained in implementing safe restraint brought this issue before Congress in 2000. As a result new regulations were adopted, and each state must comply with these new regulations. Preventing injury and death related to the use of restraint and seclusion is paramount. IDEA does not specifically define restraint and seclusion; however other legislative acts and individual states have provided definitions. The term *restraint* means any mechanical or personal restriction that immobilizes or reduces the ability of an individual to move his or her arms, legs, or head freely, not including devices, such as orthopedically prescribed devices, surgical dressings or bandages, protective helmets, or any other methods that involves the physical holding of a resident for the purpose of conducting routine physical examinations or tests or to protect the resident from falling out of bed or to permit the individual to participate in activities without the risk of physical harm (Children's Health Act of 2000).

The term *seclusion* means a behavior-control technique involving locked isolation. The term does not include a time-out. *Seclusion* is further defined as the involuntary confinement of an individual under the direction of a physician or registered nurse alone in a room that a patient is physically prevented from leaving (Maryland State Board of Education, 1981).

Guidelines and information on appropriate and inappropriate restraint and seclusion techniques issued by clinical and regulatory bodies (such as the American Psychiatric Association and the Joint Commission on Accreditation of Healthcare Organizations) are available. In addition, restraint and seclusion procedures (or any other interventions) that have been found to be best practices or, conversely, have been found to be dangerous have been widely circulated in the field. Professionals agree that the critical piece in any procedure for restraint and seclusion is the adequate training of staff implementing these procedures.

High-Stakes Testing and Accountability

The No Child Left Behind Act of 2001 (NCLB) required that, by the 2005–6 school year, states would administer annual assessments in reading and language arts and in mathematics in each of grades 3 through 5 and at least once in grades 6 through 9 and in grades 10 through 12. These assessments must be aligned with the state's rigorous academic standards and provide information about student achievement of those standards. In the 2007–8 school year, states began to administer annual assessments in science at least once in grades 3 through 5, 6 through 9, and 10 through 12. At least 95 percent of the student population must participate in the assessments. In addition, 95 percent of each identified subgroup, including special education students, must participate in these tests. Students with disabilities must take the same high-stakes tests as all general education students and be provided with access to the general education curriculum at their identified grade level. A fifth-grade student with moderate cognitive limitation who reads at a first-grade level must receive instruction in fifth-grade content and take the fifth-grade test alongside his nondisabled peers. IDEA provides for some modifications and accommodations to the testing process if they are routinely used and specified in the IEP. However, an alternative assessment is available for students with disabilities if the IEP process determines that they cannot participate in the regular assessment. These alternative assessments are available to a small, limited percentage of students with the most severe cognitive limitations. Some states, such as Maryland, have chosen to have passing a high-stakes test as part of the graduation requirement. This is not an NCLB requirement. NCLB requires that students be tested but does not require passing the tests to receive a diploma. This is a state-by-state decision.

Conclusion

Special education services have evolved over the past 30 years to include early identification of preschool age children, a broad range of services for school age children, and transition planning for those young adults aging out of the educational system. Health professionals in the community often interact with school personnel at all points of this continuum, depending on the age of the clients they serve. Even practitioners who interact with adults who have been out of the school system for years benefit the people they work with by having a working knowledge of the operations of the special education and vocational systems and how those systems affect the adults they serve. To best meet the needs of the clients of every age and the families they serve, community advocates must fully understand the special education system. Each organization working with students with disabilities brings its own expertise to the table; however, organizations often see the problems from their specific point of view. As professionals gain a better understanding of how the special education system works, the paradigms operating and the demands being placed on them, stronger collaboration and therefore better outcomes are possible.

APPENDIX. ELIGIBILITY FORM FOR STUDENTS IDENTIFIED WITH A
DISABILITY UNDER SECTION 504

Date: _____

Name: _____ DOB:_____
School:_____ Grade/Section: _____
Student ID #: _____
Name of the student's home school if different from current school: _____
_____

1. Specify the diagnosed physical or mental impairment: _____
_____

2. Cite the medical or psychological assessment report used to document the physical
or mental impairment: _____
_____

3. Check the major life activity substantially limited by the disability:
_____ Breathing   _____ Caring for Self   _____ Hearing   _____ Learning
_____ Speaking   _____ Walking   _____ Seeing   _____ Working
_____ Performing Manual Tasks
__ Other: _____
4. Specify the data for the determination of substantial limitation to the major life
activity:

History of impairment:

History of Impairment	Describe Specific Limitation

Standardized assessments (Achievement, State, Functional):

Standardized Assessment	Describe Specific Limitation

Classroom assessments (Report Card Grades, Benchmark Assessments, Milestone Assessments, Informal Assessments, Chapter Tests, Quizzes):

Classroom Assessment	Describe Specific Limitation

Teacher reports (Student Performance and Behavior):

Teacher Report	Describe Specific Limitation

5. Determine the degree to which the impairment limits the major life activity:

Consider the following:

• The extent to which the impairment limits the major life activity as a whole (i.e., all aspects of learning).

• The extent to which the impairment limits the major life activity as compared to the average student in the general population.

• The extent to which the impairment limits the major life activity not related to other factors such as motivation, immediate situation, or environment.

Check one: _____ Mild Limitation to Major Life Activity

_____ Moderate Limitation to Major Life Activity

_____ Substantial Limitation to Major Life Activity

Next Steps:

• Develop Individual Student Plan for students with a diagnosed impairment that results in a substantial limitation to a major life activity.

• Parents/guardians should receive notification of their procedural rights, including an impartial hearing, if they are in disagreement with identification, evaluation, or educational placement of their child.

Completed by:

_____

_____

_____

_____

References

Batshaw, ML (ed.) 2002. *Children with Disabilities*, 5th ed. Baltimore: Paul H. Brookes.

Board of Education of the Hendrick Hudson Central School District v. Rowley. 1982. 458 U.S. 176.

Brown v. Board of Education of Topeka. 1954. 347 U.S. 483.

Center on Positive Behavior and Interventions and Supports. 2004. *Implementers Blueprint and Self-assessment.* Eugene: University of Oregon Center on Positive Behavior and Interventions and Supports.

Children's Health Act of 2000. P.L. 106-310, 42 U.S.C. §201 et seq.

Clair EB, Church RP, Batshaw ML. 2002. Special education services. In ML Batshaw (ed.), *Children with Disabilities*, 5th ed., 589–606. Baltimore: Paul H. Brookes.

Cook L, Friend M. 1995. Co-teaching: Guidelines for creating effective practices. *Focus on Exceptional Children* 28(3): 1–15.

Council for Exceptional Children. 2002. Understanding the differences between IDEA and Section 504. Available at www.ldonline.org/article/6086.

Diana v. California State Board of Education. 1970. C-70-37 RFP, N. D. Cal.

Education for All Handicapped Children's Act. 1975. P.L. 94-142, 20 U.S.C. §1400 et seq.

Hallahan DP, Kauffman JK. 2003. *Exceptional Learners: Introduction to Special Education*, 9th ed. Boston: Allyn & Bacon.

Henley M, Ramsey RS, Algozzine RF. 2006. *Characteristics of and Strategies for Teaching Students with Mild Disabilities*, 5th ed. Boston: Allyn & Bacon.

Honig v. Doe. 1988. 484 U.S. 305.

Individuals with Disabilities Education Improvement Act of 2004. P.L. 108-446, 20 U.S.C. §1400 et seq.

Maryland State Board of Education. 1981. *Code of Maryland Regulations.* Annapolis, MD: Division of State Documents.

No Child Left Behind Act of 2001. P.L. 107-110, amendment to the Elementary and Secondary Education Act of 1965, 20 U.S.C. §6301 et seq.

Nolet V, McLaughlin MJ. 2005. *Accessing the General Curriculum: Including Students with Disabilities in Standards-Based Reform,* 2nd ed. Thousand Oaks, CA: Corwin Press.

Pennsylvania Association of Retarded Citizens v. Commonwealth of Pennsylvania. 1971/ 1972. F.Supp. 1257 (E.D. Pa. 1971) and 334 F.Supp. 1257 334 (E.D. PA 1972).

Rehabilitation Act of 1973. P.L. 93-112, 29 U.S.C. §794.

Rosenfeld SJ. 1999. Section 504 and IDEA: Basic similarities and differences. Available at www.wrightslaw.com/advoc/articles/504_ IDEA_Rosenfeld.html.

Skiba RJ. 2002. Special education and school discipline: A precarious balance. *Behavioral Disorders* 27(2): 81–97.

Smith TEC. 2001. Sections 504, the ADA, and pubic schools. *Remedial and Special Education* 22(6): 335–43.

Smith TEC, Polloway EA, Patton JR, Dowdy CA. 2008. *Teaching Students with Special Needs in Inclusive Settings,* 5th ed. Boston: Allyn & Bacon.

Turnbull HR, Turnbull AP. 1988. *Free Appropriate Public Education: The Law and Children with Disabilities,* 5th ed. Denver: Love Publishing.

U.S. Department of Education, Office of Special Education Programs. (2009). Building the Legacy: IDEA 2004. Available at http://idea.ed.gov/.

Wright PW, Wright PD. 2007. Procedural safeguards and parental notice. Available at wrightslaw.com/info/safgd.index.htm.

Wright PW, Wright PD. 2009. Discrimination: Section 504 and ADA. Available at www.wrightslaw.com/info/sec504.index.htm.

12

Pharmacotherapy

Alison A. Golombek, M.D., and
Bryan King, M.D.

CASE EXAMPLES

Kathleen is a 10-year-old girl who presents to a child and adolescent psychiatry outpatient clinic for medication follow-up. A review of her history reveals that she was diagnosed with bipolar disorder at the age of 4 owing to intense daily "meltdowns." She is currently prescribed olanzapine 10 mg daily, fluoxetine 20 mg daily, and clonidine 0.1 mg twice a day. She has had numerous medication trials over the years. Her mother reports that Kathleen often seems calmer when medications are started or increased, but that the effect generally wears off within 1 to 2 months. Kathleen has gained 30 pounds in 1 year.

Her mother states that Kathleen's temper tantrums began around the age of 2 or 3. They continue to occur daily, typically when Kathleen does not get her way or when she is separated from her mother. Her mother reports that her daughter has had longstanding problems with separation. Even in the first grade she screamed, cried, and held on to the classroom door. While she physically inched closer to the other children as the year progressed, she lost this skill over the summer and began each new school year with distress and tantrums. Her mother reports that Kathleen often seems like a younger child: she has not learned to read more than a few words, enjoys playing with first-graders, and cannot sleep in her own bed or be away from her mother without distress. She does not know whether her daughter has received intelligence or academic testing. She does not believe that Kathleen or her family ever received intervention targeted at Kathleen's temper tantrums or problems separating.

During the interview, Kathleen had difficulties focusing. Her attention was often drawn to other things in the room. Her language was only partially intelligible, and she had difficulty understanding or answering questions asked of her. She also struggled to read a book written for first-graders but enjoyed the pictures. She initially refused to give up playing with a computer toy but eventually joined her mother in reading a book. Hearing, speech and language, and neuropsychological testing was obtained. While Kathleen's hearing was intact, she demonstrated mixed receptive and expressive speech delays, a full-scale IQ of 55, and multiple deficiencies in executive function. A medical workup indicated that she was obese and had an abnormal lipid profile.

In combination with behavioral therapy and adjustments to her school curriculum, Kathleen was tapered from olanzapine and clonidine with no increase in agitation or aggression but with gradual weight loss. As her parents continued to notice problems with attention, hyperactivity, and impulsivity, she was started on a methylphenidate preparation with good results supported by serial attention deficit hyperactivity disorder (ADHD) rating scales. ▶

Christopher is a 22-year-old man with a longstanding history of developmental delay. He also has a history of seizure disorder, although recent EEGs have been unremarkable. His parents described one episode of tonic-clonic activity in early childhood but more sustained problems with momentarily "zoning out," which his teachers also noticed. Although his parents cannot recall any obvious seizures for several years, Chris continues to take carbamazepine, which was started many years ago They reported this medication was increased several months ago owing to the emergence of aggression and agitation in the context of moving to a new group home. At the time, Chris was also prescribed fluoxetine, 40 mg daily, for anxiety, and risperidone, 2 mg daily, for aggression. His parents reported that their son worries a lot about some things, such as the new group home, and sometimes picks his skin when he is upset. In the past, similar symptoms abated with fluoxetine.

Shortly after Chris's carbamazepine was increased, his parents and caregivers noted a significant change. He was unable to walk steadily and even fell once. His supported work environment supervisors observed that he was unusually tired during the day, more easily frustrated by tasks he ordinarily enjoyed, and more agitated and aggressive, yelling at staff members and coworkers.

On examination, Christopher was ataxic. He reported seeing two objects when only one was presented. He had orthostatic hypotension. A workup to determine the possibility of delirium including urine analysis and toxicology, a complete blood cell count, liver and renal function tests, and electrolytes was conducted and the results were normal. His carbamazepine level, however, was elevated. Over time, Christopher's psychiatrist, neurologist, parents, and caregivers worked to adjust his medications. He was successfully tapered from carbamazepine without seizures. Similarly, risperidone was decreased over time to 0.5 mg twice a day. Reductions beyond this dose resulted in increased agitation and aggression that abated with restored doses. However, owing to concern that this taper was initially conducted during the Christmas holidays, a subsequent trial was conducted, resulting in successful discontinuation. Reductions to fluoxetine resulted in increased anxiety symptoms and behaviors; thus, Chris continued to take fluoxetine at 40 mg with good results. ▶

Psychopharmacology in Individuals with Intellectual Disabilities

Individuals with intellectual disability (ID) may be three to six times more likely to experience some type of psychopathology (Aman et al., 2004). Studies indicate widespread use of psychotropic medications in this population, with rates of use of 20 to 50 percent for individuals living in residential communities and 25 to 33 percent for those living in the community (Harris, 2006). Furthermore, while the receipt of psychotropic medications is common, psychiatric specialists see only a minority of adults with ID (Lewis et al., 2002). Moreover, it is not uncommon for persons receiving antipsychotic medications to have no psychiatric diagnosis listed in their chart (Lewis et al., 2002). Some authors suggest that people with developmental delays may be the most overmedicated of all populations. Others observe that individuals in this population often receive only medication management despite concerns for limited efficacy and common adverse reactions, including worsening self-injurious behavior, agitation, aggression, onset of psychosis and depression, and interference with learning (Holden and Gitlesen, 2004).

Studies evaluating the efficacy of psychotropic medications for individuals with developmental disabilities are limited. Most studies are small, consist of open trials or case series, vary in outcome measure, and are short in duration. These characteristics make meta-analysis difficult if not impossible. Efforts to establish clinical consensus have been conducted in recent years, for example, with guidelines found in the *Treatment of Psychiatric and Behavioral Problems with Individuals with Mental Retardation: An Update of the Expert Consensus Guidelines for Mental Retardation / Developmental Disability* (Aman et al., 2004), which are available through www.psychguides.com. As with typically developing individuals, treatment of individuals with ID should proceed from diagnosis. Understandably, the certainty of the diagnosis of psychopathology in this population may be less clear than for typically developing populations. Multiple resources are available to assist the diagnostician in this endeavor. These include *Diagnostic Manual—Intellectual Disability: A Clinical Guide for Diagnosis of Mental Disorders in Persons with Intellectual Disability*, which is available through www.dmid.org. This resource provides *Diagnostic and Statistical Manual of Mental Disorder* (DSM) criteria with modifications when applicable for both mild-to-moderate and severe-to-profound ID (Fletcher et al., 2007).

When a specific diagnosis cannot be made with certainty or when the most appropriate diagnosis still provides limited guidance (e.g., impulse control disorder, not otherwise specified), treatment should be guided by identified target symptoms. In both cases, a functional analysis of behavior is strongly recommended. This type of evaluation identifies the context in which symptoms occur, including their nature, duration, and frequency; environmental stressors or triggers; patterns of reinforcement for both maladaptive and adaptive behaviors; and communicative intent. This information can be used to direct environmental modifications, to develop cognitive and behavioral interventions, and to track responses to therapeutic interventions, including medication strategies. After establishing baseline rates of symptoms and behaviors, tracking changes at regular intervals is critical to ensuring that an individual's symptoms are responding appropriately to a particular intervention. Rating scales such as the Aberrant Behavior Checklist (ABC) may be helpful in identifying and tracking symptoms. This checklist of 58 items is divided into five subscales: (1) Irritability, Agitation, and Crying; (2) Lethargy and Social Withdrawal; (3) Stereotypic Behavior; (4) Hyperactivity and Noncompliance; and (5) Inappropriate Speech. The Irritability subscale, often used to assess treatment intervention, is comprised of 18 items focusing on aggression, self-injury, tantrums, irritability, depressed mood, and mood lability (Aman, 1994; Aman and Singh, 1994). In addition, expert consensus recommends the institution of nonpharmacological measures before or in concert with the use of medication strategies (Aman et al., 2004). The absence of these principles is highlighted in the case of Kathleen, where tantrums and separation anxiety in the context of mental retardation (MR) and mixed language impairment are misdiagnosed as bipolar mood disorder; brief periods of improvement misinterpreted as therapeutic response; and medications are used, ineffectively, without benefit of prior or concurrent behavioral or environmental therapies.

A medical history and physical examination should also be obtained to rule out medical or neurological causes of symptoms or behavior. This effort is especially important for individuals who cannot communicate pain or other physiological distress. The side effects of medications alone or in combination, the use of over-the-counter medications, and possible drug-drug interactions should also be considered in investigating the reasons for a symptom or behavior. As in the case of Christopher, drug-drug interactions, particularly combinations of antiepileptic and other psychotropic medications, may cause toxicity. Moreover, individuals with developmental delays may be more likely to experience disinhibition with sedatives or hypnotics, side effects with stimulants, and movement disorders with neuroleptics. The prevalence of tardive dyskinesia may be as high as 35 percent in this population (Harris, 2006). Akathisia may also be more prevalent but can be difficult to detect in individuals who already appear agitated, although some rating scales may be of use (Garcia and Matson, 2008).

Persons with certain syndromes may also be more vulnerable to side effects. For instance, individuals with Down syndrome are especially sensitive to anticholinergics (Harris, 2006). Many syndromes associated with developmental delay may also be associated with cardiac defects and place an individual at greater risk of cardiac conduction abnormalities when exposed to some psychotropic medications including tricyclic antidepressants and certain neuroleptics. In addition, many psychotropic medications lower the seizure threshold, an effect that is especially problematic in a population where rates of seizure disorders may be as high as 40 percent (King et al., 1994). Last, rates of other significant physical illnesses are also elevated and often undetected in this population. A study of medical problems in 1,135 adults with ID referred for psychiatric problems revealed that 45.8 percent had undetected or inadequately treated seizures and that 12.7 percent had undiagnosed hypothyroidism (Ryan and Sunada, 1997).

Once a treatment plan has been developed, informed consent should be obtained from the individual if he or she has the capacity to give consent. If consent must be sought from other parties, a developmentally appropriate explanation of treatment with risks, benefits, and alternative should still be provided to the patient. Project MED, which can be accessed at www.projectmed.org, provides educational materials for treatment options and consent for individuals with ID (Aman et al., 2004).

Strategies for managing medication for individuals with ID also include using simple regimens with once-a-day or extended-release formulations; starting with a low dose, increasing doses slowly, and not exceeding doses typical in individuals without developmental disabilities. Frequent dose changes should be avoided if possible. To ensure adequate trials of medications, expert consensus recommends 3 to 8 weeks for antipsychotics, 1 to 3 weeks for mood stabilizers, and 6 to 8 weeks for selective serotonin reuptake inhibitors (SSRIs; Aman et al., 2004). When medications fail to adequately treat a particular symptom or behavior, it is important both to distinguish a partial response from a lack of response and to reassess the diagnosis. Changes in symptoms or behaviors from baseline as well as changes in function should be monitored regularly. Similarly, the regimen should be reassessed at least every 3 months and within 1 month of any dose change. Side effects should be monitored regularly using standardized measures if possible. Patients taking neuroleptics require regular assessment for tardive dyskinesia, weight changes, and glucose and lipid levels. The management of medications is an active process, so decreases in dose should also be considered unless contraindicated (Aman et al., 2004). This adjustment is especially true for antipsychotic agents where psychosis is not present. One study observed that even when patients have been treated for many years, a third were able to tolerate complete withdrawal and another fifth performed well on half of their typical dose without increases in maladaptive behaviors. These tapers occurred over a period of 4 months (Ahmed et al., 2000). Another study reported that 66.3 percent of 151 institutionalized individuals successfully weaned from antipsychotics were free of these medications an average of 10 years later. However, only 9 percent of those who demonstrated relapse quickly with taper or discontinuation were medication free. Moreover, subsequent attempts to taper or withdrawal in this subset were generally unsuccessful (Janowsky et al., 2006). Currently, there are medication strategies for multiple psychiatric conditions, including ADHD, anxiety, depression, and psychosis among others. Additionally, there are medication strategies that may be effective for some target symptoms such as self-injurious behavior, aggression, and insomnia.

While up to 40 percent of children and adolescents with ID demonstrate problems with attention, hyperactivity, and impulsivity, it is estimated that only 10 to 15 percent warrant a diagnosis of ADHD (Gillberg et al., 1986). Although there is insufficient evidence to suggest benefit of treatment in those individuals who do not meet criteria, studies suggest that 50 to 75 percent of those who have ADHD show significant improvement in attention, hyperactivity, and impulsivity with methylphenidate treatment (Harris, 2006). A review of studies of stimulant treatment by Handen and Gilchrist reported that methylphenidate was the most widely studied of stimulants, with more than 20 well-controlled group studies. These indicate positive response in 45 to 66 percent of individuals, which is lower than the response for typically developing children. Predictors of positive response include an IQ above 50 and higher baseline scores on parent and teacher ratings for inattention and activity. However, another study reported increased work output associated with treatment in children with lower intellectual function (Handen et al., 1994).

Studies also suggest that individuals with lower IQ demonstrate more variable response than those with normal IQ (Aman, Buican, and Arnold, 2003). Individuals with ID also demonstrate higher rates of tics and emotional lability (King, 2007), potential increased social withdrawal typically, but not always, associated with higher doses, and other side effects including decreased appetite, insomnia, possible growth suppression, depressed mood, and arrhythmias (Handen and Gilchrist, 2006). Studies of other agents have been limited. In addition to stimulants, treatment of hyperactivity with clonidine has been investigated in small studies of individuals with ID. Decreases in symptoms were noted, although half of the children studied developed drowsiness, which eventually waned. Adrenergics were also associated with sleep and appetite problems, seizures, tics, hematologic changes, and hair loss (King, 2007). At this time, expert consensus recommends stimulant therapy as the preferred treatment for hyperactivity (Aman et al., 2004). Second- and third-line treatments include atomoxetine (after two failed stimulant trials) and alpha agonists, respectively (Handen and Gilchrist, 2006).

Anxiety disorders are also common in individuals with ID and can be manifested by insomnia, agitation (including screaming and crying or clinging), compulsive or repetitive behaviors, self-injurious behaviors, and aggression. Antidepressants, anxiolytics, beta-blockers and antipsychotics all have been used to target anxiety. However, there have been no systematic trials of treatment in populations with ID (King, 2007). Expert consensus nonetheless recommends SSRIs and buspirone as preferred treatments. Some individuals, specifically those with autism spectrum disorders, may be especially sensitive to activation or disinhibition with SSRIs. Starting with low doses of medication is recommended. Additionally, individuals who exhibit side effects with SSRI treatment may benefit from a trial with buspirone. Studies suggest some efficacy in the treatment of anxiety that manifests as self-injurious behavior and aggression at doses of 15 to 45 mg daily (Ratey et al., 1989; Verhoeven and Tuinier, 1996), although increases in dose beyond this level have not been shown to increase benefit (King and Davanzo, 1996). In contrast, use of benzodiazepines is not recommended as first-line therapy (Aman et al., 2004). Individuals with ID are at greater risk for side effects of benzodiazepines, including confusion, cognitive impairment, and activation. In a study of 446 individuals with ID prescribed benzodiazepines, 17.4 percent demonstrated behavioral side effects when these medications were prescribed for behavioral or psychiatric problems, and 15.4 percent experienced adverse reactions when benzodiazepines were used in the treatment of epilepsy. However, only 2 percent of patients prescribed benzodiazepines for myoclonus or cerebral palsy experienced behaviorial side effects (Kalachnik et al., 2002). While these medications may be used effectively in some patients for acute anxiety, such as anxiety about dental appointments and other medical procedures, trials before the anticipated event are recommended to determine the nature of the effect and side effects for a particular individual. The middle seat of row 27 of a transcontinental flight is not the optimal place to perform an experiment as to whether lorazepam will help in settling an agitated patient with autism. Antipsychotics are also widely used for anxiety although such agents are not recommended as first-line therapy. If antipsychotics are used, tapers and discontinuation should be attempted after a period of time to assess ongoing need (King, 2007).

Mood disorders may be among the most common psychiatric conditions in individuals with ID and have been treated with antidepressants and mood stabilizers (Harris, 2006). Mood disorders may be detected by changes in mood from baseline. Additionally, a study of 300 adult patients evaluating symptoms of major depression, bipolar disorder, and anxiety disorder noted that sad mood, crying, and anhedonia suggested depression. Suicidality was rare (Hurley, 2008). Expert consensus recommends SSRIs as the first-line treatment for major depressive disorder. However, the use of SSRIs can be associated with aggression, suicidal ideation, and mania. As with typically developing individuals, careful monitoring of symptoms and combined psychotherapy and medication management is recommended (Harris, 2006).

For those individuals who meet the criteria for bipolar I mood disorder, divalproex or lithium alone or in combination with a newer atypical antipsychotic is recommended for mania or mixed mania and dysphoria. For depressive symptoms in the context of bipolar mood disorder, lithium alone or in combination with lamotrigine, lithium combined with an antidepressant, or divalproex with an antidepressant or lamotrigine is recommended. For psychotic depression, a mood stabilizer in combination with an atypical antipsychotic is recommended. Divalproex and lithium are both recommended for the treatment of hypomania in bipolar II disorders (Aman et al., 2004).

Schizophrenia may also occur in persons with ID at an estimated rate of 1 to 2 percent. Some syndromes, such as velocardiofacial syndrome, increase the risk for the development of schizophrenia (Harris, 2006). Expert consensus recommends an atypical antipsychotic as the first choice in the medication-compliant patient, with long-acting formulations in patients who have difficulty adhering to their treatment regimen. As with typically developing individuals, clozapine is reserved for patients who have failed numerous trials (Aman et al., 2004). Because of the necessity of frequent routine blood draws, adequate monitoring of clozapine's side effects may be particularly challenging in individuals with intellectual delay. It is also important to recognize that this population is at increased risk for tardive dyskinesia, which may be difficult to distinguish from other types of abnormal involuntary movements, such as stereotypies, that are common. Weight gain and glucose and lipid abnormalities are also a concern, especially with atypical antipsychotics. These medications require regular monitoring. Currently, risperidone is the most well-studied medication in this class for psychosis and behavioral problems (La Malfa et al., 2006).

Individuals with ID may present with self-injurious behavior and aggression. Self-injury is estimated to occur in 5 to 10 percent of this population and may also be associated with significant morbidity and mortality (Harris, 2006). In one study, up to 12 percent of deaths of people with ID were attributed to self-injurious behavior (Nissen and Haveman, 1997). Some populations are at particular risk. It is estimated that 60 percent of individuals with autism and severe ID demonstrate self-injurious behavior. Additionally, finger and lip biting is associated with Lesch-Nyhan syndrome, skin picking with Prader-Willi syndrome, and nail pulling with Smith-Magenis syndrome (Harris, 2006). Individuals with certain medical illnesses, such as constipation, ulcers, aspiration, and ear infections, are also prone to self-injurious behavior. In one study reviewed, medical illnesses were present in up to 28 percent of persons with self-injurious behavior, and significant reductions in behavior were reported when these conditions were treated (Bosch et al., 1997).

While self-injurious and aggressive behaviors may be targets of treatment, a functional evaluation is still required to understand environmental factors and triggers, patterns of reinforcement, and communicative intent. Medical and neurological causes, especially pain, potential toxicity from other medications, including barbiturates and benzodiazepines, drug-drug interactions, and underlying psychiatric diagnosis, especially anxiety and depression, should also be explored. Treatment of self-injurious behavior and aggression must address the underlying causes of these behaviors. When nonpsychopharmacological measures fail to adequately treat these behaviors, expert consensus recommends treatment with an atypical antipsychotic or an anticonvulsant or mood stabilizer, specifically divalproex or carbamazepine (Aman et al., 2004). While older antipsychotics such as thioridazine have demonstrated efficacy in treating these behaviors, there are significant concerns for cardiac conduction abnormalities sufficient to warrant a black box warning. Other older agents are also associated with increased risk of tardive dyskinesia. However, newer agents are not without risk, especially those associated with weight gain, glucose and lipid abnormalities, and gynecomastia. Despite these concerns, the use of antipsychotics in reducing target symptoms is supported by a combination of limited randomized controlled trials and prospective and retrospective studies (Deb et al., 2007). The use of antipsychotics for aggression is not without controversy. A recent study of 86 nonpsychotic adults with ID and aggression were randomized to risperidone (maximum dose of 2 mg), haloperidol (maximum dose of 5 mg), or placebo. All methods demonstrated reduction of aggression at 4 weeks with placebo outperforming both risperidone and haloperidol (Tyrer et al., 2008).

Additional agents have also been used in the treatment of self-injurious behaviors and aggression. As reviewed by Stigler and McDougle (2008), these have included antipsychotics, alpha-2 agonists, and mood stabilizers. A review of studies by Harris (2006) also reports other agents may be effective. These include serotonergic agents such as buspirone and trazodone, opioid antagonists, and beta-blockers. In contrast, medications that target GABA receptors, such as benzodiazepines, have not produced consistent results for self-injurious behavior or aggression. Similarly, the use of anticonvulsants is somewhat unclear. Although divalproex and carbamazepine are recommended by some for self-injurious behavior and aggression (Aman et al., 2004), a review of other studies of lamotrigine noted both increases and decreases in challenging behavior (King, 2007). Thus, tracking individual responses to medication is critical. Regardless of medication, treatment of self-injurious behavior and aggression must be multidimensional and address the reason such behaviors occur, especially for individuals who may be unable to communicate their physical or psychological distress in other ways.

Sleep is frequently a concern in individuals with ID. Expert consensus recommends sleep hygiene including regular routine without naps, reduced stimulations and disruptions at night, and avoidance of caffeine and other stimulating substances including medications. Sleep disorders must also be ruled out including obstructive sleep apnea (Aman et al., 2004). Melatonin is the best-studied medication for insomnia in children with ID. In doses up to 9 mg, hours of sleep, nocturnal and early morning awakenings, and sleep onset is improved (Coppola et al., 2004). These results were also supported by a randomized, double-blind, placebo-controlled trial of 51 individuals with ID and chronic insomnia (Braam et al., 2008).

Psychopharmacology in Individuals with Autism

In recent years, individuals with autism spectrum disorders have received an increasing focus with respect to psychopharmacologic interventions. The use of medications in hopes of improving behavioral symptoms and psychiatric conditions in individuals with autism is common. A study of more than 400 families revealed that 45.6 percent of individuals with autism were taking some type of psychotropic medication, including melatonin and St. John's wort. Medications used with some frequency included antidepressants (21.6%), antipsychotics (14.9%), antihypertensives (21.6%), stimulants (1.3%), and antiepileptic medication (11.3%). 10.3 percent took an over-the-counter autism preparation. Polypharmacy was also not uncommon, with 9.8 percent taking two medications, 7.7 percent taking three, and more than 3 percent taking four or more medications (Aman, Lam, and Collier-Crespin, 2003).

Despite trials of multiple medications (including antidepressants, atypical antipsychotics cholinesterase-inhibitors, naltrexone, glutamatergic agents, lamotrigine, D-cycloserine, NMDA antagonists, and oxytocin), there is no medication consistently proven effective in treating the core social and communication deficits of autism (Posey, Erickson, and McDougle, 2008). More promising have been trials targeted to specific symptoms. These symptoms include disruptive behaviors such as aggression and self-injury, repetitive behaviors, hyperactivity, and mood, anxiety, and sleep problems. Multiple agents have been examined to varying degrees to target these problems. NIH funding has significantly accelerated knowledge in this field, primarily focusing on children and adolescents. The Research Units on Pediatric Psychopharmacology (RUPP) Autism Network, created in 1997, examined risperidone and methylphenidate and is studying combined drug and behavioral treatment. In addition, the Studies to Advance Autism Research and Treatment (STAART) network, created in 2000, promises further advances in the areas of cause, diagnosis, early detection, prevention, and treatment. STAART sites have also investigated repetitive behavior and anxiety in children with autism.

As with typically developing individuals, treatment of individuals with autism should be based on psychiatric diagnosis or on a specific behavioral-pharmacological hypothesis. Any such hypothesis should include a functional analysis of the behavior or symptoms and consider problems in the context of autism, psychiatric conditions, illness and pain, current medications, psychosocial and environmental factors, and the history and efficacy of previous trials. In poorly defined conditions such as autism, targeting therapy at specific symptoms and monitoring response over time is entirely reasonable (Bostic and Rho, 2006). Identifying specific target symptoms, obtaining baseline data before a trial, and monitoring change using rating scales should guide decision making. Both a functional analysis of behavior and targeting specific symptoms are especially important in this population, as medication studies are limited and demonstrate significant variability in response. The ABC Irritability subscale may help identify target symptoms and track responses to interventions (King and Bostic, 2006). This subscale evaluates aggression, self-injurious behavior, tantrums, mood lability, depressed mood, and irritability (Aman and Singh, 1986; Aman, 1994). It is also critical to note that pharmacotherapy is rarely sufficient as an end in itself and should be augmented with other measures directed at modifying the environment and behavioral contingencies and with alternative strategies. Maladaptive behaviors exist within a context and frequently may communicate some unmet need. Moreover, they may indicate illness or pain. Last, persons with autism may be exquisitely sensitive to medications with high rates of side effects. Starting with low-doses, increasing doses slowly, avoiding frequent medication or dose changes unless there is a valid reason, and periodic attempts of a slow withdrawal are all highly recommended.

Aggression and self-injurious behavior are among the most common reasons for psychiatric referral. The etiology of these concerns is likely heterogeneous but may also reflect dysregulation of specific neurotransmitter pathways including dopaminergic, serotoninergic, adrenergic, opioid, and GABA-ergic systems Multiple agents targeting these various systems have been examined. A 2008 review of medication interventions specifically for aggression and self-injury by Parikh, Kolevzon, and Hollander revealed 21 randomized controlled trials that included well-defined subject samples and used at least one standardized assessment of aggression or self-injurious behavior as a primary outcome. These included trials for risperidone, haloperidol, methylphenidate, clomipramine, tianeptine, clonidine, naltrexone, valproate, lamotrigine, levetiracetam, secretin, and omega-3 fatty acids. Most of the results were not favorable. A randomized study of clomipramine revealed no difference in target symptoms but was associated with significant side effects. Studies of valproate, lamotrigine, and levetiracetam showed no improvement of target symptoms. Neither have studies of secretin and omega-3 fatty acids shown benefit. The use of naltrexone is less clear, with some studies indicating improvement in some domains and others demonstrating no difference from treatment with placebo (Parikh, Kolevzon, and Hollander, 2008). While children treated with clonidine (0.15 to 0.20 mg/day) demonstrated improvement on the ABC Irritability subscale, this trial was limited to eight children and also produced side effects of drowsiness, decreased activity, and hypotension in three children sufficient to warrant a reduction in dose (Jaselskis et al.,

1992). In a retrospective analysis of guanfacine in 80 children with pervasive developmental disorder, 10 of 69 children with significant aggression improved (Posey et al., 2004). Last, two small randomized controlled trials of methylphenidate reviewed revealed significant reductions in the ABC Irritability scale (Quintana et al., 1995; Handen, Johnson, and Lubetsky, 2000).

Antipsychotics are the best-studied class of medication in the treatment of irritability, aggression, and self-injury. While a randomized-controlled comparison of haloperidol and placebo revealed no significant difference on ABC Irritability scores compared with placebo and was associated with significant side effects (Remington, Sloman, and Konstantareas, 2001), a review of earlier studies found haloperidol effective in treating a range of maladaptive behaviors, although also frequently associated with dystonic reactions and dyskinesias (Stigler and McDougal, 2008). Atypical antipsychotics, including risperidone, olanzapine, quetiapine, ziprasidone, and aripiprazole have also been investigated. With the exception of risperidone, the majority of these studies were limited by size and design and produced less conclusive results than those found with risperidone. In addition, specific side effects (such as increased weight gain with olanzapine), decreased tolerability (with quetiapine) and concerns for increased QT prolongation (ziprasidone) were noted (Stigler and McDougle, 2008). Aripiprazole was also evaluated in a retrospective chart review of 32 children, ranging from 5 to 19 years of age, and diagnosed with developmental disabilities, including 24 with autism spectrum diagnoses and 18 with ID. Target symptoms included aggression, hyperactivity, impulsivity, and self-injurious behaviors. With a mean daily starting dose of 7.1ffl0.3 mg, a daily maintenance dose of 10.6ffl6.9 mg, and a duration of 6 to 15 months, improvement in target symptoms was seen in 56 percent of cases, but in only 37 percent (9 of 24) was seen in children with autism. Side effects occurred in 50 percent, included sleepiness (six children), aggression (two children) and stiffness, myalgia, or dyskinesia (three children), and resulted in discontinuation of the study in seven of 32 children. Additionally, body mass index increased from 22.5 to 24.1, with increased changes in younger children (Valicenti-McDermott and Demb, 2006).

Risperidone is now the only FDA-approved medication for children ages 5 to 16 years for treatment of the symptoms of irritability, aggression or self-injurious behavior, tantrums, or mood swings in the context of autism. Studies that support this recommendation include two randomized, placebo-controlled studies as well as two discontinuation studies (Parikh, Kolevzon, and Hollander, 2008). The RUPP study of risperidone in 2002 was an 8-week double-blind, placebo-controlled, parallel group trial of 101 children 5 to 17 years of age, followed by an open-label 16-week continuation for responders. At a mean dose of 1.8 mg/day with a dose range of 0.5–3.5 mg, this 8-week study demonstrated a 56.9 percent reduction on the Irritability scale of the ABC compared with 14.1 percent reduction with placebo. 69 percent of individuals were considered responders, compared with 12 percent who received placebo. Positive response was defined by a 25-percent reduction on the Irritability scale of the ABC and a rating of much improved or very much improved on the Clinical Global Impression (CGI) scale. Side effects were more prevalent with risperidone and included increased appetite (49% mild, 24% moderate), fatigue (59%), drowsiness (49%), drooling (17%), and dizziness (16%). While no significant extrapyramidal symptoms were noted, weight gain was significant with those treated with risperidone gaining 2.7ffl2.9 kg compared to 0.8ffl2.2 kg taking placebo (RUPP, 2002). Risperidone was also associated with reductions in the ABC subscales of Hyperactivity and Stereotypy but did not show statistically significant improvement in Lethargy and Social Withdrawal and Inappropriate Speech (McDougle et al., 2005). In contrast, a subsequent study of similar design in highly irritable children demonstrated improvements across all ABC domains including Lethargy and Social Withdrawal and Inappropriate Speech (Shea et al., 2004). A follow-up 4-month open-label phase of the study showed that the effects of treatment remained stable over time and did not require increases in dose beyond the average of 1.8 mg/day used in the first phase. The third phase assessed the effects of withdrawal (tapered at 25% per week) and found that relapse was significantly more common on placebo. However, 6 of 16 children treated with risperidone for 6 months did not relapse after withdrawal suggesting that in some patients, risperidone may be discontinued (RUPP, 2005b). Subsequent studies have produced similar results suggesting that risperidone may emerge as a standard treatment for aggression, tantrums, and self-injury in individuals with autism spectrum disorders (Scahill and Martin, 2005).

Repetitive, stereotyped, or compulsive behaviors can adversely affect the quality of life of individuals with autism as well as their families. While the etiology of these behaviors is unknown, serotonergic dysfunction has been implicated (Soorya, Kiarashi, and Hollander, 2008). In children, risperidone has been associated with a decrease in repetitive behaviors (McDougle et al., 2005). The results of SSRIs on repetitive behaviors are less promising. In a placebo-controlled double-blind crossover study of fluoxetine, modest, but statistically significant, reductions in repetitive behaviors as measured by the Child Yale-Brown Obsessive-Compulsive Scale, but not on the CGI autism score, were observed at a mean dose of 9.9ffl4.4 mg/day (Hollander et al., 2005). However, preliminary results of the large STAART citalopram trial do not support the use of citalopram for repetitive behaviors in children and adolescents with autism spectrum disorders (King, 2008). A review of studies of clomipramine in children revealed one small positive study, but subsequent studies that demonstrated only limited efficacy accompanied by significant side effects, including increased irritability, self-injury, aggression, urinary retention, fatigue, tremors, and tachycardia. At least one case of serotonin syndrome has also been reported (Soorya, Kiarashi, and Hollander, 2008).

In contrast, a review of studies of fluvoxamine, fluoxetine, risperidone, and IV oxytocin in adults have been associated in reductions of repetitive behaviors. In addition, sertraline was also investigated in an open-label study of 42 with diagnoses of autism, Asperger disorder, and pervasive developmental disorder, not otherwise specified (PDD, NOS). Full-scale IQ of participants ranged from 25 to 114 and included 28 individuals with ID. At a mean dose of 122ffl60.5 mg/day, 57 percent demonstrated improvement in repetitive and aggressive symptoms, although there was no change in social relatedness. Side effects were generally limited, although agitation caused three participants to leave the study and four participants to be treated with chloral hydrate for agitation (McDougle et al., 1998). The largest double-blind, randomized, placebo-controlled study of an SSRI, specifically citalopram, reported no significant difference in response from placebo in the treatment of repetitive behaviors in children with autism spectrum disorders (King et al., 2009). In addition, a double-blind, placebo-controlled study of 31 adults treated with risperidone at a mean dose of 2.9 mg/day demonstrated significant reductions in repetitive behaviors as well as aggression, irritability, and anxiety (McDougle et al., 2000).

Although anxiety and depression are considered common in individuals with autism, most studies examining the effects of antidepressants have focused on behavior as a primary target. A review of the efficacy and tolerability of antidepressants in 2006 reviewed three randomized controlled trials and 10 open-label trials or retrospective chart reviews and included studies of citalopram, escitalopram, fluoxetine, fluvoxamine, and sertraline. Most demonstrated improvement in global functioning and symptoms related to anxiety and repetitive behaviors. Side effects were generally mild but included behavioral activation and agitation (Kolevzon, Mathewson, and Hollander, 2006). A 2005 review of the literature of antidepressants in individuals with pervasive developmental disorders by Scahill and Martin (2005) also noted that studies were generally small with poorly defined target symptoms. Responses were variable. Adverse side effects, including agitation and behavioral activation, characterized by symptoms of hyperactivity, insomnia, and aggression among others, were reported with various agents, including fluoxetine, sertraline, and fluvoxamine. Behavioral activation appeared to be more common among younger children. They concluded that there is only limited support for the use of SSRIs in children with pervasive developmental disorders. More research targeting specific mood disorders in both children and adults is warranted.

Symptoms of hyperactivity, impulsivity, and inattention are also common in autism. In a nonclinical sample of 487 school children, ADHD symptoms were noted by both parents and teachers alike with difficulty concentrating and problems being distracted reported in approximately 50 percent and 60 percent of children, respectively. Short attention spans were noted by parents in 54 percent of children and by teachers in 47 percent. Excessive fidgeting, wiggling, and squirming were observed in about 42 percent of children. Overactivity was reported by teachers in 29 percent of cases and by parents in 41 percent of cases. Similarly, high energy levels were problematic for 30 percent of children for teachers and 44 percent for parents (Lecavalier, 2006). Multiple agents have been investigated with respect to ADHD symptoms, including stimulants, atomoxetine, alpha-2 agonists, antipsychotics, antidepressants, and other agents (Aman et al., 2008).

The best-studied medication for ADHD is methylphenidate. In addition to at least six smaller studies, the RUPP Autism Network conducted a randomized double-blind, placebo-controlled crossover trial of methylphenidate with 72 children with autism and ADHD-like symptoms. Methylphenidate was provided in dosage levels of 0.125, 0.25 and 0.50 mg/kg and was given three times a day. This study reported a response in 49 percent of children, but discontinuation owing to adverse effects, especially irritability, in 18 percent of children. These results contrast with the Multisite Multimodal Treatment Study of Children with ADHD (RUPP, 2005a) that examined 289 typically developing children. In this study, response rate was between 70 and 80 percent, the effect size larger (0.35–1.31 compared with 0.48–0.89), and only 1.4 percent of individuals discontinued treatment owing to adverse effects. In the RUPP methylphenidate study, symptoms most improved were inattention, distractibility, hyperactivity, and impulsivity. Symptoms that did not improve included irritability, lethargy, social withdrawal, stereotypies, or inappropriate speech. Of note, increased social withdrawal was associated with higher doses, a finding present in prior studies. In general, despite its clear effects, methylphenidate was found to have less positive benefit and more adverse effects in children with autism than in typically developing children (RUPP, 2005a). While methylphenidate should be considered in children with autism with features of attention deficit hyperactivity disorder, lower expectation and greater awareness of potential adverse effects is warranted. Dose levels in keeping with the lower levels of the study are also recommended for initial treatment. Last, stimulants may be associated with increased hyperactivity, sterotypies, dysphoria, or motor tics. In a review of one study, these adverse effects occurred in up to one-third of children taking a single test dose of 0.4 mg of methylphenidate (King and Bostic, 2006). Thus, careful monitoring of target symptoms and potential adverse effects is strongly recommended.

Studies of other agents used in the treatment of ADHD symptoms have been far more limited. A review of these include two small studies of amphetamine products reported worse behavior as rated on the CGI in the majority of children (Aman et al., 2008). However, both studies consisted of children between the ages of 3 and 6. Three open-label studies of atomoxetine in children with PDD and ADHD symptoms have also been conducted. The largest included 20 patients (including 10 with comorbid MR) and lasted an average of 19.5 weeks. 12 children were considered responders with reduction in hyperactivity and inattention (Jou, Handen, and Hardan, 2005). Smaller studies demonstrated improvement in target symptoms, but five of 12 children in one study terminated their participation owing to side effects that included gastrointestinal complaints (Troost et al., 2006). One double-blind, placebo-controlled, crossover trial of 16 children resulted in early termination of three children (one because of an atomoxetine-related side effect, two because the placebo arm of the research showed a lack of effect). Nine children responded to atomoxetine compared with four on placebo. In this study, side effects were mild (Arnold et al., 2006). Studies of clonidine have been small and results have been mixed (Aman et al., 2008). Studies of guanfacine include a retrospective study of 80 children with PDD ranging in age from 3 to 18 years. At a mean daily dose of 2.6ffl1.7 mg and a duration of treatment ranging from 7 to 1776 days, treatment was considered effective in only 23.8 percent (19 of 80) children for target symptoms of hyperactivity, inattention, insomnia, and tics. Children without MR responded better than those with MR (37.5% versus 17.9%) Guanfacine was well tolerated and did not produce significant changes in heart rate or blood pressure (Posey et al., 2004). In addition, there have been numerous trials of risperidone. While predominantly consisting of children and adolescents, at least one included adults. In general, response rates were high (Aman et al., 2008) including 69.4 percent among 101 participants in the RUPP trial (RUPP, 2002).

Sleep is problematic in 44 to 86 percent of children with autism. These difficulties include problems falling asleep, staying asleep, and maintaining regular sleep-wake patterns. Although the etiology of this concern is unclear, dysregulation of GABA, serotonin, and melatonin may be involved. However, behavioral and environmental causes are also implicated. In evaluating problems with sleep, sleep disorders such as obstructive sleep apnea and REM and non-REM sleep disorders must also be considered. The Pediatric Sleep Questionnaire (Chervin et al., 2000) may be of use in assessing sleep (Johnson and Malow, 2008). The treatment of problematic sleep relies heavily on sleep hygiene and should always be considered. Medication trials are limited, especially in children with autism.

There is some evidence to support the use of melatonin in this population. This includes numerous small trials in children with neurodevelopmental differences and one large retrospective trial of 100 children with autism (Anderson et al., 2008). Reduced sleep latency, improved sleep duration, and improved sleep efficiency (time in bed) were typically noted with minimal side effects. However, one study of five children with refractory epilepsy reported an increase of seizures during treatment with melatonin (Sheldon, 1998). In general, hypnotic doses typically started at 1 mg and increased by 1 mg every 2 weeks to a typical maximum of 3 mg (although doses up to 6 mg were warranted at times; Johnson and Malow, 2008).

Multiple other agents have been used to treat numerous symptoms present in children with autism spectrum disorders as well as ID more broadly. Studies supporting these interventions are generally limited and should be reviewed individually when a particular agent is considered. Caution is recommended as children and adults with intellectual and developmental disabilities often experience adverse effects, and may not be able to articulate their subjective discomfort—or may rely on behaviors for communicating their distress that are the very targets for treatment. Initiating treatments carefully, against an established baseline of behavior, and monitoring for both positive and negative effects is the current standard of care.

Conclusion

While medications may serve a useful role in the treatment of psychiatric concerns of individuals with neurodevelopmental disorders, they should not be the first or sole intervention and are often insufficient without behavioral or environmental changes guided by a functional analysis of behavior. Moreover, pharmacotherapy should begin only after pain and illness have been ruled out and established psychiatric diagnoses or specific target behaviors are identified. Symptoms should be tracked over time to monitor efficacy of treatment. Care should also be taken to assess side effects, which are more frequent in individuals with neurodevelopmental delays and may go unnoticed either because the individual is unable to articulate distress or because he or she relies on behaviors that may be the very targets of intervention to communicate distress. Last, medication strategies also should be evaluated periodically to determine if they are still necessary. In summary, while medications may help treat psychiatric disorders and symptoms in individuals with neurodevelopmental disorders, their use is limited and must be guided by careful evaluation and follow-up.

REFERENCES

Ahmed Z, Fraser W, Kerr MP, et al. 2000. Reducing antipsychotic medication in people with learning disability. *British Journal of Psychiatry* 176: 42–46.
Aman MG. 1994. Instruments for assessing treatment effects in developmentally disabled populations. *Assessments in Rehabilitation and Exceptionality* 1: 1–20.
Aman MG, Buican B, Arnold, LE. 2003. Methylphenidate treatment of children with borderline IQ and mental retardation: Analysis of three aggregated studies. *Journal of Child and Adolescent Psychopharmacology* 13: 29–40.
Aman MG, Crismon ML, Frances A, King BH, Rojahn J (eds.). 2004. *Treatment of*

Psychiatric and Behavioral Problems in Individuals with Mental Retardation: An Update of the Expert Consensus Guidelines for Mental Retardation / Developmental Disability Populations. Available at www.psychguides.com.

Aman MG, Farmer CA, Holloway J, Arnold, LE. 2008. Treatment of inattention, overactivity, and impulsiveness in autism spectrum disorders. *Child and Adolescent Psychiatric Clinics of North America* 17: 713–738.

Aman MG, Lam KS, Collier-Crespin A. 2003. Prevalence and patterns of use of psychoactive medicines among individuals with autism in the Autism Society of Ohio. *Journal of Autism and Developmental Disorders* 33(5): 527–34.

Aman MG, Singh NN. 1986. *Aberrant Behavior Checklist Manual.* East Aurora, NY: Slosson Educational Publications.

Anderson I, Kaczmarska J, McGraw SG, et al. 2008. Melatonin for insomnia in children with autism spectrum disorders. *Journal of Child Neurology* 23:482–485.

Arnold L, Aman M, Cook A, et al. 2006. Atomoxetine for hyperactivity in autism spectrum disorders: Placebo-controlled crossover pilot trial. *Journal of American Academy of Child and Adolescent Psychiatry* 45: 1196–1205.

Bosch J, Van Dyke C, Smith SM, Poulton S. 1997. Role of medical conditions in the exacerbation of self-injurious behavior: An exploratory study. *Mental Retardation* 35: 124–30.

Bostic JQ, Rho Y. 2006. Target-symptom psychopharmacology: Between the forest and the trees. *Child and Adolescent Psychiatric Clinics of North America* 15(1): 289–302.

Braam W, Didden R, Smits M, Curfs L. 2008. Melatonin treatment in individuals with intellectual disability and chronic insomnia: A randomized placebo-controlled study. *Journal of Intellectual Disability Research* 52(3): 256–64.

Chervin RD, Hedger K, Dillon JE, Pituch, KJ. 2000. Pediatric sleep questionnaire (PSQ): Validity and reliability of scales for sleep-disordered breathing, snoring, sleepiness, and behavioral problems. *Sleep Medicine* 1(1): 21–31.

Coppola G, Iervolino G, Mastrosimone M, La Torre G, Ruiu F. 2004. Melatonin in wake-sleep disorders in children, adolescents, and young adults with mental retardation with or without epilepsy: A double-blind, placebo-controlled trial. *Brain and Development* 26(6): 373–76.

Deb S, Sohanpal SK, Soni R, Unwin G, Lenotre L. 2007. The effectiveness of antipsychotic medication in the management of behavior problems in adults with intellectual disabilities. *Journal of Intellectual Disability Research* 51(10): 766–77.

Fletcher RJ, Loschen E, Stavrakaki C, First M (eds.) 2007. *Diagnostic Manual—Intellectual Disability: A Clinical Guide for Diagnosis of Mental Disorders in Persons with Intellectual Disability.* Kingston, NY: National Association for the Dually Diagnosed.

Garcia MJ, Matson JL. 2008. Akathisia in adults with severe and profound intellectual disability: A psychometric study of the MEDS and ARMS. *Journal of Intellectual and Developmental Disability* 33(2): 171–76.

Gilberg C, Persson E, Grufman M, Themner U. 1986. Psychiatric disorders in mildly and severely mentally retarded urban children and adolescents: Epidemiological aspects. *British Journal of Psychiatry* 149: 68–74.

Handen BL, Gilchrist R. 2006. Practitioner review: Psychopharmacology in children and adolescents with mental retardation. *Journal of Child Psychology and Psychiatry* 47(9): 871–82.

Handen BL, Janosky J, McAuliffe S, Breaux AM. 1994. Prediction of response to methylphenidate among children with ADHD and mental retardation. *Journal of American Academy of Child and Adolescent Psychiatry* 33: 1185–93.

Handen BL, Johnson CR, Lubetsky M. 2000. Efficacy of methylphenidate among children with autism and symptoms of attention-deficit hyperactivity disorder. *Journal of Autism and Developmental Disorders* 30: 245–55.

Harris JC. 2006. *Intellectual Disability: Understanding Its Development, Causes, Classification, Evaluation, and Treatment,* 289–332. Oxford: Oxford University Press.

Holden B, Gitlesen JP. 2004. Psychotropic medication in adults with mental retardation: Prevalence, and prescription practices. *Research in Developmental Disabilities* 25: 509–21.

Hollander E, Phillips A, Chaplin W, et al. 2005. A placebo controlled crossover trial of liquid fluoxetine on repetitive behaviors in childhood and adolescent autism. *Neuropsychopharmacology* 30(3): 582–89.

Hurley AD. 2008. Depression in adults with intellectual disability: Symptoms and challenging behavior. *Journal of Intellectual Disability Research* 52(11): 905–16.

Janowsky MD, Barnhill LJ, Khalid AS, Davis JM. 2006. Relapse of aggressive and disruptive behavior in mentally retarded adults following antipsychotic drug withdrawal predicts psychotropic drug use a decade later. *Journal of Clinical Psychiatry* 67: 1272–77.

Jaselskis CA, Cook EH, Fletcher KE, Leventhal BL. 1992. Clonidine treatment of hyperactive and impulsive children with autistic disorder. *Journal of Clinical Psychopharmacology* 12: 322–27.

Johnson KP, Malow BA. 2008. Assessment and pharmacologic treatment of sleep disturbance in autism. *Child and Adolescent Psychiatric Clinics of North America* 17: 773–85.

Jou R, Handen B, Hardan A. 2005. Retrospective assessment of atomoxetine in children and adolescents with pervasive developmental disorders. *Journal of Child and Adolescent Psychopharmacology* 15: 325–30.

Kalachnik JE, Hanzel TE, Sevenich R, Harder SR. 2002. Benzodiazepine behavioral side effects: Review and implications for individuals with mental retardation. *American Journal on Mental Retardation* 107(5): 376–410.

King BH. 2007. Background rationale for a trial of SSRI: Design and baseline characteristics. Paper presented at American Academy of Child and Adolescent Psychiatry annual meeting, Chicago.

King BH, Bostic JQ. 2006. An update on pharmacologic treatments for autism spectrum disorders. *Child and Adolescent Psychiatric Clinics of North America* 15(1): 161–75.

King BH, Davanzo PA. 1996. Buspirone treatment of aggression and self-injury in autistic and non-autistic persons with severe mental retardation. *Developmental Brain Dysfunction* 9: 22–31.

King BH, DeAntonio C, McCracken JT, Forness SR, Ackerland V. 1994. Psychiatric consultation in severe and profound mental retardation. *American Journal of Psychiatry* 151: 1802–8.

King BH, Hollander E, Sikich L, et al. 2009. Lack of efficacy of citalopram in children with autism spectrum disorders and high levels of repetitive behavior. *Archives of General Psychiatry* 66(6): 583–90.

Kolevzon A, Mathewson KA, Hollander E. 2006. Selective serotonin reuptake inhibitors in autism: A review of efficacy and tolerability. *Journal of Clinical Psychiatry* 67(3): 407–14.

La Malfa G, Lassi S, Bertelli M, Castellani A. 2006. Reviewing the use of antipsychotic drugs in people with intellectual disability. *Human Psychopharmacology Clinic and Experimental* 21: 73–89.

Lecavalier L. 2006. Behavioral and emotional problems in young people with pervasive developmental disorders: Relative prevalence, effects of subject characteristics, and empirical classifications. *Journal of Autism and Developmental Disorders* 36: 1101–14.

Lewis MA, Lewis C, Leake B, King BH, Lindeman R. 2002. Public health issues: The quality of health care for adults with developmental disabilities. *Public Health Reports* 117: 174–84.

McDougle CJ, Brodkin ES, Naylor ST, et al. 1998. Sertraline in adults with pervasive developmental disorders: A prospective open-label investigation. *Journal of Clinical Psychopharmacology* 18(1): 62–66.

McDougle CJ, Epperson CN, Pelton GH, Wasylink S, Price LH. 2000. A double-blind, placebo-controlled study of risperidone addition in serotonin reuptake inhibitor-refractory obsessive-compulsive disorder. *Archives of General Psychiatry* 57(8): 794–801.

McDougle CJ, Scahill L, Aman MG, et al. 2005. Risperidone for the core symptom domains of autism: Results from the study by the Autism Network of the Research Units on Pediatric Psychopharmacology. *American Journal of Psychiatry* 162: 1142–48.

Nissen JM, Haveman MJ. 1997. Mortality and avoidable death in people with severe self-injurious behavior: Results of a Dutch study. *Journal of Intellectual Disability Research* 41: 252–57.

Parikh MS, Kolevzon A, Hollander E. 2008. Psychopharmacology of aggression in children and adolescents with autism: A critical review of efficacy and tolerability. *Journal of Child and Adolescent Psychopharmacology* 18(2): 157–78.

Posey DJ, Erickson CA, McDougle CJ. 2008. Developing drugs for core social and communication impairment in autism. *Child Adolescent Psychiatric Clinics of North America* 17(4): 787–801.

Posey, DJ, Puntney JI, Sasher TM, et al. 2004. Guanfacine treatment of hyperactivity and inattention in pervasive developmental disorders: A retrospective analysis of 80 cases. *Journal of Child and Adolescent Psychopharmacology* 14(2): 233–41.

Quintana H, Birmaher B, Stedge D, et al. 1995. Use of methylphenidate in the treatment of children with autistic disorder. *Journal of Autism and Developmental Disorders* 25: 283–94.

Ratey JJ, Sovener R, Mikkelsen E, Chmielinski HE. 1989. Buspirone therapy for maladaptive behavior and anxiety in developmentally disabled persons. *Journal of Clinical Psychiatry* 50: 382–84.

Remington SG, Sloman L, Konstantareas M. 2001. Clomipramine versus haloperidol in the treatment of autistic disorder: A double-blind placebo-controlled, crossover study. *Journal of Clinical Psychopharmacology* 21: 440–44.

Research Units on Pediatric Psychopharmacology. 2002. Risperidone in children with autism and serious behavioral problems. *New England Journal of Medicine* 347: 314–21.

Research Units on Pediatric Psychopharmacology. 2005a. Randomized, controlled, crossover trial of methylphenidate in pervasive developmental disorders with hyperactivity. *Archives of General Psychiatry* 62: 1266–74.

Research Units on Pediatric Psychopharmacology. 2005b. Risperidone treatment of autistic disorder: Longer-term benefits and blinded discontinuation after 6 months. *American Journal of Psychiatry* 162: 1361–69.

Ryan R, Sunada K. 1997. Medical evaluation of persons with mental retardation referred for psychiatric assessment. *General Hospital Psychiatry* 19: 274–80.

Scahill L, Martin A. 2005. Psychopharmacology. In FR Volkmar, R Paul, A Klin, D Cohen. (eds.), *Handbook of Autism and Pervasive Developmental Disorders*, 3rd ed., 2:1102–17. Hoboken, NJ: Wiley.

Shea S, Turgay A, Carrol A, et al. 2004. Risperidone in the treatment of disruptive behavioral symptoms in children with autistic and other pervasive developmental disorders. *Pediatrics* 114: e634–41.

Sheldon S. 1998. Pro-convulsant effects of oral melatonin in neurologically disabled children. *Lancet* 351: 1254.

Soorya L, Kiarashi J, Hollander E. 2008. Psychopharmacologic interventions for repetitive behaviors in autism spectrum disorders. *Child and Adolescent Psychiatric Clinics of North America* 17: 753–71.

Stigler KA, McDougle CJ. 2008. Pharmacotherapy of irritability in pervasive developmental disorders. *Child and Adolescent Psychiatric Clinics of North America* 17: 739–52.

Troost P, Steenhuis M, Tuynman H, et al. 2006. Atomoxetine for attention-deficit/hyperactivity disorder symptoms in children with pervasive developmental disorders: A pilot study. *Journal of Child and Adolescent Psychopharmacology* 16: 611–19.

Tyrer P, Oliver-Africano PC, Ahmed Z, et al. 2008. Risperidone, haloperidol, and placebo in the treatment of aggressive challenging behavior in patients with intellectual disability: A randomized controlled trial. *The Lancet* 371: 57–63.

Valicenti-McDermott MR, Demb H. 2006. Clinical effects and adverse reactions of off-label use of aripiprazole in children and adolescents with developmental disabilities. *Journal of Child and Adolescent Psychopharmacology* 16(5): 549–60.

Verhoeven WM, Tuinier S. 1996. The effect of buspirone on challenging behavior in mentally retarded patients: An open prospective multi-case study. *Journal of Intellectual Disability Research* 40: 502–8.

13

Behavioral Interventions

Craig H. Kennedy, Ph.D.

Problematic behaviors that may sometimes be associated with developmental disabilities (DDs) include self-injury, aggression, and destruction of property (Luiselli, 2006). The most frequent forms of self-injury include head hitting, biting, slapping, eye gouging, and skin picking. Aggressive acts toward others range widely in topography but are characterized as behaviors likely to cause physical harm to another person. Destruction of property refers to damaging items such as windows, furniture, clothing, and so on. These behaviors place people with DDs at increased risk for more restrictive school and residential placements. Indeed, along with multiple health and physical disabilities, se-vere behavior problems is the most frequently cited reason for institutional placement of youth and adults with DDs (McConkey et al., 2007).

The prevalence of behavior problems in persons with DDs is controversial and varies across studies. This controversy is primarily as a result of defini-tional issues relating to what constitutes a "behavioral problem" but is also due to the age and location of the population sampled. For example, boys and men with developmental delay are 50 percent more likely to engage in prob-lem behaviors than are girls and women, behavioral problems begin to in-crease about 5 years of age and continue to increase into early adulthood, and a higher prevalence of behavioral disorders occur in institutional set-tings (Rojahn and Esbensen, 2002). The last variable is due to not only place-ment bias but also to these settings' being associated with increases in prob-lem behavior among individuals not previously displaying such symptoms

(Robertson et al., 2005). However, as community-based placement has become the preferred approach for providing support, studies have become less varied in prevalence rates over the past decade. The current, best prevalence estimate of behavioral problems in people with DDs in community-based settings is 15 percent (Emerson et al., 2001).

Patterns of Behavioral Problems

Of those individuals engaging in problem behavior, most engage in more than one form. That is, most people with behavioral disorders evidence some combination of self-injury, aggression, and property destruction. For example, a person might engage in biting herself and hitting others or in multiple forms of self-injury. Often these behaviors are topographically distinct and not related to any clear underlying pathology other than the DD (Wacker et al., 2006; Sturmey, 2007). This observation is important because it frames how behavioral problems are assessed and treated.

Historically, researchers and clinicians treated problem behaviors based on their topographical nature. For example, certain interventions were used to treat self-injury, others to treat aggression, and still others to treat property destruction. Unfortunately, treatment success was sporadic and unpredictable (Axelrod, 1987; Mace, 1994; Munk and Repp, 1994). Beginning in the 1970s, researchers noted that problem behaviors may be a form of communication directed toward others in a person's environment (Carr, 1977). This led researchers to assess the effects of a person's behavioral problems on his or her social environment and what those behaviors may be communicating to others (Carr and Durand, 1985). In addition, as part of this functional assessment approach it became clear that multiple types of behavior could serve a similar communicative effect. This led to the development of behavior problems comprising a response class. A *response class* is any set of behaviors that produce a similar effect on the environment (Catania, 2007). An example of this would be an adult who hits himself in the face but also bites others and rips clothing. If all of these behaviors produce the same consequence (e.g., gaining negative attention from others), then they are functionally equivalent and form a response class.

The combined conceptualization of problem behavior as occurring as a form of communication and in response classes has shaped how these behaviors are treated using contemporary behavioral interventions. Problem behaviors among people with DDs are typically assessed to see what kinds of behavior comprise a response class and how those behaviors function in terms of communication. Because response classes necessarily focus on the consequences of behavior, how a person's environment is altered by problem behavior becomes an important aspect in assessment and intervention. Similarly, because behavioral problems are often communicative in nature, the social milieu in which the behaviors occur is also a focus.

Behavioral problems are currently classified into one of five mutually exclusive functional categories: (1) negative reinforcement, (2) positive reinforcement, (3) automatic reinforcement, (4) multiply determined, or (5) undifferentiated (Hanley, Iwata, and McCord, 2003; Asmus et al., 2004). *Negative reinforcement* involves behavioral problems engaged in to avoid or escape people, places, or things. An example would be an adolescent who engages in face slapping and spitting to avoid academic instruction or the people and places associated with academic instruction. *Positive reinforcement* involves behavioral problems engaged in to obtain people, places, or things. For example, the same adolescent's face slapping and spitting could occur to gain attention from parents or siblings, particularly in settings where the behaviors cannot be ignored (e.g., a shopping mall or grocery store). *Automatic reinforcement* involves behavioral problems engaged in because of the sensory consequences produced. Using the same adolescent and behaviors as an example, face slapping and spitting may occur for the proprioceptive stimulation each behavior produces. *Multiply determined* functions involve any combination of the three previous reinforcement types. For example, the face slapping and spitting may be negatively reinforced by avoiding instruction and positively reinforced by adult attention. Finally, an *inconclusive function* is noted if no clear behavioral outcome is identified.

Behavioral epidemiologic studies provide estimates of the frequency with which these behavioral functions are encountered in the DDs. Table 13.1 shows the results of the two largest clinical studies estimating the prevalence of different behavioral functions. In children the most frequent behavioral functions are negative reinforcement or positive reinforcement or the combination of two reinforcing functions (i.e., multiply determined; Asmus et al., 2004). In adults the most frequent behavioral functions are negative, positive, or automatic reinforcement as individual functions (Iwata et al., 1994). Only 5 percent of behavioral disorders occur for some other reason (see Symons, 2002; Kennedy and O'Reilly, 2006).

Table 13.1. Summary of functional behavioral assessment outcomes
(percentage of sample)

Behavioral function	Iwata et al. (1994)[1]	Asmus et al. (2004)[2]
Negative reinforcement	38	27
Positive reinforcement	26	14
Automatic reinforcement	26	7
Multiply determined	5	48
Inconclusive	5	4

[1]Institutionalized adult population
[2]Community-based child population

Functional Assessment of Problem Behaviors

Assessing the functions of problem behaviors involves a process referred to as *functional behavioral assessment,* or FBA, which is designed to identify the environmental events associated with behavioral problems. Typically, a series of increasingly complex assessment techniques are used until a clear hypothesis regarding why problem behaviors are occurring is achieved. Once the behavioral functions have been identified, then intervention is based on these findings (discussed in the next section). The most commonly used sequence of assessments include: (1) record reviews or interviews, (2) descriptive assessments, and (3) experimental analyses.

The first step in conducting an FBA is to clearly identify and define what behaviors are of primary concern. This involves a two-stage process: deciding what behaviors are considered problematic and operationally defining those behaviors. Operationalizing problem behavior involves defining the response in terms of observable physical characteristics. That is, referring to specific aspects of a problem behavior rather than a more general and vague label (see Wolery, Bailey, and Sugai, 1988; Sulzer-Azaroff and Mayer, 1990).

Record Reviews and Interviews

Once problem behaviors have been identified and defined, record reviews and interviews are conducted to identify variables that predict the occurrence and nonoccurrence of events associated with the behavioral problems. Record reviews typically involve health records, educational and vocational documents, psychological assessments, and any other information that may contribute to an understanding of why problem behaviors are occurring. Interviews can involve care providers answering open-ended questions or completing questionnaires (O'Neill et al, 1996; Alberto and Troutman, 2002; Miltenberger, 2003). The focus of record reviews and interviews is to find out more information about the origins of the problem behavior, when the behaviors occur and do not occur, and what environmental events occur before and after problem behaviors. Establishing what behavior-environment patterns exist often suggests specific reasons for the problem behavior occurring (i.e., reinforcer functions). If the reasons are clear, a hypothesis regarding behavioral function is identified at this point (e.g., attention from siblings as positive reinforcement) and clinicians may proceed to developing an intervention plan. However, if hypotheses regarding behavioral functions are questionable or there may be multiple behavioral functions, then clinicians often proceed to descriptive assessments.

Descriptive Assessments

This assessment approach involves the direct observation of problem behavior in the environments in which the person who engages in them lives, works, or recreates. The goal of descriptive assessments is to develop possible correlations between antecedent and consequent events that may be related to behavioral problems. Often these events can be identified from record reviews and interviews, but sometimes critical events are not identified until the behaviors are observed in the environments in which they occur. A range of data collection protocols have been developed to conduct descriptive assessments, but all share a common focus on collecting direct observation data on the antecedents and consequences relating to the problem behaviors (Bijou, Peterson, and Ault, 1968; Touchette, MacDonald, and Langer, 1985; O'Neill et al., 1996; T. Thompson, Felce, and Symons, 1999). By directly observing what occurs before and after problem behavior, one can make further refinements regarding hypotheses of the functional properties of behavior. Because behavioral interventions are based on functional consequences, identifying plausible sources of reinforcement and the types of stimuli that are reinforcing is critical.

Experimental Analyses

In instances when descriptive assessments in conjunction with record reviews and interviews do not yield clear hypotheses regarding sources of reinforcement, then experimental analysis of problem behavior can be used. Experimental analysis, as the name implies, is a small-scale experiment using some type of single-case design (Kennedy, 2005). Conditions are explicitly arranged allowing for the testing of specific reinforcement contingencies in relation to problem behavior (Iwata et al., 1994; Wacker et al., 2004). This FBA technique exposes problem behavior to experimentally arranged environments to test hypotheses regarding antecedents and consequences. For example, social attention might be made contingent on problem behavior or demands may be withdrawn contingent on problem behavior. By conducting experimental analyses, a precise set of hypotheses can be tested in relation to the occurrence of problem behavior to gain additional information about why behaviors are occurring. The information from the earlier FBA techniques is used to increase the contextual validity of the experimental analysis conditions.

As a collection, the FBA techniques just reviewed are designed to identify environmental events having functional effects on the occurrence of problem behavior. Clinicians typically use record reviews and interviews in conjunction with descriptive assessments. If additional clarity or refinement is needed to understand why problem behavior is occurring, then experimental analyses may also be conducted. However, the overall goal is to develop clear hypotheses regarding why problem behaviors are occurring so behavioral interventions can be derived from this functional assessment information.

Behavioral Intervention Plans

The results of the FBA are used to define the nature of the behavioral intervention by matching the intervention to the behavioral function (Repp, Felce, and Barton, 1988; Sigafoos, Arthur, and O'Reilly, 2003; Luiselli, 2006). For example, if access to items serving as positive reinforcers is identified as the basis for the behavioral problem, then functional communication training (Durand, 2002) can be used to teach alternative forms of appropriate communication to access the preferred events. This could also be combined with an extinction procedure in which instances of the problem behaviors do not result in the preferred event (R. H. Thompson and Iwata, 2005). Other function-specific interventions would be used for behavioral problems that are negatively reinforced. A combination of these procedures would be used for an individual whose behavioral problems are multiply determined. For automatic reinforcement, the current basis of treatment is to provide an enriched environment that produces stimulation similar to the behavioral problem itself (Rapp, 2006). Finally, for instances of undifferentiated outcomes, current intervention approaches focus on noncontingent reinforcement to reduce behavioral problems (Carr and LeBlanc, 2006).

The effectiveness of FBA-based interventions has been demonstrated in hundreds of highly controlled small-*N*, single-case design experiments. These studies have shown the effectiveness of these function-specific interventions and have allowed for the refinement of methods for matching interventions to behavioral functions (DeLeon, Rodriguez-Catter, and Cataldo, 2002; Kahng, Iwata, and Lewin, 2002; Hanley, Iwata, and McCord, 2003; Wacker, Berg, and Harding, 2006). The FBA-based approach itself has become the "gold standard" for assessment and intervention in behavioral problems for persons with DDs (e.g., Council for Children with Behavioral Disorders, 2002; American Association on Mental Retardation, 2004; National Association of School Psychologists, 2005).

As noted earlier, the specific intervention selected will be based on the hypothesized environmental variable maintaining problem behavior. For example, if a person's problem behavior is negatively reinforced by escaping the demands made by authority figures (e.g., teachers, job coaches, parents and other care providers), then the intervention should focus on strategies associated with this behavioral function. Potential strategies could include teaching the person alternative responses for requesting assistance or a break, care providers providing attention for only compliance, and so on. What is critical about interventions is that the hypothesized maintaining variable be the focus of the procedure.

Selecting an intervention depends on the hypothesized function of the problem behavior. Perhaps the most important guidelines in selecting an intervention are (1) matching the intervention to the hypothesized behavioral function, (2) selecting "behavior pairs" (i.e., emphasizing a desirable behavior to replace the undesirable behavior), (3) emphasizing the efficiency and usefulness of the alternative, desirable behavior, (4) providing consistent delivery of the intervention across people, settings, and days, and (5) allowing the intervention enough time to have an impact on problem behavior.

It is beyond the scope of this chapter to exhaustively list different types of behavioral interventions. For a more comprehensive listing, the following books are suggested for in-depth reference: Carr et al. (1994), O'Neill et al. (1996), Durand (2002), Sigafoos, Arthur, and O'Reilly (2003), and Luiselli

(2006). However, listed and described below are several general types of interventions that have been empirically demonstrated to be effective. The behavioral interventions are classified into two general types: proactive interventions and consequence-based interventions. *Proactive interventions* focus on using behavioral strategies that will preclude the person with DDs from engaging in problem behavior. *Consequence-based interventions* focus on the response-reinforcer relations maintaining the problem behavior by either altering reinforcement contingencies or teaching alternative skills to achieve the same type of reinforcement. Typically, clinicians use both proactive and consequence-based interventions in combination. Some examples of both types of interventions are listed below.

Proactive Interventions

- *Meaningful activities.* Are the activities being given to a person useful to him and relevant to his daily life? For example, does instruction directly teach an individual how to successfully use objects or activities he frequently encounters (e.g., making retail purchases, using a computer, preparing a meal)?
- *Frequent variation in activities.* Do the activities a person is exposed to vary from time to time and day to day? For example, are "hands-on" instruction and exploratory learning approaches interspersed with paper-and-pencil and lecture presentations for job training sessions?
- *Actively providing choices.* Does a person actively choose the focus and content of activities? For example, does an adult help select what recreation activities she is going to engage in?
- *Frequent attention for appropriate behavior.* Does a person receive attention from care providers primarily for engaging in appropriate behavior? For example, is an individual's engaging in an activity positively commented on by care providers (or does he or she receive attention only when acting out)?
- *Frequent access to peers without disabilities.* Does the person with DDs have regular, daily opportunities to interact and develop relationships with peers who do not have disabilities? For example, are adults with disabilities regularly participating in community activities and interacting with peers without disabilities during a typical day?
- *Age-appropriate activities.* Are the activities being given to a person

something that her same-age peers without disabilities frequently use? For example, are the books and magazines she has access to the same as those read by her peers without disabilities? An emphasis on age-appropriate activities also increases the range of materials the person is allowed access to.

- *Predictable routines.* Is a person able to understand and predict what activities he is being asked to engage across the day? For example, is the work schedule reviewed in the morning with the individual and does the student keep an individual schedule? Or, is the student's schedule adapted to make it more concrete so changes from one activity to another can be understood (e.g., picture books, tangible objects)?
- *Awareness and appropriate action regarding health conditions.* Does the person have any identified or suspected health conditions and is it being actively treated? For example, is there a treatment plan for an adult who has asthma that affects how he feels? People with DDs should regularly receive check-ups from a health care professional, especially before the development of a behavior management plan to assess for the existence of potential medical conditions causing problem behavior (e.g., migraine headaches, toothaches, constipation).

Consequence-Based Interventions

- *Functional communication training.* Functional communication training focuses on replacing problem behavior with appropriate behavior. Once the function of a problem behavior is identified, a more desirable response is taught to the person that serves a similar function. For example, if a person yells at others to gain attention, teaching the person to raise her hand to request adult attention can be taught. This procedure typically results in a rapid reduction in problem behavior and a similarly rapid increase in the newly learned form of communication (Durand, 2002).
- *Social skills training.* Teaching social skills involves providing a person with the ability to act in a socially appropriate manner in order to obtain specific events (e.g., interacting with peers). Social skills training typically includes discussing social skills, role playing, feedback, modeling, and practice (Lewis, 1994).
- *Extinction.* Extinction is the elimination of a reinforcer that has previ-

ously been identified as maintaining the problem behavior. The technique is effective because it removes the behavioral basis for an individual to engage in a particular response. Either positive or negative reinforcers can be involved in an extinction procedure (R. H. Thompson and Iwata, 2005). This technique is typically paired with some type of reinforcement procedure for more desirable behavior (e.g., functional communication training).

- *Differential reinforcement.* Differential reinforcement of other behavior and differential reinforcement of incompatible behavior are well-established behavioral change strategies. Differential reinforcement works by providing positive reinforcement for desirable behavior, while ignoring (i.e., extinguishing) problem behavior. When using this technique it is critical to identify meaningful, naturally occurring reinforcers to use to promote positive behavior (Sulzer-Azaroff and Mayer, 1990).
- *Time-out.* Time-out is the removal of a positive reinforcer contingent on the occurrence of a problem behavior. Like differential reinforcement, time-out is a well-established technique for reducing problem behavior. However, it is also the most misunderstood. Importantly, if misused, it will actually increase the occurrence of problem behavior. Time-out works only if the person is being removed from a positively reinforcing situation (as defined above). If the student is being removed from a situation that is not positively reinforcing, then the intervention is actually negatively reinforcing the problem behavior (i.e., increasing the response; Solnick, Rincover, and Peterson, 1977). If a time-out technique has been in place for an extended period of time, other procedures need to be considered (i.e., if time-out is going to be effective, its effects should be rapid).
- *Behavioral momentum.* Behavioral momentum was developed primarily for increasing compliance with requests. The intervention requires that a caregiver make three to four requests of the person with DDs that she typically will complete (e.g., answering a brief question), provide praise for completing each request, and then make the request that she is not complying with. The result is high levels of compliance (Kennedy, Itkonen, and Lindquist, 1995).
- *Problem-solving training.* Problem-solving training involves teaching a person a set of effective coping skills to use during problematic situa-

tions (e.g., social conflicts). This technique involves teaching a person to recognize problem situations, generate possible solutions, decide which solution would constructively resolve the situation, and then implement the solution (Spivack and Shure, 1974).

- *Contingency contracting.* Contingency contracting is a technique that arranges for a person to receive rewards for completing work and acting appropriately. It can be either a written or verbal contract between an adult and an individual with DDs. The contract specifies "if, then" relations between expected performance and the consequences for desired and problem behavior (Sulzer-Azaroff and Mayer, 1990).
- *Self-monitoring.* Self-monitoring involves teaching a person to first discriminate some aspect of her behavior (e.g., using appropriate social skills), then monitor its occurrence; when a specified number of target behaviors have occurred, the person receives some type of reinforcer. Typically, the behavior to be monitored is a socially desirable behavior that is incompatible with problem behavior (Mooney et al., 2005).

Monitoring Progress and Decision Making

Once the environmental variables associated with problem behavior have been identified and a behavioral intervention has been designed, a system should be developed for monitoring progress. It is important to monitor occurrences of both problem behavior and more desirable behavior. A monitoring system allows for the regular documentation of the occurrence of problem behavior during the time period of intervention. This step is an essential component of any behavioral intervention for accountability and to allow for data-based decision making regarding the effectiveness of the intervention (see Kennedy, 2005). The most important aspects of a monitoring system are that it be easy to use and accurate.

To construct a monitoring system, the following components must be followed: (1) problem behaviors must be operationally defined; (2) a dimension of each behavior must be identified so that it can be measured (i.e., frequency, rate, duration, latency, inter-response time, or celeration); (3) a measurement strategy must be selected to record the occurrence of problem behaviors (i.e., permanent product, time-sampling, or interval-sampling be used to record behavior); (4) decisions regarding when, where, and who will collect data need to be determined (e.g., will data be collected every day, once per day, or once per week?); (5) a set of procedures need to be arranged for analyzing the information collected (i.e., the type of graphic display to be used); and, (6) regular times need to be scheduled regarding when the care providers will summarize and assess the data (e.g., initially once per day, then changing to weekly summaries).

Part of effectively managing problem behavior is the use of data-based decision making. By systematically monitoring the occurrence of problem behavior, one can more accurately assess the rate of responding. One important benefit of data-based decision making is that it facilitates the assessment of the overall effectiveness of behavioral interventions. As has been noted throughout this chapter, the basis of any intervention is the development of hypotheses regarding the environmental events maintaining problem behavior. For the intervention to be successful, it should be maintained along with the proactive behavioral support strategies.

However, given the nature of hypotheses (i.e., they are the best estimation of why problem behavior is occurring), in some instances initial hypotheses may be incorrect. This will be indicated by only partial reductions in the frequency of problem behavior (or increases). If this occurs in the context of consistently delivered interventions occurring across a period of several weeks, the initial hypothesis regarding problem behavior may be inaccurate or only partly correct.

Such an occurrence should not be viewed as a treatment failure; instead, it should be seen as a refinement in the understanding of the problem behavior. For example, if it was originally hypothesized that behavior was maintained by negative reinforcement in the form of escaping from demands and that proves incorrect, then this one variable has been eliminated as a source of behavioral problems. The development of behavioral interventions shares many similarities with solving a problem and should be viewed as an iterative process.

Given this understanding of why hypotheses are sometimes accurate and sometimes need to be further refined, the next course of action is to reassess the original hypothesis. However, more than that needs to be done before new intervention procedures are developed. If the results of the intervention do not have the impact that was desired, the FBA process needs to begin again. Beginning again at this point is necessary because several weeks may have elapsed since the initial assessment, and conditions may have changed since the process was originally begun. Once proactive behavioral support strategies have been reassessed, if necessary, the behavioral intervention can be redesigned within the context of the knowledge gained from the initial intervention process.

Conclusion

Selecting and developing interventions for problem behavior requires five steps: (1) operationalizing problem behavior, (2) assessing the function of problem behavior, (3) selecting an intervention, (4) developing a monitoring system, and (5) monitoring intervention effects. Following this strategy, and altering hypotheses when necessary, the behavioral support strategies outlined in this chapter provide the basis for decreasing the occurrence of problem behavior, increasing the occurrence of socially important behavior and thereby increasing the ability of the individual with DDs to remain in the least-restrictive community setting possible.

References

Alberto PA, Troutman AC. 2002. *Applied Behavior Analysis for Teachers*, 6th ed. Saddle River, NJ: Prentice Hall.

American Association on Mental Retardation. 2004. *Position Statement: Behavioral Supports*. Washington, DC: American Association on Mental Retardation.

Asmus JM, Ringdahl JE, Sellers JA, et al. 2004. Use of a short-term inpatient model to evaluate aberrant behavior: Outcome data summaries from 1996 to 2001. *Journal of Applied Behavior Analysis* 37: 283–304.

Axelrod S. 1987. Functional and structural analyses of behavior: Approaches leading to reduced use of punishment procedures? *Research in Developmental Disabilities* 8: 165–78.

Bijou SW, Peterson RF, Ault MH. 1968. A method to integrate descriptive and experimental field studies at the level of data and empirical concepts. *Journal of Applied Behavior Analysis* 1: 175–91.

Carr EG. 1977. The motivation of self-injurious behavior: A review of some hypotheses. *Psychological Bulletin* 84: 800–816.

Carr EG, Durand VM. 1985. Reducing behavior problems through functional communication training. *Journal of Applied Behavior Analysis* 18: 111–26.

Carr EG, Levin L, McConnachie G, et al. 1994. *Communication-Based Intervention for Problem Behavior*. Baltimore: Paul H. Brookes.

Carr EG, LeBlanc LA. 2006. Noncontingent reinforcement as antecedent behavioral support. In J Luiselli (ed.), *Antecedent Assessment and Intervention: Supporting*

Children and Adults with Developmental Disabilities in Community Settings, 147–63. Baltimore: Paul H. Brookes.

Catania AC. 2007. *Learning*, 4th ed. New York: Prentice Hall.

Council for Children with Behavioral Disorders. 2002. *Position Paper on School Discipline Policies for Students with Significantly Disruptive Behavior*. Alexandria, VA: Council for Exceptional Children.

DeLeon IG, Rodriquez-Catter V, Cataldo MF. 2002. Treatment: Current standards of care and their research implications. In SR Schoeder, ML Oster-Granite, T Thompson (eds.), *Self-Injurious Behavior: Gene-Brain-Behavior Relationships*, 81–92. Washington, DC: American Psychological Association.

Durand VM. 2002. *Severe Behavior Problems: A Functional Communication Training Approach*. New York: Guilford Press.

Emerson E, Kiernan C, Alborz A, et al. 2001. The prevalence of challenging behaviors: A total population study. *Research in Developmental Disabilities* 22: 77–93.

Hanley GP, Iwata BA, McCord BE. 2003. Functional analysis of problem behavior: A review. *Journal of Applied Behavior Analysis* 36: 147–85.

Individuals with Disabilities Education Improvement Act of 2004, P.L. 108-446, 118 Stat. 2647.

Iwata BA, Dorsey MF, Slifer KJ, Bauman KE, Richman GS. 1994. Toward a functional analysis of self-injury. *Journal of Applied Behavior Analysis* 27: 197–209. (Originally published in 1982)

Iwata BA, Pace GM, Dorsey MF, et al. 1994. The functions of self-injurious behavior: An experimental-epidemiological analysis. *Journal of Applied Behavior Analysis* 27: 215–40.

Kahng SW, Iwata BA, Lewin AB. 2002. The impact of functional assessment on the treatment of self-injurious behavior. In SR Schoeder, ML Oster-Granite, T Thompson (eds.), *Self-Injurious Behavior: Gene-Brain-Behavior Relationships*, 119–32. Washington, DC: American Psychological Association.

Kennedy CH. 2005. *Single-Case Designs for Educational Research*. Boston: Allyn & Bacon.

Kennedy CH, Itkonen T, Lindquist K. 1995. Comparing interspersed requests and social comments as antecedents for increasing student compliance. *Journal of Applied Behavior Analysis* 28: 97–98.

Kennedy CH, O'Reilly ME. 2006. Pain, health conditions, and problem behavior in people with developmental disabilities. In TF Oberlander, FJ Symons (eds.), *Pain in Children and Adults with Developmental Disabilities*, 121–38. Baltimore: Paul H. Brookes.

Lewis TJ. 1994. A comparative analysis of the effects of social skill training and teacher-directed contingencies on social behavior of preschool children with disabilities. *Journal of Behavioral Education* 4: 267–81.

Luiselli JK (ed.). 2006. *Antecedent Assessment and Intervention: Supporting Children and Adults with Developmental Disabilities in Community Settings*. Baltimore: Paul H. Brookes.

Mace FC. 1994. The significance and future of functional analysis methodologies. *Journal of Applied Behavior Analysis* 27: 385–92.

McConkey R, Abbott S, Walsh PN, Linehan C, Emerson E. 2007. Variations in the social inclusion of people with intellectual disabilities in supported living schemes and residential settings. *Journal of Intellectual Disabilities Research* 51: 207–17.

Miltenberger RG. 2003. *Behavior Modification: Principles and Procedures*. Independence, KY: Wadsworth Publishing.

Mooney M, Ryan JB, Uhing BM, Reid R, Epstein MH. 2005. A review of self-management interventions targeting academic outcomes for students with emotional and behavioral disorders. *Journal of Behavioral Education* 14: 203–21.

Munk DD, Repp AC. 1994. The relationship between instructional variables and problem behavior: A review. *Exceptional Children* 60: 390–401.

National Association of School Psychologists. 2005. *Position Statement on Students with Emotional and Behavioral Disorders*. Bethesda, MD: National Association of School Psychologists.

O'Neill RE, Horner RH, Albin RW, Storey K, Sprague JR. 1996. *Functional Assessment and Program Development for Problem Behavior: A Practical Handbook*. Independence, KY: Wadsworth Publishing.

Rapp J. 2006. Toward an empirical method for identifying matched stimulation for automatically reinforced behavior. *Journal of Applied Behavior Analysis* 39: 137–40.

Repp AC, Felce D, Barton LE. 1988. Basing the treatment of stereotypic and self-injurious behaviors on hypotheses of their causes. *Journal of Applied Behavior Analysis* 21: 281–89.

Robertson J, Emerson E, Pinkney L, et al. 2005. Treatment and management of challenging behaviours in congregate and noncongregate community-based supported accommodation. *Journal of Intellectual Disabilities Research* 49: 63–72.

Rojahn J, Esbensen AJ. 2002. Epidemiology of self-injurious behavior in mental retardation: A review. In SR Schroeder, ML Oster-Granite, T Thompson (eds.), *Self-Injurious Behavior: Gene-Brain-Behavior Relationships*, 41–78. Washington, DC: American Psychological Association.

Sigafoos J, Arthur M, O'Reilly M. 2003. *Challenging Behavior and Developmental Disability*. Baltimore: Paul H. Brookes.

Solnick JV, Rincover A, Peterson CR. 1977. Some determinants of the reinforcing and punishing effects of timeout. *Journal of Applied Behavior Analysis* 10: 415–24.

Spivack G, Shure M. 1974. *Social Adjustment of Young Children: A Cognitive Approach to Solving Real-Life Problems*. San Francisco: Jossey-Bass.

Sturmey P. 2007. *Functional Analysis in Clinical Treatment*. New York: Academic Press.

Sulzer-Azaroff B, Mayer R. 1990. *Applying Behavior Analysis Procedures with Children and Youth*. New York: Holt, Rinehart, & Winston.

Symons F. 2002. Self-injury and pain: Models and mechanisms. In SR Schroeder,

ML Oster-Granite, T Thompson (eds.), *Self-Injurious Behavior: Gene-Brain-Behavior Relationships*, 223–34. Washington, DC: American Psychological Association.

Thompson RH, Iwata BA. 2005. A review of reinforcement control procedures. *Journal of Applied Behavior Analysis* 38: 257–78.

Thompson T, Felce D, Symons F. 1999. *Behavioral Observation: Technology and Applications in Developmental Disabilities*. Baltimore: Paul H. Brookes.

Touchette PE, MacDonald RF, Langer SN. 1985. A scatter plot for identifying stimulus control of problem behavior. *Journal of Applied Behavior Analysis* 18: 343–51.

Wacker DP, Berg WK, Harding JW. 2006. The evolution of antecedent-based interventions. In JK Luiselli (ed.), *Antecedent Assessment and Intervention: Supporting Children and Adults with Developmental Disabilities in Community Settings*, 3–30. Baltimore: Paul H. Brookes.

Wacker DP, Berg W, Harding J, Cooper-Brown L. 2004. Use of brief experimental analyses in outpatient clinic and home settings. *Journal of Behavioral Education* 13: 213–26.

Wolery M, Bailey DB, Sugai GM. 1988. *Effective Teaching: Principles and Procedures of Applied Behavior Analysis of Exceptional Students*. Boston: Allyn & Bacon.

PART V ◆

SPECIAL
ISSUES

14

Ethical and Legal Issues

Judith M. Levy, M.S.W., M.A., and
Maureen van Stone, J.D., M.S.

A major shift in the public perception of the rights of people with disabilities occurred in the early 1960s and 1970s. Up until that time, many people with disabilities were sent away from their family of origin and lived regimented existences in institutions. Regardless of where they lived, they were believed to be incapable of living independently or of making important decisions that affected their lives.

This shift of opinion initially concerned the perception of children with disabilities. The community at large was exposed to more children with disabilities and also no longer accepted the conventional wisdom about what was best for them. At first it seemed to be entirely the result of advances in medical technology that saved infants and children who would otherwise have died at birth or following an illness or traumatic injury. However, other factors were at work as well. These included the European experience with adverse outcomes for children institutionalized after World War II, the work of John Bowlby and Rene Spitz on institutionalized children, a growing awareness of the importance of the mother-child relationship, and studies demonstrating the positive outcomes for children with trisomy 21 raised with their families versus foster placement. Studies addressing what was thought to be the negative impact on family members of institutionalizing a family member with DDs demonstrated that this assessment was not a foregone conclusion. It was suggested that the effect on a mother of committing her child to an institution might be equally or more deleterious (Antommaria, 2006).

Person-Centered Planning

The disability community today is strong, and its members advocate for self-determination, inclusion, integration, and normalization in every facet of life across the age span. In all aspects of life, persons with disabilities want to be treated as individuals and involved in determining the course of their lives, the choices they have, and those they make. Although informed consent is generally thought of related to medical decision making, it is, of course, related to all decisions. Currently, best practice involves attempting to follow the "choice" of even the most profoundly affected individual. "Nothing about me without me!" is the battle cry. Whenever possible and whatever the issue, the individual with the disability leads the discussion and privacy laws (Health Insurance Portability and Accountability Act, 1996) as well as an expectation of ethical practice prevail.

Respecting an individual includes respecting that person's culture. Cultural values and norms about people with disabilities and medical conditions vary greatly from country to country and even within the United States. It is important to understand the cultural beliefs that individuals hold in order to help them achieve their goals. Arthur Kleinman (Fadiman, 1997) has written extensively on the subject of sensitizing doctors and other professionals who help people to cultural differences in matters of health and sickness. He suggests that those in the helping professions ask their patients the following questions:

- What do you call the problem?
- What do you think has caused the problem?
- Why do you think it started when it did?
- What do you think the sickness does? How does it work?
- How severe is the problem? Will it have a short or long course?
- What kind of treatment is necessary and what do you hope the results will be?
- What are the chief problems the condition has caused?
- What do you fear most about the illness?

In this way, the physician will understand the patient's perception of the problem and will be able to work toward reasonable goals. A slight modification would assist in learning an individual's perceptions of many other choices he or she must make. In a related matter, there remains considerable misunderstanding in the community at large about the rights of adults with developmental disabilities to make their own decisions unless proven incompetent in a court of law. Although this is changing, parents, in particular, frequently think that their decision-making responsibilities should continue after their child reaches the age of majority no matter what their child's level of functioning is. Parents may also be frustrated by service providers who interpret the law superficially by expecting all except the most profoundly disabled to understand every aspect of a decision rather than assessing their adult child's understanding of the decision to be made.

In 2002, the American Association on Mental Retardation, now the American Association on Intellectual and Developmental Disabilities, developed a new classification and system of supports for people with mental retardation. Given an individual's intelligence and adaptive skills, the person has strengths, limitations, and needs in certain environments that require varying levels of support for the person to pursue legitimate interests. Persons with disabilities may need help occasionally and in specific circumstances, or they may need support in all aspects of their lives. Any supports should be provided in the least-restrictive, most normalized manner.

CASE EXAMPLE

Larry is a 45-year-old man with moderate mental retardation of unknown origin whose language skills are similar to those of an 8-year-old child. He is his own guardian. He is communicative but concrete in his thinking. For the past 20 years, he has lived in a group home in the community with three other residents, attends work daily, and participates in recreational and family activities regularly. Support staff and family members assist him in taking care of himself as necessary. Until recently his major health problem has been obesity. Lately he has been feeling poorly, so he sees his general practitioner who conducts an evaluation and finds that he has an enlarged prostate. The general practitioner refers Larry to a urologist, who prescribes a medication. Larry takes it religiously but ultimately the doctor recommends surgery to relieve his symptoms. He is anxious and depressed about his physical condition and potential surgery. His doctor refers him to a psychiatrist for medication but the psychiatrist is concerned that he will not be able to understand well enough to give informed consent. What is the best way to help Larry make a decision about the medication and the surgery? ▶

Ethics 101

In the *Principles of Biomedical Ethics* (2001), Tom Beauchamp and James Childress discuss their evolving thinking about the principles of respect for the autonomy of persons, nonmaleficence, beneficence, and justice. Autonomy requires that we show respect for the views and decisions of others, which are based on their personal values. Informed consent is derived from this principle. The elements of informed consent are providing information, understanding and appreciating of the information by the individual for him- or herself, and having the ability to make a voluntary choice. Nonmaleficence requires that "one ought not to inflict evil or harm" on another person (Beauchamp and Childress, 2001). Whereas nonmaleficence requires that we refrain from some actions, "beneficence requires taking action by helping—preventing harm, removing harm, and promoting good." Interpreted broadly this could include refraining from causing physical or psychological injury or promoting other people's pursuing legitimate interests, such as those concerning living and working arrangements, friendships and recreational activities, and allowing them to make their own decisions if they have the ability to do so. Ask what a person's interests are and what the person considers harmful or helpful, learn how the person's perception differs from your own, and whether there are others whose interests count. Conflict may occur when values differ but this does not mean that there is a right or wrong answer. Paternalism is defended as beneficent because one person presumes to know what is best for another. Justice involves treating people fairly according to their needs and using consistent standards, avoiding decisions based purely on diagnosis or disabilities, and distributing scarce resources fairly. Person-centered planning and people-first language are examples of the application of all four of the principles.

Decision-Making Capacity of Individuals

Both the law and morality require that competent adults, at least 18 years of age, give informed consent for their own medical care. With few exceptions, health care professionals must obtain informed consent from the parents or guardians of individuals under the age of 18. The discussion between the health care professional and the individual should include any materials, diagrams, illustrations, videos, and question-and-answer sessions that are needed to help explain the illness or treatment in a meaningful way. If alternative treatments or no treatment is an option for the individual, the health care professional should explain these options and why they are not recommending a particular course of action. In terms of material risks, the health care professionals should explain the effect of the treatment on the life expectancy. The health care professional working with the individual must balance the need for information and the details of the information with the risk of the individual becoming overwhelmed, confused, or anxious. Thus, the appropriate test is not what the physician in the exercise of his medical judgment thinks a patient should know before acquiescing in a proposed course of treatment; rather, the focus is on what data the patient requires to make an informed decision.

Griso and Appelbaum (1998) designed the MacArthur Competence Assessment Tool (MacCAT), a structured interview schedule for assessing the decision-making abilities of individuals to determine their capacity to give informed consent for medical treatment. A mental status exam will give some information but is not seen as the final word in such a determination. But currently there is "no standardized decision-making capacity assessment tool for people with intellectual or developmental disabilities" (Kingsbury, 2007). In relation to the case example, if Larry felt pressured by his doctor to agree to the recommended course of treatment, he might make an irrational decision based on fear and misunderstanding. This would be disrespectful of his autonomy, could be harmful, and is unjust because it is not standard practice to pressure patients into acquiescence.

Decision-making capacity is related to actual functioning in a specific decision-making context, one's cognitive abilities and affective states and it can change. The degree to which a person must understand and appreciate the information is directly correlated with the severity of the consequences. Assessment of an individual's decision-making capacity can involve formal standardized tools such as the MacCAT or another standardized clinical interview. Family and caregivers who know the individual well can provide invaluable information about the individual's values, religious beliefs, past decisions, and past statements. Individuals may have strong skills in one life domain but not others. It is important to try to increase the potential of the individual to make a decision by increasing functional abilities or decreasing the decision-making demands of the situation. In Larry's case, the help of trusted friends and relatives, and the anti-anxiety and antidepressant medications may increase his functional abilities. "The health care provider is required to give . . . information in terms understandable to the patient but is not required to give extensive technical information" (Hurley and O'Sullivan, 1999). This is an example of decreasing the demands of the situation. Removing barriers is a part of respecting Larry's autonomy. If he needs help from others, it should be provided, including assistive technology or interpretive services, repeated conversations, and increased time to make the decision, if possible.

What does Larry understand about his medical and psychological conditions? His general practitioner, urologist, and psychiatrist need to team up and develop a plan to facilitate Larry's decision-making capacity. He functions well in his daily routine and has considerable support. Respecting his autonomy is a given, unless he demonstrates that he cannot make these decisions and he would suffer harm. It is beneficent and just. The first conversation should be about the positive effect medication could have on his mood and abilities and should provide information about possible medication side effects as well as why a certain medication is being recommended over another or no medication. All of us make major decisions somewhat differently but most of us involve others in the decision-making process. People with limited decision-making capacity require support as well.

Decision-Making Alternatives

The Health Care Decisions Act of the state of Maryland does not define the term *incapacity*; however; it sets forth the process that must be followed for a physician (including psychiatrist) to make a certification of incapacity. Health care professionals may consider the level of competency depending on whether the treatment poses a greater or lower risk to the patient (e.g., surgery or antibiotics). Declaring a person "incompetent" and assigning a court-appointed guardian should be a last resort because it deprives a person of many rights and may or may not be in person's best interest. Other regulated options, varying from state to state, include the appointment of a health care agent through an advance directive or living will or a surrogate. A frequently overlooked option for people with cognitive disabilities, the appointment of a health care agent (primary and secondary), is a less restrictive and more normalized option. If an individual is able to understand the need for assistance in making future medical decisions it is possible, without court involvement, to appoint a health care agent for medical and mental health treatment. It respects the autonomy of the individual because only a person with capacity to understand can appoint his own health care agent. Surrogates are generally assigned from a hierarchy of family and friends, after two physicians determine that the individual with developmental disabilities cannot understand the decision to be made. Some of the thorniest ethical questions arise because some people have only paid care providers in their lives because family and friends are deceased or do not prefer to help in that manner. The care providers may therefore be put in a position of making health care and other decisions, which set up a conflict of interest.

CASE EXAMPLE

Sarah, age 55, is malnourished and "nonverbal" because cerebral palsy has affected her oral motor and swallowing abilities. Her doctor recommends a feeding tube so that she will gain weight. Her caregiver tells the doctor that if Sarah gains weight, she will not be able to lift her. Should this sway the doctor's treatment recommendations? Should this person be permitted to make such decisions? This would clearly be a harmful decision for Sarah, whose condition might worsen. In this example, it may be beneficial for Sarah to have a court-appointed guardian or health-care agent to represent her best interests. The involvement of the guardian or agent decreases the likelihood that any conflict of interest is introduced to this situation either by the caregiver or by the doctor. ▶

Decision-Making Capacity in the Transition from School Years to Adulthood

If more-restrictive assistance is necessary, limited guardianship for medical purposes, finances, or, in some instances, more general authorizations may be necessary. In that context, the team who works with a child who is on the verge of adulthood should identify appropriate measurable postsecondary goals based on transition assessments related to training, education, employment, and, where appropriate, independent living skills, beginning not later than the first individualized education plan (IEP) to be in effect when the child turns 16, or younger if the IEP team determines it is appropriate, and updated annually thereafter. The IEP must reflect the courses of study needed to assist the adolescent in reaching the goals and must include a statement that the young person has been informed of his or her rights under this title, if any, that will transfer to the individual on reaching the age of majority. The federal statute and regulations articulate that "if the participating agency, other than the local educational agency, fails to provide the transition services described in the IEP, then the local educational agency must reconvene the IEP team to identify alternative strategies to meeting the transition objectives in the child's IEP" (Individuals with Disabilities Education Act, 2004; Code of Federal Regulations, 2006).

IEP teams should consider multiple components when developing a transition plan for a young person with a disability including a career education curriculum (e.g., selecting and planning occupational choices, exhibiting appropriate work behaviors, and seeking, securing, and maintaining employment), postsecondary educational activities (e.g., effective study habits, job tryouts, college accommodations, identifying and applying for postsecondary schools), independent living (e.g., home economics, money management, daily living, housing options, and community-based curriculum), eligibility for adult services (e.g., vocational rehabilitation, advocacy groups, and nonprofit organizations,; community participation (e.g., leisure, recreation, social, and personal skills), and vocational placement options (e.g., adult day programs, rehabilitation facilities, supported employment, sheltered workshop, etc.). It is critical that the IEP team involves members who are knowledgeable about services available in the community, about the least restrictive environment, and about how to engage other public agencies in the transition planning for an adolescent with a disability.

When young people with a disability transition from high school to a postsecondary institution they face all of the issues that students without disabilities face, plus other issues directly related to their disability. It is imperative that adolescents learn early on in the transition process to take ownership of their disability, be an equal member of the decision-making process, be their own best advocate and lead an independent, self-sufficient life to the maximum extent possible. If individuals begin taking ownership of their disability in high school, it will increase their chances of being successful at a postsecondary institution and becoming an effective advocate on their own behalf. Members of the person's IEP team should conduct a functional vocational assessment, a portfolio assessment, achievement or psychometric tests, order a neuropsychological evaluation or an ecological, or curriculum-based vocational assessment (National Information Center for Children and Youth with Disabilities, 1990). If a young person with a disability receives appropriate transition services through the IEP process, he or she may be prepared to enter postsecondary education and access those services to which the individual is entitled under federal law.

Autonomy and the Law

Section 504 of the Rehabilitation Act of 1973

Section 504 of the Rehabilitation Act of 1973 states that "no otherwise qualified person with a disability in the United States . . . shall, solely by reason of . . . disability, be denied the benefits of, be excluded from participation in, or be subjected to discrimination under any program or activity receiving federal financial assistance" (Rehabilitation Act, 1973). In terms of postsecondary education, a qualified person with a disability is one who meets the requisite academic and technical standards required for admission or participation in the postsecondary institution's programs and activities and who may need modifications, accommodations, or auxiliary aids to enable him or her to participate in and benefit from the programs or activities. Colleges and universities receiving federal financial assistance must not discriminate in the recruitment, admission, or treatment of students. These institutions must make changes, when appropriate, to ensure that the academic program is accessible to the greatest extent possible to all students with disabilities. These may include adaptations in the way specific courses are conducted, the use of auxiliary equipment and support staff, and modifications in academic requirements. The postsecondary institution has the flexibility in selecting the specific aid or service it provides, as long as it is effective for the student who will use them. Some modifications may include removing architectural barriers; providing readers for learning disabled or otherwise developmentally disabled individuals or blind persons, interpreters and note takers, or extra time; allowing examinations to be proctored, read orally, dictated, or typed; changing testing formats; using alternative forms for course mastery; and permitting the use of computer software programs or other assistive technological devices. For a student with a disability to access these modifications, it is critical that the student self-advocate and bring his or her needs to the attention of the appropriate college or university personnel. The care network of people with developmental disabilities should also advocate when appropriate.

Under Section 504 of the Rehabilitation Act, colleges and universities are prohibited from limiting the number of students with disabilities who are admitted to their institution, making preadmission inquiries as to whether a student has a disability, or use admissions tests or criteria that inadequately measure the academic qualifications of students with disabilities because appropriate accommodations were not made for them. Once a student is enrolled in a postsecondary institution, the college or university cannot exclude a qualified student from any course of study, limit the student's eligibility for financial assistance on the basis of a disability, or counsel a student toward a more restrictive career. Furthermore, colleges and universities must not measure student achievement using modes that adversely discriminate against a student with a disability or establish policies, practices, and procedures that may adversely affect students with disabilities.

For students with disabilities to gain access to modifications, accommodations, or auxiliary aids, the students must self-identify and provide documentation to the college or university. This may be a challenge for some students who have never had to advocate on their own behalf. To best prepare for facing this challenge after an adult graduates from high school or exits special education in the public school system, the IEP team should include goals and objectives in the transition plan that relate to increasing the individual's ability to advocate on his or her own behalf and how assistance with advocating may be provided. It is imperative that students with disabilities, as well as their parents and service providers, research the requirements of the postsecondary institution in order to ensure compliance with the policies.

The Americans with Disabilities Act of 1990

The Americans with Disabilities Act of 1990 (ADA) provides protection from discrimination for individuals on the basis of disability through employment in the public and private sectors, transportation, public accommodations, services provided by the state and local government, and telecommunication relay services and upholds and extends the standards for compliance set for in Section 504 of the Rehabilitation Act of 1973 to employment practices, communications, and all policies, procedures, and practices that affect the treatment of students with disabilities in postsecondary institutions. As a result of ADA, the public's attention is focused on disability access to institutions of higher education, specifically the institution's facilities, programs, and employment.

Colleges or universities should make reasonable accommodations within the employment process to ensure nondiscrimination on the basis of a disability. Institutions should be prepared to accommodate persons with disabilities qualified to work in campus offices and departments in all aspects of employment, including, but not limited to, recruitment, application, hiring, benefits, promotion, evaluation, termination and for employee grievances.

Conclusion

This chapter speaks to the current standard of practice in the field of developmental disabilities from the ethical and legal perspectives. People with disabilities and their families are rightfully demanding a place at the table when decisions are made that concern them. Previously it was parents who fought for the rights of their children, however, individuals entering adulthood are learning to fight for their own rights to self-determination in all areas of their lives. Both ethics and the law support this, from the Developmental Disabilities Assistance and Bill of Rights Act of 2000 to the body of laws that affect the education of children with disabilities.

The ethical and legal issues presented in this chapter are meant to introduce readers to some of the complex issues facing persons with disabilities from childhood to adulthood. It is important that health care professionals learn some of the basic issues affecting this population and explore the issues that they will be confronted with in their professional roles.

References

Americans with Disabilities Act. 1990. P. L. 101-336, 42 U.S.C. §12101 et seq.
Antommaria A. 2006. Who should survive? One of the choices on our conscience:

Mental retardation and the history of contemporary bioethics. *Kennedy Institute of Ethics Journal* 16(3): 205–24.

Beauchamp T, Childress J. 2001. *Principles of Biomedical Ethics,* 5th ed. Oxford: Oxford University Press.

Code of Federal Regulations. 2006. Special Education / Personnel Development to Improve Services and Results for Children with Disabilities. Title 34, Chapter 1, Part 104.

Developmental Disabilities Assistance and Bill of Rights Act of 2000. P.L. 106-402, 42 U.S.C. §15001 et seq.

Fadiman A. 1997. *The Spirit Catches You and You Fall Down.* New York: Farrar, Straus and Giroux.

Grisso T, Appelbaum PS. 1998. *MacArthur Competence Assessment Tool.* Sarasota, FL: Professional Resource Exchange.

Health Care Decisions Act. 1993. §5-601 et seq. (Maryland)

Health Insurance Portability and Accountability Act. 1996. P.L. 104-191, U.S.C. 290dd–292.

Hurley A, O'Sullivan J. 1999. *Informed Consent for Health Care: A Guide to Consent.* Washington, DC: American Association on Mental Retardation.

Individuals with Disabilities Education Improvement Act. 2004. P.L. 108-446, 20 U.S.C. §1400 et seq.

Kingsbury LAC. 2007, March 29. Conversations for the End-of-Life: Reaching Out to Special Needs Populations [workshop]. Silver Spring, MD: Holy Cross Home Care and Hospice.

National Information Center for Children and Youth with Disabilities. 1990. "Vocational assessment: A guide for parents and professionals," *Transition Summary* 6: 1–16.

Rehabilitation Act. 1973. P.L. 93-112, 29 U.S.C. §794.

15

Advocacy

Lee Combrinck-Graham, M.D.

Individuals with developmental disabilities (DDs) need advocates to promote the lifetime objective that all of us share: to become functioning adults who participate in and contribute to their communities. Specifically, we hold the goal for individuals to function as independently as possible, to be contributing members of communities, and to have opportunities to make choices and decisions for themselves. As with all individuals, people with DDs continue to grow and change and adapt, so advocacy is an ongoing process. It continues to have broad political and economic objectives for persons with DDs and their families. In addition, individuals with DDs require advocacy for specific objectives based on their developmental stage as well as their particular conditions. And because many individuals with DDs are not able to advocate for themselves, they need others to advocate for them. Advocates for individuals with disabilities are necessary to keep these individuals from being relegated to a silent, suffering, and understimulated minority (Gleidman and Roth, 1980).

This chapter will examine all of these aspects of advocacy, particularly emphasizing the role of the health care and mental health care professionals in advocating and promoting advocacy.

Levels of Advocacy

There are at least five levels of advocacy, and all should be in operation for any individual with a DD:

- the family and the individual advocating for themselves
- the caregivers and service providers
- the extended family, friends, and involved members of the community
- advocates for the distinct categories of DD (e.g., Rett syndrome, Asperger syndrome, Down syndrome, etc.)
- local, state, and federal sources of program definition, mandates, and funding

Advocacy Begins at the Time of Diagnosis

As soon as someone identifies that an individual's development is compromised in some way, even in the communication of the diagnosis, needs for care, and prognosis, the individual and family members should also be given basic tools for advocating. These tools will be based on the professional's communication of hope and expectation, not necessarily that the person will "recover" and develop "normally" but that the person will develop and will become a functioning member of a community. With these expectations, family members can begin to prepare for identifying and building a community for the individual and ensuring that the individual's potential for contributing is developed as much as possible (Klein and Schive, 2001).

Let us assume that we are starting with a young child, possibly a newborn, more likely an infant or a toddler. Usually the parents identify that something is different about their child. When parents express concerns to their pediatrician they are initiating advocacy for their child. Once a disability has been identified family members (usually parents) need to ask what can be done and who can do it. These are the parents' first acts of advocacy for their child, and as advocates they will have to ask these questions repeatedly as their family member develops.

In the lives of most individuals with a DD, parents, and other family members are the most important advocates. For some parents, being an advocate evolves naturally, and this has been more necessary when their children were affected with disabilities that were not well known or were more challenging to community systems such as medical and educational supports. In such cases, parents have taken on the role of continuously asking questions and even of demanding help. As one parent of an infant with multiple congenital defects commented, "I have learned that all doctors are [difficult] until proven otherwise." The eloquence of Featherstone (1980), mother of a child with multiple handicaps, Dorris (1989), adoptive father of a child with fetal alcohol syndrome, and the contributors in Klein and Schive (2001) speak to the often endless quests for answers and help that parents pursue for their children.

However, some parents do not advocate in this way for their children. Sometimes this is because they don't recognize a problem (perhaps they have disabilities themselves) or deny the problem and try to protect their child. These families need far more advocacy assistance from professionals who identify difficulties and then need to direct parents to needed support services. Sometimes it becomes the individual with a disability who is the chief advocate, as happened to Robison, after discovering as an adult that he had Asperger disorder and then attempting to learn more about himself in this framework, as well as about others (Robison, 2007). Klein followed up his 2001 book with one reporting from the perspective of adults with disabilities, subtitled "What Adults with Disabilities Wish All Parents Knew" (Klein and Kemp, 2004).

Health care professionals should become advocates, identifying, putting into place, and seeking funding for the kinds of services that will be necessary to help the individual. However, sometimes the health care professionals, feeling defeated or not knowing what to do, may simply try to withdraw. This often happens when parents ask their pediatrician if their child is all right. Many pediatricians will say, "He'll grow out of this," and often children do grow out of whatever their parents were concerned about. However, parents may have to insist if they continue to believe that something is not right. In the optimal situation, when a disability is identified, the pediatrician will help to identify and advocate for services, and as a service team is assembled, the members of that team should also serve as advocates.

Ordinarily a team requires a coordinator so that each team member's advocacy for his or her service necessity doesn't collide with or eclipse another's. Often doctors are designated as team coordinators, and many are good at it, because they are conversant with the different biopsychosocial aspects and how to integrate them. But many doctors may not be effective facilitators of team functioning, may not have a broad knowledge of available and effective intervention possibilities, and may not have the time or skill to manage the necessary interpersonal matters that need to be attended to.

CASE EXAMPLE

At a meeting of parents talking about the special needs of their children, one mother of premature twins, each with a set of serious and complex handicaps, reported that the schedule of therapies for the twins were so packed that following it was impossible and exhausting. She called a meeting of all the individuals who cared for the twins. These caregivers sat around her kitchen table and heard from one another. When the members of the team realized what each one of them had been requiring and how much it added up to, many of them burst into tears. Following that, they all began to work together to plan the twins' care. ▶

In this case, the mother coordinated the team. Many parents can do this and should be supported to thus advocate for their children. It is important to recognize the special effectiveness of a parent team coordinator, because it is the parents who live daily with the problems and the progress. However, many parents don't have the time or skills to perform this function, and someone else has to do so. In many areas there are designated teams with designated managers. This kind of model seems to be a good one until there are necessary deviances from the regular lineup of team members and routine for managing different services. Then it is probably better to have a team leader who emerges naturally. Organizational systems have rules and regulations that may limit their flexibility or even their ability to consider a full range of possibilities, while leaders emerging from the community are less likely to be limited by "red tape" and may therefore perceive and pursue a wider range of possibilities.

An organization from Canada, Planned Lifetime Advocacy Network (PLAN), helps to develop networks around individuals with disabilities in which members of the network assume responsibility for fostering different aspects of the individual's life, taking care of financial, residential, and physical needs while taking care of social, educational, and recreational aspects at the same time. Natural members of networks may include families and service providers but also could include unrelated people in the community who share a common interest and are committed to engaging with the individual over time. The intention of PLAN is that the advocacy network is for life and that networkers assume responsibility and transfer this responsibility to the individual with disabilities over the course of his or her lifetime (Etmanski, 2000).

Advocacy Changes through the Life Cycle

Table 15.1 describes objectives in several realms for each developmental stage and who are the natural advocates. As is described in chapter 2 on the life cycle approach to DDs, individuals with DDs do go through the same stages as "regular" individuals, though the timing and degree of accomplishment may be different. Thus, given the overall objective of advocacy, to promote lifetime functioning as contributing members of communities, it is necessary to recognize what is required socially and educationally to meet them.

The table emphasizes the importance of specific objectives in the social, educational, and emotional and personal adjustment areas. For infants, these objectives are centered on ways of experiencing one's self in the world, of differentiating self from other, and of having some predictability or stability. Physicians and other service providers can advise family members about types of services available. They are the first advocates, to shape the expectation that people will be involved with the individual with disabilities, interacting and responding.

It is also evident from the table which social, emotional, and educational objectives apply at different stages of the life of an individual with DDs. Those who should be advocating for them are listed in the last column. These are natural advocates working to enhance the individual's competence, independence, and inclusion, all of which lead to self-esteem and a sense of productivity and making a contribution.

In every developmental period, continued efforts at "habilitation" must be made. This involves working on skills that are necessary to be as independent as possible. It means not giving up on working on better speech articulation or increasing money skills even in young adults who seem to have hit a level of competence that some would define as the best they can do. These efforts have to be offered in what more than 70 years ago, Vygotsky (1933 /1966) referred to as the "zone of proximal development," an area that is close to what the individual has already achieved but pushes a bit beyond it with the teacher's help. As we don't stop exercising the limbs of a person with paralysis, we should not stop exercising parts of the brain of individuals with intellectual disabilities. Thus, exposure to education that is relevant to what the individual is doing or wants to do is necessary and must be advocated for.

Table 15.1. Advocacy through the life cycle: Developmental objectives

Stage	Social objective	Emotional personal adjustment	Educational objective	Advocates
Infancy	Involvement Stimulation Warmth Reciprocity	Sense of being loved and cared for Secure attachment	Sensorimotor activation Stimulation	Family Professionals
Preschool	Widening circle of involvement, includes family friends, professionals, and other children	Sense of participation	Physical control Locomotion Self-care Communicating needs	Family Professionals Service providers Family friends
School-age	Inclusion, Involvement with peers Special Olympics as example of involvement and skill development	Sense of competence	Learning skills at capacity	Family Educational system Professionals Service providers Family friends
Adolescence	Attendance at performances, athletic events, parties, dances Mentor or Big Brother/Sister	Sense of maturing Growing independent Making decisions Making some contribution	Focus on work skills Learn about body and sexuality and how to express and manage	Family Educational/vocational system Professionals Service providers Family friends Friends' families

Adulthood	Social and leisure activities Having a community of peers Adult mentors Being in a neighborhood Succeeding at job or work	Sense of contributing Making one's own way Having meaningful and valued work Possibly forming partnerships	Focus on normalization Managing work, leisure, self-care, routines, and vacations Habilitation	Family Vocational system (e.g., job finders and coaches) Recreation facilities Friends Neighbors Work associates
Older adulthood	Leisure activities Continuing value in social groups and function as a neighbor	Sense of community Reflection on the value of one's life	Possible retirement and time management Managing personal health Habilitation	Family Service providers Coordinating staff Recreation facilities Friends Neighbors Work associates

Case Examples

A 13-year-old boy with intellectual disabilities has both gross and fine motor problems. In addition, he continues to be confused about the objectives of team sports, though he wants to be part of the team. The physical therapist in the school states that physical therapy (PT) is no longer necessary on his IEP, because he is so big, she can't manage him. The occupational therapist (OT) says that he has achieved maximum benefit from her services. However, all agree to "adaptive PE (physical education)" where he is specifically oriented during team sports. The teacher physically orients him to the direction of play in floor hockey and he scores a goal! The enthusiasm of his teammates reinforces his success and his interest in future activities. The PE teacher also invites him to attend early morning practice with the team. He becomes a member of a group of students for the early morning practice. The PE intervention advocated for membership in a social group and helped him to use his physical skills more appropriately in the process of playing. But who was there to advocate for the continuing value of PT and OT for him?

An adult with intellectual disabilities has always had trouble with reading. He wants to learn how to read. Someone has to advocate for his finding a suitable reading teacher and funding it.

A man in his 50s can't feed himself. While feeding him, shouldn't his support staff also continue to try to help him hold the utensil and put it into his mouth? Does his support staff member need some instruction or strategies for stimulating more independence in his feeding himself?

These are some examples of the ongoing needs throughout the life cycle always striving for acquiring new skills for independence.

Advocacy in the Public Arena

Another level of advocacy goes beyond the individual to families, helping them to advocate for their family members and for groups of people with DDs. Advocacy at these levels is for the purposes of expanding information and knowledge and for increasing funding and resources for the education, housing, and continued development of these members of the group (individuals with disabilities and their families). Usually such advocacy efforts are initiated and led by family members. But professionals are essentials for this. Professionals may encourage parents to move forward with certain requests or demands, may testify, and may provide advocates with information to strengthen their cases.

An example of this is the remarkable work of the American Association of Mental Retardation (which recently changed its name to the American Association of Intellectual and Developmental Disabilities). In their 2006 book, *What Is Mental Retardation?* Switzky and Greenspan examine the changes in definition of what is necessary to open the most effective access to the services and supports needed by individuals with these disabilities.

The following is one parent's account of her discovery of her son's disability, searching for a name, description, and definition, advocating for proper schooling and proper funding, and ultimately advocating at the state level for recognition of his condition in a state agency designated to provide resources for support of individuals who have DDs. Her story is of an individual who started without knowledge but had the drive to insist on information, getting appropriate services, as well as identifying and recruiting other families to the tasks. Her account combines advocating for her child from the time of recognizing that something was different and continuing into his adulthood with advocating for herself and other family members' rights to be informed and receive support for themselves. Here is her story.

Tom's Story

Mrs. C. reports that when their son, Tom, was 4 or 5 months old, she and her husband noticed that he was floppy and that his physical development was slow. Their pediatrician thought he would grow out of it. When Tom was not walking at 18 months, finally their pediatrician referred them to a developmental pediatrician, who acknowledged that something was different and referred them to a neurologist, who said he had "benign hypotonia." When at 18 months he seemed to be more occupied with light switches than with other children in the playgroup, the parents knew something was wrong and returned to the developmental pediatrician. At this point it was agreed that something was wrong, but no one had a diagnosis. Nevertheless he was referred to Birth to Three (a federally funded program under the Education for

All Handicapped Children Act) and received weekly work on gross and fine motor skills as well as some social interaction through a circle time.

When Tom was 3, the developmental pediatrician referred him to nursery school. He identified and gave the parents the names of several local schools. Tom had been speaking since 10 months and had been able to recognize numbers and letters at 3 years old. He attended a preschool, but after the first year the staff recommended that he continue in the 3-year-old group, because he was not socializing. When a teacher made a visit to his home, Tom wanted to show her his favorite things. Lined up on the dining room floor were a mixer, a toaster, a blender, and an electric can opener. About this time he started with echolalia, began to mix up pronouns, and was repeating questions.

The developmental pediatrician referred him to a psychologist who didn't know what to do, and to a child guidance clinic where a therapist saw him three times and didn't think therapy would help. However the therapist referred him to a psychiatrist. This psychiatrist said, "I've seen other children like this." He recognized Tom's pattern of development and behavior as atypical pervasive developmental disorder (PDD). The parents' persistent search for a diagnosis and appropriate services had finally led them to a provider who gave a name to their son's disabilities and would further be able to help them identify the most helpful kind of school setting.

When Tom was ready for kindergarten, the psychiatrist referred the family to two schools, and they visited them both. One was private, and the school system wouldn't pay for it. The other was a regional educational resource that happened to be in the community where the family lived. It was a special school for children with emotional and other special needs. It operated year-round for a maximum of 2 years.

During his time there, Tom's mother started a group called "Family Focus" that met monthly at the school. This group was encouraged by the principal and led by one of the social workers. Tom's mother also developed a resource guide for parents. At one time during Tom's time at the school there was a plan to charge parents or bill insurance for the school, and Tom's parents and the parents of another child researched the names of lawyers who specialized in special education issues. The attorney they engaged indicated that "social therapy is a part of education," effectively denying that the school experience could be billed to health insurance.

When Tom was 7, he had to enter the public school system, and because the options for "severely emotionally disturbed" children (as he was classified) were not good in the city where they lived, the parents opted to move to another town. There they visited several classrooms and chose one based on the teacher they thought would be the best fit for Tom. It was self-contained for eight to nine students with mixed emotional, attention, and learning problems. He remained in this classroom through fifth grade. He was mainstreamed in some academic subjects but needed the special class for focus, as he was "zoning out" in mainstream classes, even with an aide in the classroom. Some of the youngsters in his special class are still his friends.

At 10½, Tom began to exhibit temper tantrums and sadness. His mother sought out the psychiatrist who had first seen him and persuaded him to work with her son even though the psychiatrist insisted that he was not taking any new patients. He prescribed Ritalin and an antidepressant. The depression seemed to be in the context of Tom realizing that he was different, and his brother, who was almost 3 years younger, was teasing him. Tom's depression seemed to improve with the medication and greater success in school. His recognition of his difference continued to be a challenge for him and his network, as we shall see.

Tom's mother says that in planning for middle school there was a "face-off." At the pupil planning meeting, the school authorities stated that there were no self-contained classes in the middle schools as there were "no children that needed them." Tom's mother had become friendly with the mother of one of his classmates, and she was experiencing the same frustration that Tom's mother had about her son. They set up a joint pupil planning meeting, included the fathers (who showed up in suits and ties) and invited the psychiatrist to participate. The school system responded and set up a classroom. Amazingly, it turned out that there *were* other children who required a self-contained class. Tom continued to be somewhat isolated but did have one or two friends. The school program included a "lunch bunch" with the social worker for weekly socializing.

Tom remained in this classroom for 3 years. In the eighth grade, he attended the class trip to Washington. Only then did the school personnel realize that he couldn't walk fast enough to keep up with the group, and the vice principal ended up walking with him, trailing behind the group.

While Tom was in middle school, a couple of parents in the town had formed a group, Parents of Children with Special Needs, and Tom's mother was one of the original members. It was an opportunity to trade tips and stories on dealing with school administrators, helping their children with social situations, and many other things. The school administrator took notice of the group and decided to make a Special Education Advisory Committee to meet with the Special Education Director monthly. He arranged for the meetings in school facilities and helped to distribute flyers of meetings for children to take home to their parents. He also got the school system to help to pay for a monthly newsletter. In the public library, the group set up a special area with books and articles related to disabilities and special education issues. They invited specialists to give talks. Tom's mother wrote articles for a local newsletter, *The Legal Beagle,* summarizing legal issues and outcomes of lawsuits gleaned from the national special education news.

Tom's mother refers to the middle school years as the "joiner" years. The parents' group was great, but she was still looking for more help with Tom's particular disability. She joined the founding of a local Children and Adults with ADD, became a recording secretary, and even helped to facilitate their support groups. But Tom didn't have just ADD. She joined National Alliance for the Mentally Ill Children and Adolescent Network. The founder was an energetic wife of a physician at a local academic center whose daughter has autism. The meetings were fascinating, but the emphasis was on mental illness, not on Tom's specific disabilities. She went to one meeting of Autism Association of America, but found they were dealing with children much more severely affected than Tom. In fact, Tom came with her to a meeting to hear a young adult with autism who was speaking. He took a tag that said, "My name is" and added, "Tom. I am not autistic." He was developing an awareness of how he was different from other kids. They also joined Children and Adults with Learning Disabilities. Though his "learning disability" might be classified as "nonverbal learning disability," he had little trouble with academic learning. Nevertheless, there was attention to social skill deficits in this group, and that was helpful.

Finally, Tom's mother met another mother whose son had the same diagnosis, atypical PDD. They started an atypical PDD support group and put notices in local papers and flyers in libraries and supermarkets. They got 12 people to attend the first meeting. The group grew. It started as a support group, but then invited guest speakers. It was the first group of its kind in their state for families of "higher-functioning" people with autism.

Tom's mother was tireless in her search for information and copied materials to distribute at meetings. At that time there was still a dearth of information. Attendance at the meetings soared to 100 people when there was a speaker from the local university that included doctors, therapists, special education specialists, special education attorneys, and other professionals. Many of these "advocates" attended to learn, and to speak, and many referred parents to the group.

When the fourth edition of the *Diagnostic and Statistical Manual of Mental Disorders* came out, and Asperger disorder was in it, more children were being identified with this problem. Years later, of course, there is an abundance of material about these disabilities.

Tom set up a home page for the group on the Internet, and there was correspondence with people all over the world, giving advice and making referrals. The two original founders, Tom's mother and her friend, were invited to speak at a number of national conventions. Networking was terrific.

Another parent, having attended some of the group meetings, had formed a similar group in a neighboring county that grew rapidly, as well. This woman is still an untiring advocate. She cofounded the Connecticut Autistic Spectrum Resource Center, and then she and her codirector (another parent) took advocacy courses and became experts in special education law.

Tom's special education was well established by the time he reached high school. He had regular history and math and special gym and resource room. The gym teacher engaged Tom as the video specialist for varsity basketball games, and his friend became the team manager.

Socialization has continued to be an area of difficulty. One of his teachers found a girl who "wouldn't mind" if Tom asked her on a date. He was willing to invite her to a dance, insisting, "It's not a date." They went to three or four dances together, but after he graduated from high school, she wanted to follow up, but he never called back.

The major challenge for high school was the transition from school to what was supposed to happen next. There were new federal requirements mandating that school systems provide transitional education program, but they were new. School personnel didn't know how to do it and didn't have funding for it. Tom's mother spoke at a couple school board meetings asking for funds for a transitional coordinator.

For Tom, the questions were what was he going to do, and what training did he need to make it possible? He had vocational testing that led to a suggestion that he could be a "sandwich board carrier" or a "cigarette vendor."

Tom's parents recognized that this was outmoded and highly disrespectful. As part of the transition process he was supposed to get experience in the community, but he was given work only in the school, such as helping out in the library. At the end of his junior year consultants from the Bureau of Rehabilitation Services were brought in, and he was referred to a local agency providing services to adults with DDs. He was given a couple of vocational assignments, data entry, bagging groceries, and store clerk. He was good at the data entry, but the others were both physically taxing and required interaction with people that was uncomfortable for him.

At the time he was supposed to graduate, there was a standoff with the special education director. The parents claimed that the school system hadn't fulfilled their obligations to provide Tom with community experience and were about to let him go without a proper transition. The special education director responded by saying, then, that Tom could not graduate with his class. Tom had already attended rehearsals and had his cap and gown, but even with the intervention of a congressional representative, the special education director prevailed, and Tom was not allowed to go through the ceremony with his class.

Tom got a job as a pharmacy technician. Though he was terrific at the pharmacy part, he couldn't do the counter work. He was slow and hated the pressure. Finally he got a job working in office services at his mother's office until the company downsized and his mother left.

Tom has a driver's license and was involved in an accident that was not his fault. He had a leg injury that further limits his mobility. He received an insurance settlement that allows him to support himself in his own apartment. He does not have an official job but spends a lot of time on the computer and is a source of information about many things to his family and some friends. He does not date. He loves Japan and did plan and travel on a trip to Japan, by himself.

The challenge for families with individuals with disabilities in the PDD spectrum in the state of Connecticut was that there is a Department of Mental Retardation (DMR) that serves individuals with PDD only if their tested IQ is below 70. The founder of the Autistic Spectrum Resource Center (see above) and Tom's mother, among others, began a campaign to get this agency to serve individuals with PDD regardless of IQ level, noting that it is a DD. They went to meetings with the commissioner and began to get their state representative to introduce a bill. The first bill, in the mid-1990s, did not get out of committee. However, the parent advocates have been tireless at getting their local congress people to reintroduce the bill. Step by step, and not giving up, this group has had measurable success. The legislature appointed a 2-year Advisory Commission to study the lack of services for nonretarded adults. Tom's mother was elected cochair and traveled monthly to the state capital for meetings. The commissioner of DMR has been ordered to come up with a plan to implement recommendations that the department include services to nonretarded individuals with PDD. He did so, but faltered on the subject of funding. The work continued, with the advocate from ASRC holding legislative breakfasts giving media briefings, and organizing a letter-writing campaign, and then hiring busses to take people to the capitol to testify in favor of the bill.

There is now a pilot to provide comprehensive services, including vocational and residential support, for 25 people in one area of Connecticut. Another bill worked to have the Department of Disability Services (DMR renamed) apply for a Medicaid waiver to fund and expand the program. It has passed!

Conclusion

Here are the steps necessary to become an advocate.

First: Keep in mind the objective that a person with disabilities, like everyone else, needs to be a contributing member of a community, and this requires being involved in a community and having some recognized attributes and skills that contribute.

Second: Listen to the parents, family members, other caregivers, and, most important, to the person with the developmental disability.

Third: Be familiar with strivings and conflicts that characterize each stage of the individual's development to properly identify what is normal and what needs intervention.

Fourth: Identify everyone who is involved in supporting the individual's growth to grasp the system of care or resource network and to be sure that there is collaboration not conflict in the system.

Fifth: Identify resources and supports for the parents, family members, and caregivers so that they can continue to advocate for their family member.

Sixth: Be prepared to appear in person, when necessary, to advocate for the individual's care and services both in community settings and in larger political settings.

Last: Always continue to advocate for the individual's striving for independence and the community's inclusion, because these individuals continue to grow, change, adapt, and face new challenges. Family members are natural advocates, but they cannot be effective without the support, guidance, and resources of professionals. Psychiatrists and other mental health professionals can be particularly effective in helping to differentiate disability from illness, treat illness, and find resources for optimal functioning. Though it is tempting to evaluate individuals with disabilities solely as individuals, also viewing them in the context of their communities and the momentum of personal development leads to a richer and more effective form of advocacy for a lifetime of achievement.

REFERENCES

Dorris M. 1989. *The Broken Cord*. New York: Basic Books.
Etmanski A. 2000. *A Good Life*. Vancouver, BC: Orwell Cove and Planned Lifetime Advocacy Network.
Featherstone H. 1980. *A Difference in the Family: Life with a Disabled Child*. New York: Basic Books.
Gleidman J, Roth W. 1980. *The Unexpected Minority: Handicapped Children in America*. New York: Harcourt, Brace, Jovanovich.
Klein SD, Kemp JD. 2004. *Reflections from a Different Journey: What Adults with Disabilities Wish All Parents Knew*. New York: McGraw-Hill.
Klein SD, Schive K (eds.). 2001. *You Will Dream New Dreams: Inspiring Personal Stories by Parents of Children with Disabilities*. New York: Kensington.
Robison JE. 2007. *Look Me in the Eye: My Life with Asperger's*. New York: Crown.
Switzky HN, Greenspan S. 2006. *What Is Mental Retardation?* Washington, DC: American Association for Mental Retardation.
Vygotsky, LS. 1966. "Play and its role in the mental development of the child," *Voprosy psikhologii [Soviet Psychology]*, no. 6. (Originally published 1933)

Appendix · Developmental Disabilities Resources

Organizations

ACCSES
1501 M Street, NW, 7th Floor
Washington, DC 20005
phone: 202-466-3355
fax: 202-466-7571
www.accses.org

Alliance for Healthy Homes
50 F Street, NW, Suite 300
Washington, DC 20001
phone: 202-347-7610
fax: 202-347-0058
www.afhh.org

American Academy of Child and Adolescent Psychiatry
www.aacap.org

American Association on Intellectual and Developmental Disabilities
(formerly American Association on Mental Retardation)
444 North Capitol Street, NW, Suite 846
Washington, DC 20001-1512
phone: 202-387-1968; 800-424-3688
fax: 202-387-2193
www.aamr.org

American Psychiatric Association
1000 Wilson Boulevard
Arlington, VA 22209-3901
phone: 703-907-7300
www.psych.org

Americans with Disabilities Act
  1201 Pennsylvania Avenue, NW, Suite 300
  Washington, DC 20004
  www.adawatch.org

APSE
  1627 Monument Avenue
  Richmond, VA 23220
  phone: 804-278-9187
  fax: 804-278-9377
  www.apse.org

Arc of the United States
  1010 Wayne Avenue, Suite 650
  Silver Spring, MD 20910
  phone: 301-565-3842; 800-433-5255
  fax: 301-565-3843; 301-565-5342
  www.thearc.org

Asperger Syndrome Coalition of the United States, Inc.
  P.O. Box 49267
  Jacksonville Beach, FL 32240-9267

Asperger Syndrome Education Network
  9 Aspen Circle
  Edison, NJ 08820
  phone: 732-321-0800
  www.aspennj.org

Autism Network for Hearing and Visually Impaired Persons
  7510 Oceanfront Avenue
  Virginia Beach, VA 23451
  phone: 804-428-9036
  fax: 804-428-0019

Autism Research Institute
  4182 Adams Avenue
  San Diego, CA 92116
  phone: 619-281-7165
  fax: 619-563-6840
  www.autism.com

Autism Society of America
  7910 Woodmont Avenue, Suite 300
  Bethesda, MD 20814-3067
  phone: 301-657-0881; 800-328-8476
  fax: 301-657-0869
  www.autism-society.org

Autism Speaks (formerly National Alliance for Autism Research)
    2 Park Avenue, 11th Floor
    New York, NY 10016
    phone: 212-252-8584
    fax: 212-252-8676
    www.autismspeaks.org

Best Buddies
    100 Southeast Second Street, Suite 2200
    Miami, FL 33131
    phone: 305-374-2233; 800-89-BUDDY
    fax: 305-374-5305
    www.bestbuddies.org

Center for the Study of Autism
    P.O. Box 4538
    Salem, OR 97302
    phone: 503-692-3104
    fax: 219-662-0638

Centers for Disease Control and Prevention
    1600 Clifton Road
    Atlanta, GA 30333
    phone: 404-639-3311; 404-639-3534; 800-311-3435
    www.cdc.gov

Childhood Lead Poisoning Prevention Program
    1600 Clifton Road
    Atlanta, GA 30333
    phone: 404-639-3311; 404-639-3534; 800-311-3435
    www.cdc.gov/nceh/lead/lead.htm

Coalition to End Childhood Lead Poisoning
    2714 Hudson Street
    Baltimore, MD 21224-4716
    phone: 410-534-6447; 800 370-5323
    www.leadsafe.org

Contra Costa Child Care Council
    1035 Detroit Avenue, Suite 200
    Concord, CA 94518
    phone: 925-676-5442
    www.cocokids.org

Council for Exceptional Children
  1110 North Glebe Road, Suite 300
  Arlington, VA 22201
  phone: 888-232-7733
  fax: 703-264-9494
  www.cec.sped.org

Cure Autism Now
  5455 Wilshire Boulevard, no. 715
  Los Angeles, CA 90036
  phone: 888-8AUTISM
  www.cureautismnow.org

Easter Seals, Inc.
  233 South Wacker Drive, Suite 2400
  Chicago, IL 60606
  phone: 800-221-6827
  www.easterseals.com

FASlink: Fetal Alcohol Disorders Society
  2448 Hamilton Road
  Bright's Grove, Ontario
  Canada N0N 1C0
  phone: 519-869-8026
  www.faslink.org

FASLink: Fetal Alcohol Syndrome
  2448 Hamilton Road
  Bright's Grove, Ontario
  Canada N0N 1C0
  phone: 519-869-8026
  www.acbr.com

Fetal Alcohol Syndrome World Canada
  250 Scarborough Golf Club Road
  Toronto, Ontario
  Canada M1J 3G8
  phone: 416-264-8000
  www.fasworld.com

Hydrocephalus Association
  870 Market Street, Suite 705
  San Francisco, CA 94102
  phone: 415-732-7040; 888-598-3789
  fax: 415-732-7044
  www.hydroassoc.org

Inter-National Association of Business, Industry and Rehabilitation
P.O. Box 15242
Washington, DC 20003
phone: 202-543-6353
www.inabir.org

Learning Disabilities On Line
WETA Public Television
2775 S. Quincy Street
Arlington, VA 22206
fax: 703-998-2060
www.ldonline.org

Living Arrangements for the Developmentally Disabled, Inc.
3603 Victory Parkway
Cincinnati, OH 45229
phone: 513-861-5233
www.laddinc.org

More Advanced Autistic People
P.O. Box 524
Crown Point, IN 46307
phone: 219-662-1311
fax: 219-662-0638
www.maapservices.org

National Association of Councils on Developmental Disabilities
225 Reinekers Lane, Suite 650–B
Alexandria, VA 22314
phone: 703-739-4400-
fax: 703-739-6030
www.nacdd.org

National Autism Hotline / Autism Services Center
605 Ninth Street
Prichard Building
P.O. Box 507
Huntington, WV 25710-0507
phone: 304-525-8014
fax: 304-525-8026

National Council for Support of Disability Issues
Haymarket, VA 20169
www.ncsd.org

National Council on Alcoholism and Drug Dependence
  22 Cortlandt Street, Suite 801
  New York, NY 10007-3128
  phone: 212-269-7797
  fax: 212-269-7510
  HOPELINE: 800-NCA-CALL (24–hour affiliate referral)
  www.ncadd.org

National Fragile X Foundation
  P.O. Box 37
  Walnut Creek, CA 94597
  phone: 800-688-8765
  fax: 925-938-9315
  www.fragilex.org

National Institute on Alcohol Abuse and Alcoholism
  5635 Fishers Lane, MSC 9304
  Bethesda, MD 20892-9304
  phone: 301-443-3860
  fax: 301-480-1726
  www.niaaa.nih.gov

National Organization on Fetal Alcohol Syndrome
  900 17th Street, NW, Suite 910
  Washington, DC 20006
  phone: 202-785-4585; 800-66NOFAS
  fax: 202-466-6456
  www.nofas.org

Office of the Surgeon General
  U.S. Department of Health and Human Resources
  5600 Fishers Lane, Room 18-66
  Rockville, MD 20857
  phone: 301 443-4000
  fax: 301 443-3574
  www.surgeongeneral.gov

Parent to Parent USA
  www.p2pusa.org

People First of Oregon
  P.O. Box 12642
  Salem, OR 97309
  phone: 503-362-0336
  fax: 503-585-0287
  www.people1.org

Self-Advocate Leadership Network
   Human Services Research Institute
   7420 S.W. Bridgeport Road, Suite 210
   Portland, OR 97224
   phone: 503-924-3783
   fax: 503-924-3789
   www.hsri.org

Self Advocates Becoming Empowered
   P.O. Box 30142
   Kansas City, MO 64112
   www.sabeUSA.org

Special Olympics
   1133 19th Street, NW
   Washington, DC 20036
   phone: 202-628-3630
   fax: 202-824-0200
   www.specialolympics.org

Substance Abuse and Mental Health Services Administration
   Treatment Facility Locator
   phone: 800-662-HELP
   www.findtreatment.samhsa.gov

TASH
   1025 Vermont Avenue, NW, Floor 7
   Washington, DC 20005
   phone: 202-263-5600
   fax: 202-637-0138
   www.tash.org

U.S. Environmental Protection Agency
   www.epa.gov

Voice of the Retarded
   5005 Newport Drive, Suite 108
   Rolling Meadows, IL 60008
   phone: 847-253-6020
   fax: 847-253-6054
   www.vor.net

Publications

"Children with Prenatal Drug and/or Alcohol Exposure"
   ARCH National Resource Center for Respite and Crisis Care Services
   www.archrespite.org/archfs49.htm

"Fetal Alcohol Syndrome"
   KidsHealth
   http://kidshealth.org/parent/medical/brain/fas.html

"Fetal Alcohol Syndrome"
   League for the Prevention of Alcohol Related Fetal Brain Injury
   www.worldprofit.com/mafas.htm

"Illicit Drug Use during Pregnancy"
   March of Dimes
   www.marchofdimes.com/professionals/14332_1169.asp

Glossary

The words below are defined as they pertain to the fields of special education and developmental disabilities.

autism A developmental disability, generally evident before age 3, that significantly affects verbal and nonverbal communication, social interaction, and educational performance

deaf-blindness Concomitant hearing and visual impairments, the combination of which causes such severe communication and other developmental and educational needs that they cannot be accommodated in special education programs solely for students with deafness or blindness

deafness A hearing impairment so severe that the student is impaired in processing linguistic information through hearing, with or without amplification, that adversely affects educational performance

emotional disturbance A condition exhibiting one or more of the following characteristics, displayed over a long period of time and to a marked degree that adversely affects educational performance:

- an inability to learn that cannot be explained by intellectual, sensory, or health factors
- an inability to build or maintain satisfactory interpersonal relationships with peers or teachers
- inappropriate types of behavior or feelings under normal circumstances
- a general pervasive mood of unhappiness or depression
- a tendency to develop physical symptoms or fears associated with personal or school problems.

hearing impairment An impairment in hearing, whether permanent or fluctuating, that adversely affects educational performance but is not severe enough to be included under the definition of deafness

mental retardation Significantly subaverage general intellectual functioning that exists concurrently with deficits in adaptive behavior and manifested during the developmental period and adversely affects educational performance

multiple disabilities Concomitant impairments (such as mental retardation-blindness, mental retardation-orthopedic impairment, etc.) the combination of which causes such severe educational needs that they cannot be accommodated in special education programs solely for one of the impairments. The term does not include deaf-blindness.

orthopedic impairment A severe orthopedic impairment that adversely affects educational performance

other health impairment Having limited strength, vitality, or alertness or a heightened alertness to environmental stimuli due to chronic or acute health problems such that one or more of these conditions adversely affects educational performance

specific learning disability A disorder in one or more of the basic psychological processes involved in understanding or in using language, spoken or written, that may manifest in an imperfect ability to listen, think, speak, read, write, spell, or do mathematical calculations, including conditions such as perceptual disabilities, brain injury, minimal brain dysfunction, dyslexia, and developmental aphasia. Learning problems that are primarily the result of visual, hearing, or motor disabilities, of mental retardation, of emotional disturbance, or of environmental, cultural, or economic disadvantage are not included in this category.

speech or language impairment A communication disorder, such as stuttering, impaired articulation, language impairment, or a voice impairment, that adversely affects educational performance

traumatic brain injury An acquired injury to the brain caused by an external physical force that results in total or partial functional disability, psychosocial impairment, or both and adversely affects educational performance

visual impairment An impairment in vision that, even with correction, adversely affects performance. The term includes both partial sight and blindness.

Sources for the glossary are edservices.ccps.org/specialED/index.html and 34 *Code of Federal Regulations* §300.7(c)(10).

Index

Page numbers in *italics* indicate figures and tables.